T0306051

"The book is an outstanding resource for any teacher, student, medical doctor, coach, physiotherapist, athlete and patient willing to extend his/her knowledge in a broad range of existing hypoxic strategies to improve various pathological states and sport performance."

Louise Deldicque, *Professor in Exercise Physiology and*
Sport Nutrition at UCLouvain, Belgium

HYPOXIA CONDITIONING IN HEALTH, EXERCISE AND SPORT

While severe hypoxia has detrimental health consequences, the controlled application of hypoxia can be protective and holds great promise as a performance-enhancing and therapeutic intervention. *Hypoxia Conditioning in Health, Exercise and Sport: Principles, Mechanisms and Applications* delivers an understanding of systemic and molecular mechanisms involved in hypoxia adaptations and examines the most promising forms of hypoxia conditioning with a view to create performance-enhancing strategies for athletes, as well as offering an examination on clinical applications for numerous pathologies.

This cutting-edge book examines how positive physiological adaptations not only acutely enhance tolerance to hypoxia but can also induce sustained health benefits. This has enabled the development and refinement of approaches utilizing hypoxia, strategies also termed hypoxia conditioning, to improve health and performance outcomes.

By linking research with recommendations for real-world situations, this volume will serve as an invaluable resource for students, academics, exercise science professionals, and sports medicine specialists, especially those in environmental physiology and coaching subjects.

Olivier Girard is a professor at the University of Western Australia, researching the mechanisms and adaptations that influence health and performance during exercise in adverse environmental conditions (heat and altitude). (https://www.oliviergirard.com/)

Johannes Burtscher is a neurobiologist investigating oxygen availability and consumption in humans and animals, with a focus on mitochondrial physiology in the brain and in brain-aging.

Martin Burtscher is a retired professor in sports science and sports medicine at the University of Innsbruck, Austria.

Grégoire Millet is a professor in exercise and environmental physiology at the University of Lausanne, Switzerland.

HYPOXIA CONDITIONING IN HEALTH, EXERCISE AND SPORT

Principles, Mechanisms and Applications

Edited by Olivier Girard, Johannes Burtscher, Martin Burtscher, and Grégoire Millet

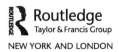

NEW YORK AND LONDON

Designed cover image: Getty images

First published 2025
by Routledge
605 Third Avenue, New York, NY 10158

and by Routledge
4 Park Square, Milton Park, Abingdon, Oxon, OX14 4RN

Routledge is an imprint of the Taylor & Francis Group, an informa business

ISBN: 978-1-032-51574-8 (hbk)
ISBN: 978-1-032-51572-4 (pbk)
ISBN: 978-1-003-40287-9 (ebk)

DOI: 10.4324/9781003402879

Typeset in Sabon
by SPi Technologies India Pvt Ltd (Straive)

CONTENTS

FIGURES

TABLES

CONTRIBUTORS

Sébastien Baillieul
Grenoble Alpes University, HP2
Laboratory, INSERM U1300 and
Grenoble Alpes University Hospital
Grenoble, France

Tom Behrendt
Department for Sport Science
Otto von Guericke University
Magdeburg
Magdeburg, Germany

François Billaut
Département de kinésiologie
Université Laval
Québec, QC, Canada

Franck Brocherie
Laboratory Sport, Expertise and
Performance (EA 7370)
Research Unit, French Institute of
Sport (INSEP)
Paris, France

Johannes Burtscher
Institute of Sport Sciences, Faculty
of Biology and Medicine
University of Lausanne
Building Synathlon, Lausanne,
Switzerland

Martin Burtscher
Department of Sport Science
University of Innsbruck
Innsbruck, Austria

Sarah Carter
Faculty of Health, Exercise and
Sports Science
Charles Darwin University
Darwin, NT 0810, Australia

Marie Chambion-Diaz
Atherosclerosis, Thrombosis and
Physical Activity, LIBM UR7424
Université Claude Bernard Lyon 1,
Université de Lyon, Faculty of
Medicine
Lyon, France

Bryna Chrismas
School of Sport, Exercise and
Health Sciences
Loughborough University, National
Centre for Sport and Exercise
Medicine (NCSEM)
Loughborough, United Kingdom

Annalisa Cogo
Altitude Pediatric Asthma Centre in
Misurina
Pio XII Institute
Belluno, Italy

Tadej Debevec
Faculty of Sport
University of Ljubljana
Ljubljana, Slovenia

H. Fred Downey
University of North Texas Health
Science Center
Fort Worth, United States

Tobias Dünnwald
Institute of Sports Medicine, Alpine
Medicine and Health Tourism (ISAG)
UMIT TIROL—Private University
for Health Sciences and Health
Technology
Hall in Tyrol, Austria

Chris Esh
Aspetar, Orthopaedic and Sports
Medicine Hospital
FIFA Medical Centre of Excellence
Doha, Qatar
and
School of Sport, Exercise and
Health Sciences

Loughborough University, National
Centre for Sport and Exercise
Medicine (NCSEM)
Loughborough, United Kingdom

Raphael Faiss
Institute of Sport Sciences
University of Lausanne
Switzerland

Olivier Girard
School of Human Sciences (Exercise
and Sport Science)
University of Western Australia
Perth, WA, Australia

Oleg S. Glazachev
Department of Human Physiology,
Institute of Clinical Medicine
I.M. Sechenov First Moscow State
Medical University
Moscow, Russia

Mohammed Ihsan
Scientific Conditioning Centre
Elite Training and Technology
Division
Hong Kong Sports Institute
Hong Kong

Bengt Kayser
Institute of Sport Sciences
University of Lausanne
Lausanne, Switzerland

Bastien Krumm
Institute of Sport Sciences
University of Lausanne
Switzerland

Nadezhda P. Lyamina
Moscow Centre for Research and
Practice in Medical Rehabilitation
Restorative and Sports Medicine
Moscow, Russia

Svetlana V. Lyamina
Moscow State University of
Medicine and Dentistry
Moscow
Russia

Robert T. Mallet
Department of Physiology and
Anatomy
University of North Texas Health
Science Center
Fort Worth, Texas, United States

Eugenia Manukhina
University of North Texas Health
Science Center
Fort Worth, United States
and
Institute of General Pathology and
Pathophysiology
Moscow, Russia

Konrad Mayer
Charité - Universitätsmedizin Berlin
Berlin, Germany

Grégoire Millet
Institute of Sports Sciences (ISSUL)
University of Lausanne
Lausanne, Switzerland

Gustavo R. Mota
Department of Sport Sciences,
Institute of Health Sciences
Federal University of Triângulo
Mineiro
Uberaba, Brazil

Gino Panza
John D. Dingell Veterans Affairs
Medical Center
Detroit, MI, United States
and
Department of Health Care
Sciences, Program of Occupational
Therapy
Wayne State University, Detroit, MI,
United States

Vincent Pialoux
Atherosclerosis, Thrombosis and
Physical Activity
LIBM UR7424, Université Claude
Bernard Lyon 1
Université de Lyon, Faculty of
Medicine
Lyon, France

Antoine Raberin
Institute of Sport Sciences
University of Lausanne
Switzerland

Lutz Schega
Department of Sport Science, Chair
for Health and Physical Activity
Otto-von-Guericke University
Magdeburg
Magdeburg, Germany

Brendan R. Scott
Murdoch Applied Sports Science
Laboratory, Discipline of Exercise
Science
Murdoch University
Perth, Australia
and
Centre for Healthy Ageing
Murdoch University
Perth, Australia

Markus Tannheimer
Department of Sport and
Rehabilitation Medicine
University of Ulm
Ulm, Germany
and
Department of General and Visceral
Surgery
Krankenhaus Blaubeuren
Blaubeuren, Germany

Lee Taylor
School of Sport, Exercise and
Health Sciences
Loughborough University, National
Centre for Sport and Exercise
Medicine (NCSEM)
Loughborough, United Kingdom
Sport and Exercise Discipline
Group, Faculty of Health
University of Technology Sydney
Moore Park, NSW, Australia
and
Human Performance Research
Centre
University of Technology Sydney
(UTS)
Sydney, Australia

Vadim E. Tseilikman
Scientific and Educational Center
"Biomedical Technologies", School
of Medical Biology
South Ural State University
Chelyabinsk 454080, Russia
Zelman Institute of Medicine and
Psychology

Novosibirsk State University
Novosibirsk 630090, Russia
and
Institute of Sport Sciences, Faculty
of Biology and Medicine
University of Lausanne
Building Synathlon, Campus
Dorigny, 1015, Lausanne,
Switzerland

Samuel Verges
Univ. Grenoble Alpes, Inserm
Grenoble Alpes University Hospital,
HP2 laboratory
Grenoble, France

Randall L. Wilber
United States Olympic &
Paralympic Committee
Colorado Springs, Colorado, United
States

Lei Xi
Pauley Heart Center, Department of
Internal Medicine
Virginia Commonwealth University
Richmond, Virginia, United States

Fei Zhao
John D. Dingell Veterans Affairs
Medical Center
Detroit, MI, United States
and
Department of Health Care
Sciences, Program of Occupational
Therapy
Wayne State University
Detroit, MI, United States

PREFACE

Dear reader,

As obligate aerobes, humans need oxygen to survive. A significant reduction in ambient oxygen availability is perilous, and near-complete depletion of usable oxygen (anoxia) leads to death within minutes. The fear of suffocation is a primordial human emotion, making the suggestion to intentionally lower ambient oxygen levels to promote health at first appear absurd. Yet, this is the main premise of the present book.

To grasp this concept, it is necessary to consider specific notions that underlie the reasoning of many chapters in this book: the *hypoxic dose*, *hormesis*, and *acclimatization/adaptation*. These concepts are discussed in greater detail in Chapter 1. First, it is necessary to consider how changes in ambient oxygen availability occur and acknowledge that the degree of reduction determines the outcomes. Oxygen conditions range from "normal" in plain air at sea level ("normoxia") to the absence of oxygen (anoxia). While this book briefly addresses interventions involving higher-than-normal oxygen availability ("hyperoxia"), its main focus is on lower-than-normal oxygen ("hypoxia") levels. Hypoxia can result from the modulation of two main factors, the concentration of oxygen and the partial pressure of oxygen. The Earth's atmosphere maintains a relatively homogeneous oxygen concentration of about 20.9%, regardless of location, whether it's a beach next to the Atlantic Ocean (close to 0 m above sea level) or the summit of Mount Everest (8,848 m). However, lower concentrations of oxygen in inspired air ("normobaric hypoxia") are commonly applied, such as in "hypoxic training" for athletes by artificially reducing the inspired oxygen concentration in hypoxia chambers/tents or face masks. With increasing terrestrial altitudes, the factor that does change and influences the oxygen we can extract from the air is barometric pressure.

As terrestrial altitude rises, barometric pressure decreases, and in accordance with Dalton's law, the partial pressure of oxygen decreases as well. A lower partial pressure of oxygen in the ambient air produces "hypobaric hypoxia." Both normobaric and hypobaric hypoxia lead to lower oxygen uptake in humans and therefore reduced oxygen saturation in the blood.

The "hypoxic dose" encompasses various components that define the severity of a hypoxia exposure. An essential component is the (1) intensity, which refers to the oxygen concentration (ranging from 0% and 20.9%, or up to 100% for a "hyperoxic dose") or partial pressure of oxygen (between 0 mmHg and 160 mmHg, or more for hyperoxic doses). Nonetheless, to define the hypoxic dose, the (2) duration of exposure is also important. Intensity and duration are defining parameters for the outcomes of hypoxia exposure, determining whether it is harmful. These parameters are further influenced by exposure patterns, such as whether the exposure is (3) continuous or repeated ("intermittent"), and in the case of the latter, they depend on the (4) frequency of exposure, as well as the (5) temporal patterns of changing normoxic and hypoxic periods. Finally, individual resilience to hypoxia varies greatly, which means that the same hypoxic dose may exert very different effects on different individuals.

Hormesis characterizes a common feature of various stressors (chemical, metabolic, environmental, psychogenic, etc.) and simply means that an excessive stress can be harmful but mild stress may even be beneficial. As long as the dose remains small enough not to exceed the capacity of an individual to manage this stress, the activated defense mechanisms may actually increase the affected individuals' resilience to future stressors. In essence, hormesis aligns with the sentiment articulated by the German philosopher Friedrich Nietzsche: "What doesn't kill me, makes me stronger."

In hypoxic environments (such as high altitude), various organ and molecular systems contribute to increasing tolerance to hypoxia through a process termed "acclimatization" by initiating protective physiological responses in healthy humans. In this book, the physiological consequences of these hypoxia responses are sometimes referred to as "adaptations." It is important to note that some authors restrict the term "adaptations" to genetic adaptations, such as mutations or genetic polymorphisms that influence survival in hypoxic surroundings, especially in the context of high-altitude adaptations. When controlled hypoxia exposures are used to systematically induce hypoxia responses to improve health or performance, it is referred to as "hypoxia conditioning". While hypoxia conditioning is a broad term encompassing any intervention involving (ambient) hypoxia, our focus is specially on protocols involving mild intermittent hypoxic episodes interspersed with normoxic or hyperoxic "resting" phases. Chapter 2 of this book outlines the systemic and molecular mechanisms that enable humans to respond to and adapt to intermittent hypoxia, both physiologically and metabolically.

Chapter 3a and 3b introduce examples of techniques related to hypoxia conditioning, namely ischemic (pre-)conditioning and training with voluntary hypoventilation. The following Chapter 4 marks the conclusion of the first section of the book, focusing on definitions and techniques, by providing a historical overview of altitude training and hypoxia conditioning.

Sections 2–7 (comprising Chapters 5 to 14) are dedicated to exploring clinical applications of hypoxia conditioning. Despite considerable preclinical evidence and scattered clinical trials suggesting significant health benefits and eventual clinical applications, we have not yet reached a definite conclusion stage. Therefore, the aim of these sections is to outline the current knowledge, ongoing progress, and indicate next steps. Various classes of diseases are covered, including neurological and psychiatric (Chapters 5–7), pulmonary/respiratory (Chapter 8), metabolic (Chapters 9 and 10), cardiovascular (Chapters 11 and 12), musculoskeletal (Chapter 13) and generally age-related diseases (Chapter 14).

Subsequently, Section 8 (Chapters 15–18) explores the use of hypoxia/altitude for performance enhancement. This includes hypoxia-based methods for the preparation of sojourns in hypoxic environments (Chapter 15), and enhancing athletic performance in various sports (Chapters 16–18) is discussed.

Section 9 deals with risks and some ethical considerations related to hypoxia interventions (Chapters 19–20).

The final Section 10 touches on a highly complex topic, the detailed investigation of which has only just begun. It provides an outlook on the combination of hypoxia with different environmental stressors, primarily focusing on air temperature (Chapter 21) and hyperoxia (Chapter 22). These stressors elicit distinct as well as overlapping responses, inducing adaptations that may either complement or inhibit each other. Understanding these complex interactions will eventually pave the way for the development of highly efficient environmental stimuli-based strategies as a novel class of treatments for many diseases and performance enhancement. It will also help to reduce risks in conditions characterized by various extreme environmental factors (e.g., in extreme sports competitions/challenges).

In conclusion, we take immense pride in successfully bringing together numerous world-renowned researchers in the field of hypoxia conditioning and altitude training to provide this book. We hope that this collaborative effort will contribute to improving the acceptance of research in the health- and performance-promoting applications of hypoxia. The growing commercial interest in hypoxia applications serves as an additional incentive to enhance our understanding of related strategies, their specific benefits and risks, and to provide optimized protocols tailored for well-defined target groups.

We also want to highlight another major problem in hypoxia conditioning research, aside from acceptance, which is the lack of uniform terminology.

Hypoxia conditioning is investigated in various cell types, organ systems, models, and diseases, and the communication between these research fields is historically relatively limited. This results in heterogeneous terminology and unharmonized protocols and experimental approaches. In this book, we aimed to prioritize clarity of terminology and outline necessary steps for advancing hypoxia conditioning research in the future. However, the attentive reader may observe differences in terminology throughout the chapters in this book and even more so when delving into the referenced original research. For example, intermittent hypoxia is also occasionally termed cyclic or episodic hypoxia. According to the hormesis-principle, high-frequency, severe intermittent hypoxia (characterizing diseases like obstructive sleep apnea) induces mostly maladaptive responses, while lower doses of intermittent hypoxia are largely associated with beneficial, adaptive responses. The controlled use of intermittent hypoxia aiming to improve health or performance is called (relatively) interchangeably intermittent hypoxia conditioning (IHC), acute intermittent hypoxia, mild intermittent hypoxia (MIH), intermittent hypoxia exposure (IHE) or intermittent hypoxia training (IHT), depending on research field or group. IHT sometimes denominates combinations of intermittent hypoxia and exercise protocols (but sometimes also merely passive exposure).

Whichever terms are used, the utilization of controlled intermittent hypoxia for health benefits is an emerging promising strategy for a lot of exciting applications, as this book hopefully demonstrates.

Wishing you a pleasant and enriching read,

The editors: Olivier, Johannes, Martin, Grégoire

SECTION 1

1

HYPOXIA

The Basics

Tadej Debevec and Grégoire Millet

1.1 Hypoxia—What, how and why

1.1.1 Importance of oxygen availability and sensing

Constant oxygen (O_2) availability is crucial for maintaining systemic and local physiological homeostasis in humans and most other mammals [1]. Human cells require stable and continuous O_2 delivery for survival, optimal function, and adenosine triphosphate (ATP) generation within the oxidative phosphorylation pathway. Accordingly, maintaining a stable O_2 supply plays a crucial role in survival, and energy production and has far-reaching consequences for long-term health and well-being. Throughout evolution, humans developed O_2 sensing mechanisms and efferent systems to counteract deviations in O_2 endogenous availability [2]. The former hinges predominantly on peripheral chemoreceptors (carotid bodies) capable of sensing variations in the O_2 (and importantly also CO_2) partial pressures. The afferent adaptation responses, detailed in the subsequent section, are activated via neuronal activity and are, at least acutely, manifested via modulation of cardiorespiratory mechanisms, predominantly regulation of respiration and cardiac output. Changes in O_2 availability trigger a sustained transcriptional response, which can lead to altered expression of many (as much as 1,000) genes and accordingly also modulate long-term genetic adaptations [2]. The hypoxia-inducible factor(s) (HIF) pathway represents one of the key transcription modulators involved in altered gene expression in response to lower endogenous O_2 availability [3]. While the HIF pathway has been extensively studied in the framework of long-term physiological and cellular effects resulting from variations in O_2 availability [4], it should be noted that other transcription factors

DOI: 10.4324/9781003402879-2

(e.g., Nuclear factor kappa-light-chain-enhancer of activated B cells (NF-κB), Cyclic adenosine monophosphate response element binding protein and so forth) are also involved in the long-term modulation of cellular responses [5].

These orchestrated physiological and cellular adaptations to both decreased (hypoxia) and increased (hyperoxia) O_2 availability primarily aim to restore physiological homeostasis. However, in addition to beneficial modulation, these adjustments can lead to maladaptation, resulting in detrimental consequences. Notably, hyperoxia is often employed to manage or treat various pathological conditions associated with prolonged systemic and local hypoxia (e.g., chronic obstructive pulmonary disease, heart failure) [6]. On the other hand, hyperoxia also finds important applications in high-performance sport and intermittent hypoxic/hyperoxic conditioning. Despite the potential benefits of acute O_2 supplementation, it is essential to consider the potential detrimental effects, particularly during prolonged hyperoxic exposures. Excessive production of reactive oxygen species during such exposures can result in O_2 toxicity–related lung and nervous system damage [6, 7]. Given that the focus of this book is on hypoxia conditioning, the following sections mainly address the beneficial and potential detrimental effects of both intermittent and continuous reduced O_2 availability in the context of health and performance.

1.1.2 Hypoxia—Key definitions and adaptation overview

Hypoxia is commonly defined as a condition in which O_2 availability falls below normal values at either systemic or local tissue cell levels. It can result from environmental (exogenous) and/or internal (endogenous) factors. Despite different definitions, from a mechanistic standpoint, hypoxia can arise from (1) reduced environmental O_2 availability (e.g., altitude exposure) or impaired O_2 extraction in the alveoli (e.g., diffusion limitations); (2) inability of convective O_2 transfer, due to reduced O_2 carrying capacity of the blood (e.g., anemia) or compromised cardiovascular system capacity (e.g., sickle cell disease, hypothermia); and/or (3) inability of cells to utilize the delivered oxygen (e.g., due to poisoning). Regarding subsequent physiological effects, the key element of hypoxic exposure is the overall hypoxic dose, modulated by hypoxia intensity, duration, and intermittency (discussed in detail in Section 1.1.3). To facilitate the readers' understanding of subsequent sections and employ standardized terminology [8], Table 1.1 outlines key terms and concepts employed in the context of hypoxic physiological adaptation and conditioning.

In healthy humans, the most prevalent cause of hypoxia is environmental altitude exposure. This type of exposure is also widely employed in the framework of hypoxic training and conditioning. As detailed in Chapter 4, altitude physiology has a rich history of research and practical application, with written reports dating back to as early as the first century CE. However, scientific development and investigation of altitude physiology have been

TABLE 1.1 Key terms and concepts

Term	Definition
Acclimation	Physiological and functional adaptation obtained in laboratory-based or artificial environments
Acclimatization	Physiological and functional adaptation obtained in a natural environment
Acute exposure	Initial exposure phase with a duration between a few seconds to a day
Chronic exposure	Prolonged exposure following the sub-acute phase with a duration between a few days to years and beyond
Hyperbaric exposure	Increased ambient pressure condition
Hyperoxia	Increased partial pressure of inspired oxygen (external) and/or increased tissue oxygenation (internal)
Hypobaric	Reduced ambient pressure condition
Hypoxemia	Reduced arterial blood partial pressure of oxygen
Hypoxia	Reduced partial pressure of inspired oxygen (external) and/or reduced tissue/cellular oxygenation (internal)
Intermittent exposure	Cyclic and/or repetitive exposures
Normobaric	Normal ambient pressure condition
Sub-acute exposure	Exposure lasting between one and a few days

predominantly conducted in the last two centuries, primarily for aviation, military, industrial, and leisure applications [9].

Exposure to increased terrestrial altitude provokes a reduction in ambient (barometric) pressure, subsequently reducing the partial pressure of O_2 (PO_2). As PO_2 is a key determinant of convective O_2 delivery, this reduction significantly decreases O_2 availability throughout the whole O_2 cascade. Depending on the severity of altitude or hypoxic exposure and the subsequent reduction in PO_2, arterial PO_2 (P_AO_2) is reduced at each step of the cascade, from the alveoli, through the bloodstream (arteries and capillaries), to the cell cytosol [10]. Systemic hypoxemia, at least acutely, limits oxidative energy production within all cells, ultimately leading to reduced aerobic capacity and exercise capacity [11].

The reduced O_2 availability is predominantly sensed by type I glomus cells of the carotid and aortic bodies. This initiates compensating mechanisms, acutely manifesting as increased minute ventilation (also termed hypoxic ventilatory response) coupled with pulmonary vasoconstriction as well as augmented cardiac output (primarily through increased heart rate) [2]. Concomitantly, reduced PO_2-related renal tissue hypoxia likely induces augmented erythropoietin production. This, in turn, sub-acutely leads to increased red blood cell production, ultimately increasing O_2 blood carrying capacity via an increase in total hemoglobin mass and simultaneous plasma volume reductions. The intricate interplay of factors also involves adjustments in mitochondrial energy and nitric oxide metabolism, angiogenesis, and vasodilation, predominantly governed by the stabilization of HIF pathway(s) and subsequent gene induction [12]. The adaptation kinetics are significantly modulated by the altitude of residence which is a key component of the overall hypoxic dose. To harmonize and specify definitions, Table 1.2 outlines altitude range definitions along with the corresponding expected O_2-related environmental parameters.

While the outlined acclimatization mechanisms serve to maintain an optimal physiological milieu, the effector responses are sometimes exaggerated, resulting in maladaptation and altitude/hypoxia-related illnesses [15]. One of the most common conditions is acute mountain sickness, characterized by nonspecific symptoms including headache, nausea, malaise, and dizziness. It typically manifests within the first two days of ascent to altitudes above 2,500 m in unacclimatized and susceptible individuals. Although self-limiting and normally resolving within a day or two, it can potentially progress to more serious conditions, which can be fatal and occur at altitudes above 3,000 m. Pulmonary edema is characterized by dyspnea and chest congestion, predominantly underlined by excessive hypoxic pulmonary vasoconstriction. Cerebral edema is marked by ataxia and decreased consciousness, primarily caused by increased fluid accumulation and swelling of the brain. Regardless of the cause, both conditions require immediate medical attention and/or evacuation to lower altitudes or higher PO_2 environments. These conditions usually develop with continuous acute and subacute exposures and are not relevant in the framework of short-term intermittent conditioning. Finally, susceptibility to these conditions and overall acclimatization capacity vary among individuals with factors such as age [16], biological sex [17], and premature birth [18] as well as chronic disease–associated physiological limitations being important modulators.

TABLE 1.2 Altitude range definitions and corresponding environmental parameters

Classification	Altitude(s) (m)	BP (mmHg)	PO_2 (mmHg)	P_IO_2 (mmHg)	F_IO_2 (%)
Near sea level	0–500	760–800	160–150	149–140	20.9–20
Low altitude	500–2,000	800–605	150–125	140–117	20–16.5
Moderate altitude	2,000–3,000	605–537	125–110	117–103	16.5–14.8
High altitude	3,000–5,500	537–395	110–82	103–72	14.8–10.2
Extreme altitude	> 5,500	< 395	< 82	<72	<10.2

Note: BP, Barometric pressure; PO_2: Partial pressure of ambient O_2; P_IO_2: Partial pressure of inspired O_2; F_IO_2: Fraction of inspired O_2 corresponding to targeted values at sea level (normobaria). PO_2, P_IO_2, and F_IO_2 values are recalculated based on data from [13]. Altitude ranges are defined according to the proposed classification from [14].

These factors, therefore, require consideration in the framework of hypoxic adaptation and conditioning.

1.1.3 Hypoxic dose—The key driver of physiological adaptation

Exposure of humans to various environmental factors provokes a dose-modulated response, typically following the hormesis principle of stimulatory effects up to a certain level and inhibitory effects beyond [19]. Accordingly, defining and targeting an optimal hypoxic dose is crucial within the framework of hypoxia conditioning to maximize physiological benefits while minimizing harmful consequences. The overall hypoxic dose is defined by three parameters: (1) hypoxia intensity (defined by the level of reduction in PO_2 and/or P_AO_2), (2) hypoxia duration (defining the duration of a particular hypoxic exposure), and (3) hypoxia frequency (encompassing the number of repetitions in an intermittent hypoxic exposure scenario). In addition, factors such as hypoxia type (hypobaric or normobaric), hypoxic pattern (considering combinations with other factors such as hyperoxia and temperature), and timing of hypoxic exposures (effects of circadian and seasonal cycles) are known to modulate the subsequent effects of a particular hypoxic dose and should be taken into consideration. For example, ample evidence shows that, in healthy humans, a relatively small hypoxic dose is sufficient to provoke measurable ventilatory acclimatization (heightened hypoxic ventilatory response). Conversely, a significantly greater hypoxic dose is required to result in importantly augmented hematological adaptation (i.e., increased hemoglobin mass).

Various attempts have been made to define or calculate the hypoxic dose and thereby characterize the dose-response relationships with numerous hypoxia-related physiological adaptations. These efforts are grounded in two complementary approaches—one trying to quantify the "external" exogenous hypoxic load and the other the "internal" endogenous hypoxic stress. The external exogenous load can be simply defined by the amount of time spent at a certain altitude or hypoxic. Recently, new exposure metrics have been developed, such as "kilometer hours," defined as exposure elevation times total exposure duration [20], and accumulated altitude exposure that is calculated multiplying the altitude elevation and the number of residence days [21]. Novel metrics aiming to quantify the internal hypoxic dose include "saturation hours" that consider the duration of particular capillary oxygen saturation (S_pO_2) during hypoxic exposure [22], and SpO_2 to F_IO_2 ratio index [23] that takes into account the external and consequent internal load.

A major benefit of aiming to implement the actual internal hypoxic dose is undoubtedly related to the significant individual variability in response to standardized hypoxic stimuli. There is ample evidence indicating that the magnitude of most physiological responses to hypoxia varies significantly between individuals [24, 25]. Although the exact underpinnings of this variance remain unclear, they are probably related to differences in peripheral chemoreceptor sensitivity [26] and genetic signatures [27]. Accordingly, the characterization of the exact internal and particularly internal hypoxic dose, along with individualized approaches, seems paramount in the framework of hypoxic conditioning. This approach should provide the development of optimized protocols on the one hand and enable the proper scrutiny of the individual effects of the employed protocol on the other.

1.2 Normobaric versus hypobaric hypoxia

1.2.1 Real versus simulated altitude with contemporary technological approaches

Logistical challenges connected with high-altitude sojourns and the limited availability of suitable altitude locations in many world regions have led to the extensive development of alternative technological methods enabling altitude simulation. These methods are particularly relevant for various acute and sub-acute intermittent hypoxic conditioning and training modalities that may be impractical to execute at terrestrial altitudes. Given that PO_2 levels change as a function of variations in BP and/or F_IO_2, achieving the same level of environmental hypoxia can theoretically be accomplished by manipulating either of those factors [28]. From a technological perspective, there are two main modes or means of inducing hypoxia (e.g., PO_2 reduction)—namely, hypobaric (HH) and normobaric hypoxia (NH). HH is induced by lowering BP either via ascent to a higher terrestrial altitude or artificially using hypobaric chambers (simulated HH). On the other hand, NH is usually generated by reducing F_IO_2 using portable or stationary hypoxic air generators. These devices use different technological approaches (e.g., oxygen filtration, vacuum pressure swing adsorption, and similar) to generate hypoxic air. Depending on their capacity, they can be used for individual applications (via masks and/or tents) or for building hypoxic facilities (e.g., hypoxic rooms and hotels). Bottled precision hypoxic mixtures represent an alternative NH application method, often used in research and conditioning settings. For hypoxic conditioning, terrestrial altitude remains the method of choice, mostly for sub-acute and chronic exposures, as hypobaric chambers are often difficult to access, challenging to maintain, and primarily used for research and specific purposes. On the other hand, for acute and sub-acute hypoxic conditioning, NH that predominantly uses hypoxicators is favored due to its ease of transitions from hypoxic to normoxic (and oftentimes hyperoxic) exposures at the same location. Besides logistical advantages, the lower cost of NH applications makes simulated NH strategies more feasible and accessible to a larger population.

The physiological reasoning for using NH as a surrogate for HH exposures is based on the "equivalent air altitude" model, suggesting that exposure to the same PO_2, whether achieved by reducing F_IO_2 or BP, should result in relatively similar physiological responses [28]. However, as outlined in a subsequent section, a growing body of evidence challenges this assumption and suggests that numerous physiological responses crucial for adaptation to hypoxia or altitude may differ between HH and NH.

1.2.2 Are normobaric and hypobaric hypoxia comparable?

Early studies that challenged the physiological equivalence of HH and NH showed that HH can provoke greater high-altitude illness severity [29] and detailed differential ventilatory [30, 31] and fluid balance [32] responses between the two. Subsequently, numerous studies have been conducted on the topic, and the majority of those, with key findings summarized in Table 1.3, have supported the notion that HH might represent a greater physiological stimulus than NH at the same PO_2. While the exact underpinning mechanisms remain unclear, it has been hypothesized that the HH-related change in BP can independently provoke greater pulmonary vasoconstriction [30] and result in greater physiological dead space within the respiratory system [31]. It must be

TABLE 1.3 Key studies investigating physiological differences between normobaric and hypobaric hypoxia at the same P_IO_2

Parameter	Outcome	Study
Respiration	↑ V_E & ↓ S_pO_2	[30]
	↑ V_E & ↓ S_pO_2	[31]
	↔ V_E & S_pO_2	[37]
NO metabolism	↓ eNO	[38]
AMS	↑ AMS incidence	[39]
	↔ AMS	[37]
Sleep quality	↑ AHI & ↑ periodic breathing	[40]
Redox balance	↑ OS & ↓ AO	[41]
	↑ OS	[42]
	↑ OS	[43]
Postural stability	↓ postural stability	[44]
Exercise performance	↓ Time trial	[45]
	↓ Time trial	[46]
Hematological adaptation	↔ HBmass	[47]
Cerebral	↔ Cerebral perfusion	[48]

Note: ↑: Increased in HH as compared to NH; ↓: Decreased in HH as opposed to NH; ↔: No significant difference between HH and NH; V_E: Minute ventilation; S_pO_2: Capillary oxygen saturation; eNO: Exhaled nitric oxide; AMS: Acute mountain sickness; AHI: Apnea-hypopnea index; OS: Oxidative stress; AO: Antioxidant capacity; HBmass: Hemoglobin mass.

noted, however, that the topic of HH and NH equivalency has been extensively debated [33–36] and still lacks a final consensus. It seems conceivable that some of the equivocal findings regarding responses of various physiological parameters might indeed be related to methodological issues and insufficient control of all relevant environmental factors.

Regardless of the foregoing and given the clear importance of BP in PO_2 modulation, seasonal and daily variations in BP at the same terrestrial altitude also warrant mention. While reported by West et al. [49] and more recently analyzed using one year of BP variation data from different altitude locations in Switzerland [35], significant variations in BP and corresponding "simulated" altitude changes were observed. The maximal daily variations were ≈ 250 m, and the maximal yearly variations were ≈ 500 m at the same altitude location. Accordingly, these changes need to be considered both when using HH conditioning and when comparing study outcomes between HH and NH.

Overall, despite varying opinions, the presented data underscore the importance of considering potential differences between the HH and NH. When implementing both HH and NH conditioning, any changes in BP (as well as F_IO_2) need to be considered while defining the targeted and actual hypoxic dose. Moreover, the exact reporting of all relevant environmental parameters (e.g., exposure altitude, BP, PO_2, and F_IO_2) and, when directly comparing HH versus NH, exact matching of PO_2 should become the norm for future research and applied work in this area.

Abbreviations

AHI	apnea-hypopnea index
AMS	acute mountain sickness
AO	antioxidant capacity
ATP	adenosine triphosphate
BP	barometric pressure
cAMP	cyclic adenosine monophosphate
CO_2	carbon dioxide
eNO	exhaled nitric oxide
F_IO_2	fraction of inspired O_2
HBmass	haemoglobin mass
HH	hypobaric hypoxia
HIF	hypoxia-inducible factor(s)
NF-κB	nuclear factor kappa-light-chain-enhancer of activated B cells
NH	normobaric hypoxia
O_2	oxygen
OS	oxidative stress
P_AO_2	arterial partial pressure of O_2

P_IO_2 partial pressure of inspired O_2
PO_2 partial pressure of ambient O_2
S_pO_2 capillary oxygen saturation
V_E minute ventilation.

References

1. Samanta, D., N.R. Prabhakar, and G.L. Semenza, *Systems biology of oxygen homeostasis.* Wiley Interdiscip Rev Syst Biol Med, 2017. **9**(4).
2. Cummins, E.P., M.J. Strowitzki, and C.T. Taylor, *Mechanisms and consequences of oxygen and carbon dioxide sensing in mammals.* Physiol Rev, 2020. **100**(1): p. 463–88.
3. Kaelin, W.G., Jr. and P.J. Ratcliffe, *Oxygen sensing by metazoans: The central role of the HIF hydroxylase pathway.* Mol Cell, 2008. **30**(4): p. 393–402.
4. Prabhakar, N.R. and G.L. Semenza, *Adaptive and maladaptive cardiorespiratory responses to continuous and intermittent hypoxia mediated by hypoxia-inducible factors 1 and 2.* Physiol Rev, 2012. **92**(3): p. 967–1003.
5. Cummins, E.P. and C.T. Taylor, *Hypoxia-responsive transcription factors.* Pflugers Arch, 2005. **450**(6): p. 363–71.
6. Brugniaux, J.V., et al., *Highs and lows of hyperoxia: Physiological, performance, and clinical aspects.* Am J Phys Regul Integr Comp Phys, 2018. **315**(1): p. R1–R27.
7. Singer, M., et al., *Dangers of hyperoxia.* Crit Care, 2021. **25**(1): p. 440.
8. Panza, G.S., J. Burtscher, and F. Zhao, *Intermittent hypoxia: A call for harmonization in terminology.* J Appl Physiol, 1985. **135**(4): p. 886–90, 2023.
9. West, J.B., *Early history of high-altitude physiology.* Ann N Y Acad Sci, 2016. **1365**(1): p. 33–42.
10. Brown, J.P. and M.P. Grocott, *Humans at altitude: Physiology and pathophysiology.* Continuing Education in Anaesthesia Critical Care & Pain, 2012. **13**(1): p. 17–22.
11. Wehrlin, J.P. and J. Hallen, *Linear decrease in .VO2max and performance with increasing altitude in endurance athletes.* Eur J Appl Physiol, 2006. **96**(4): p. 404–12.
12. Luks, A.M., *Physiology in medicine: A physiologic approach to prevention and treatment of acute high-altitude illnesses.* J Appl Physiol (1985), 2015. **118**(5): p. 509–19.
13. Gallagher, S.A. and P.H. Hackett, *High-altitude illness.* Emerg Med Clin North Am, 2004. **22**(2): p. 329–55, viii.
14. Bartsch, P. and B. Saltin, *General introduction to altitude adaptation and mountain sickness.* Scand J Med Sci Sports, 2008. **18 Suppl 1**: p. 1–10.
15. Luks, A.M., E.R. Swenson, and P. Bärtsch, *Acute high-altitude sickness.* Eur Respir J, 2017. **26**(143): p. 160096.
16. Levine, B.D., J.H. Zuckerman, and C.R. deFilippi, *Effect of high-altitude exposure in the elderly: The Tenth Mountain Division study.* Circulation, 1997. **96**(4): p. 1224–32.
17. Beidleman, B.A., et al., *Predictive models of acute mountain sickness after rapid ascent to various altitudes.* Med Sci Sports Exerc, 2013. **45**(4): p. 792–800.
18. Debevec, T., et al., *Premature birth: A neglected consideration for altitude adaptation.* J Appl Physiol (1985), 2022. **133**(4): p. 975–8.

19. Calabrese, E.J. and M.P. Mattson, *Hormesis provides a generalized quantitative estimate of biological plasticity.* J Cell Commun Signal, 2011. **5**(1): p. 25–38.
20. Garvican-Lewis, L.A., K. Sharpe, and C.J. Gore, *Time for a new metric for hypoxic dose?* J Appl Physiol (1985), 2016. **121**(1): p. 352–5.
21. Beidleman, B.A., et al., *New metric of hypoxic dose predicts altitude acclimatization status following various ascent profiles.* Phys Rep, 2019. **7**(20): p. e14263.
22. Millet, G.P., et al., *Commentaries on viewpoint: Time for a new metric for hypoxic dose?* J Appl Physiol (1985), 2016. **121**(1): p. 356–8.
23. Soo, J., et al., *The use of the SpO(2) to FiO(2) ratio to individualize the hypoxic dose in sport science, exercise, and health settings.* Front Physiol, 2020. **11**: p. 570472.
24. Friedmann, B., et al., *Individual variation in the erythropoietic response to altitude training in elite junior swimmers.* Br J Sports Med, 2005. **39**(3): p. 148–53.
25. Chapman, R.F., J. Stray-Gundersen, and B.D. Levine, *Individual variation in response to altitude training.* J Appl Physiol, 1998. **85**(4): p. 1448–56.
26. Vizek, M., C.K. Pickett, and J.V. Weil, *Interindividual variation in hypoxic ventilatory response: Potential role of carotid body.* J Appl Physiol (1985), 1987. **63**(5): p. 1884–9.
27. Simonson, T.S. and A. Malhotra, *Variability in hypoxic response: Could genetics play a role?* J Physiol, 2020. **598**(10): p. 1805–6.
28. Conkin, J. and J.H. Wessel, 3rd, *Critique of the equivalent air altitude model.* Aviat Space Environ Med, 2008. **79**(10): p. 975–82.
29. Roach, R.C., J.A. Loeppky, and M.V. Icenogle, *Acute mountain sickness: Increased severity during simulated altitude compared with normobaric hypoxia.* J Appl Physiol, 1996. **81**(5): p. 1908–10.
30. Loeppky, J.A., et al., *Ventilation during simulated altitude, normobaric hypoxia and normoxic hypobaria.* Respir Physiol, 1997. **107**(3): p. 231–9.
31. Savourey, G., et al., *Normo- and hypobaric hypoxia: Are there any physiological differences?* Eur J Appl Physiol, 2003. **89**(2): p. 122–6.
32. Levine, B.D., et al., *Role of barometric pressure in pulmonary fluid balance and oxygen transport.* J Appl Physiol, 1988. **64**(1): p. 419–28.
33. Millet, G.P., R. Faiss, and V. Pialoux, *Point: Counterpoint: Hypobaric hypoxia induces/does not induce different responses from normobaric hypoxia.* J Appl Physiol, 2012. **112**(10): p. 1783–4.
34. Richalet, J.P., *CrossTalk opposing view: Barometric pressure, independent of PO2, IS NOT the forgotten parameter in altitude physiology and mountain medicine.* Phys J, 2020. **598**(5): p. 897–99.
35. Millet, G.P. and T. Debevec, *CrossTalk proposal: Barometric pressure, independent of PO2, is the forgotten parameter in altitude physiology and mountain medicine.* J Physiol, 2020. **598**(5): p. 893–96.
36. Richard, N.A. and M.S. Koehle, *Differences in cardio-ventilatory responses to hypobaric and normobaric hypoxia: A review.* Aviat Space Environ Med, 2012. **83**(7): p. 677–84.
37. Richard, N.A., et al., *Acute mountain sickness, chemosensitivity and cardio-respiratory responses in humans exposed to hypobaric and normobaric hypoxia.* J Appl Physiol, 2013. 116(7): p. 945–52.
38. Hemmingsson, T. and D. Linnarsson, *Lower exhaled nitric oxide in hypobaric than in normobaric acute hypoxia.* Respir Physiol Neurobiol, 2009. **169**(1): p. 74–7.

39. DiPasquale, D.M., et al., *Hypoxia, hypobaria, and exercise duration affect acute mountain sickness.* Aerosp Med Hum Perform, 2015. **86**(7): p. 614–9.

40. Heinzer, R., et al., *Comparison of sleep disorders between real and simulated 3,450-m altitude.* Sleep, 2016. **39**(8): p. 1517–23.

41. Ribon, A., et al., *Exposure to hypobaric hypoxia results in higher oxidative stress compared to normobaric hypoxia.* Respir Physiol Neurobiol, 2016. **223**: p. 23–7.

42. Faiss, R., et al., *Ventilation, oxidative stress and nitric oxide in hypobaric vs. normobaric hypoxia.* Med Sci Sports Exerc, 2013. **45**(2): p. 253–60.

43. Debevec, T., et al., *Prooxidant/antioxidant balance in hypoxia: A cross-over study on normobaric vs. hypobaric "live high-train low".* PLoS One, 2015. **10**(9): p. e0137957.

44. Degache, F., et al., *Hypobaric versus normobaric hypoxia: Same effects on postural stability?* High Alt Med Biol, 2012. **13**(1): p. 40–5.

45. Beidleman, B.A., et al., *Cycling performance decrement is greater in hypobaric versus normobaric hypoxia.* Extrem Physiol Med, 2014. **3**: p. 8.

46. Saugy, J.J., et al., *Cycling time trial is more altered in hypobaric than normobaric hypoxia.* Med Sci Sports Exerc, 2016. **48**(4): p. 680–8.

47. Hauser, A., et al., *Similar hemoglobin mass response in hypobaric and normobaric hypoxia in athletes.* Med Sci Sports Exerc, 2016. **48**(4): p. 734–41.

48. DiPasquale, D.M., et al., *Evidence for cerebral edema, cerebral perfusion, and intracranial pressure elevations in acute mountain sickness.* Brain Behav, 2016. **6**(3): p. e00437.

49. West, J.B., et al., *Barometric pressures at extreme altitudes on Mt. Everest: Physiological significance.* J Appl Physiol Respir Environ Exerc Physiol, 1983. **54**(5): p. 1188–94.

2

MECHANISMS OF INTERMITTENT HYPOXIA HEALTH BENEFITS

Johannes Burtscher, Oleg S. Glazachev and Robert T. Mallet

2.1 Background

As obligate aerobes, humans are utterly dependent upon an uninterrupted supply of atmospheric oxygen. While many biochemical processes require oxygen, rendering the molecule indispensable for cellular functioning, mitochondrial oxidative phosphorylation consumes the lion's share of inspired oxygen to maintain the Gibbs free energy of ATP hydrolysis. Although glycolysis yields a modest amount of ATP, oxidative phosphorylation is the predominant ATP producer. Tissues with high energy demand, including brain, heart, exercising skeletal muscle, and kidney, are especially dependent on a continuous oxygen supply. Consequently, oxygen deficiency (i.e., hypoxia) imperils cells, organs, and the organism and plays a pivotal role in many diseases. In fact, hypoxia is either a cause, co-conspirator, or consequence of most pathologies, some of which will be discussed in later chapters. But reliance on oxygen incurs risks. A powerful oxidant, oxygen can extract electrons from its environment, transforming it into potentially cytotoxic reactive oxygen species (ROS) capable of damaging biomolecules and compromising cellular function. Consequently, aerobic organisms exist in a narrow, dynamic equilibrium between the threats of too little (hypoxia) and too much oxygen (hyperoxia) and must adapt to changes in inspired oxygen to maintain optimal oxygen supply.

Oxygen supply–demand balances vary among tissues and are partly determined by oxygen concentration in the inspired air or transported in the blood oxygen content, versus tissue oxygen demand, which changes according to varies with cellular activity; thus, during intense exercise the oxygen demand of working skeletal muscle massively exceeds its resting oxygen demand.

DOI: 10.4324/9781003402879-3

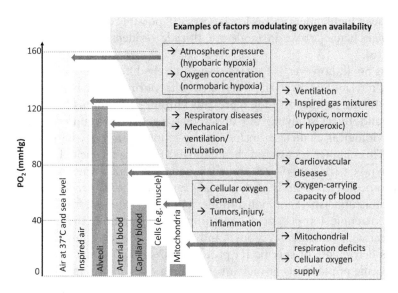

FIGURE 2.1   Partial pressure of oxygen (PO₂) across the "oxygen cascade" and examples of factors modulating oxygen availability.

Figure 2.1 depicts the partial pressure gradient of oxygen at sea level, from the atmosphere to the ultimate oxygen consumers, the mitochondria. These values vary across tissues and are perturbed by several factors, including inspiratory hypoxia, increased oxygen demand ("functional hypoxia"), or diseases. Pulmonary and cardiovascular diseases may interfere with systemic oxygen supply, and tumors, trauma, or inflammatory events may impose local hypoxia.

Recently, it has been proposed that in certain diseases impaired oxygen utilization (for example due to mitochondrial defects) can cause "functional hyperoxia," a consequence of oxygen supply exceeding cellular oxygen-consuming capacity [1]. Several mitochondrial diseases (such as Leigh syndrome) may produce such conditions, and environmental hypoxia has proven to be beneficial in animal models of such diseases [1–4]. In addition, epidemiological studies reported health benefits and reduced mortality from numerous diseases in long-term moderate-high altitude residents [5]. Reduced mortality from all diseases, especially cardiovascular diseases and some cancers (e.g., colon and breast cancer), has been documented in people living at moderate altitudes in alpine countries such as Switzerland [6] and Austria [7, 8], compared to lowland populations. While the mechanistic basis of these effects is not fully understood and many other parameters (e.g., geoclimatic and socioeconomic differences between the observed populations) may play a role, hypoxia likely contributes by inducing protective adaptations. One study demonstrated improved cerebral substrate delivery and dynamic autoregulatory function of the neurovascular unit in Andean highlanders versus lowlanders [9], possibly explaining the reduced risk of ischemic stroke in moderate altitude residents reported in another study [6].

This book, however, is focused on an entirely different hypoxia paradigm: cyclic, intermittent hypoxia, alternated with normoxia or hyperoxia exposures. Living at high altitude represents chronic, continuous hypoxia exposure, and those studying the underlying mechanisms confront daunting methodological challenges including the aforementioned confounding factors. This chapter focuses on the adaptive mechanisms elicited by intermittent hypoxia (IH) exposures and their potential health benefits. Controlled IH protocols enable study of the actual effects of hypoxia *per se*, free of other environmental aspects of high altitude, and represent more feasible interventions for clinical applications. As outlined in Chapter 1, the hypoxic dose together with individual responses and vulnerabilities determines the benefits versus detriments of specific IH protocols. Defining optimal hypoxic doses for specific populations or individuals is a major challenge for clinical application of IH. Subsequent chapters will address this matter specifically for individual applications. Here, we discuss potential benefits of IH utilizing health-promoting hypoxic doses. Such protocols directed toward improving health and physical performance, or symptoms and progression of diseases, are termed *intermittent hypoxia conditioning*.

2.2 Cellular responses and adaptations to hypoxia and reoxygenation

Cellular responses to hypoxia primarily aim at (1) maintaining vital biochemical and metabolic functions to avoid injury, energetic crisis, and cell death; and (2) improving resilience to the dangers of hypoxia and subsequent reoxygenation, itself associated with excessive ROS formation and oxidative stress. Both hypoxia and reoxygenation can damage mitochondria and trigger the release of inflammatory molecules. Functional and metabolic adaptations protecting cells from hypoxia-reoxygenation increase anaerobic ATP production capacity, capillary density, and oxygen-carrying capacity of the blood [10, 11]. The hypoxia-inducible transcription factors (HIFs) play pivotal roles in orchestrating these responses and the subsequent adaptations. Of the three known HIFs, characterized by their distinct α subunits, HIF-1 and HIF-2 are best understood, and their role in cellular hypoxia responses is well-established. HIF-3 likely is a regulator of HIF-1 and HIF-2 [12].

HIFs are regulated by and interact with many other factors. Transcriptionally, their levels are modulated by the transcription factors nuclear factor erythroid 2-related factor 2 (Nrf2), nuclear factor-κB (NF-κB), and specific protein 1 (SP1). The posttranslational regulation of HIFs primarily depends on oxygen availability (Figure 2.2) but is also influenced by microRNAs, long

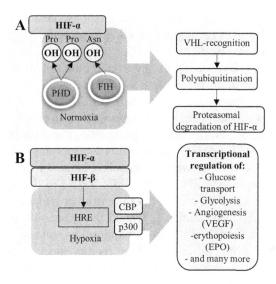

FIGURE 2.2   Oxygen concentration regulates the stability of the α-subunits of hypoxia inducible factors (HIFs). In normoxia, HIF-α subunits are hydroxylated (OH) continuously by prolyl hydroxylases (PHD) and factor inhibiting HIF (FIH). Hydroxylation allows recognition by the Von Hippel-Lindau protein (VHL), resulting in poly-ubiquitination and proteasomal degradation of HIF-α. In hypoxia, the hydroxylase activities decline, allowing HIF-α accumulation. Upon dimerization of HIF-α with constitutive HIF-β subunits, the HIF dimer transactivates hypoxia responsive elements (HREs) and recruits co-activators like CREB binding protein (CBP) or p300 to gene promoters to regulate the transcription of hypoxia-regulated genes.

noncoding RNAs, and angiotensin II [13]. Moreover, HIFs interact with many signaling pathways, including the Wnt signaling pathway, and pathways related to mammalian target of rapamycin (mTOR), Myc/Notch, and the sphingosine system, to just name a few [12, 14].

The α-subunits of the dimeric HIF proteins are continuously synthesized and degraded in normoxic conditions. High oxygen availability enables oxygen, α-ketoglutarate, and ferrous iron-dependent hydroxylation of proline residues in HIF α-subunits by prolyl hydroxylases (PHDs), permitting α-subunit binding by Von Hippel-Lindau proteins, polyubiquitination, and proteasomal degradation [13]. Similar to PHDs, factor inhibiting HIF-1 (FIH-1) hydroxylates HIFs, albeit at different residues, and inactivation of FIH-1 requires greater reductions in oxygen availability.

In hypoxia, the reduced oxygen concentrations stabilize HIF-α subunits, whereupon they combine with constitutively expressed β-subunits, forming the HIF heterodimers (Figure 2.2) that orchestrate complex transcriptional responses to hypoxia by binding hypoxia response elements (HREs) in the promoters of HIF target genes and recruiting co-activators such as cyclic AMP response element-binding protein (CBP) or p300 [15–18]. Although the paralogues HIF-1 and HIF-2 have partially overlapping functions, bind the same HREs, and participate in the regulation of angiogenesis, fatty acid metabolism, and immune responses, some of their functions are isoform-specific [19, 20]. While HIF-1 regulates glucose transport, effects a metabolic switch from oxidative energy metabolism to glycolysis, and is responsible primarily for adaptations to acute hypoxia, HIF-2 mediates especially adaptations of the circulating blood to chronic hypoxia, including induction of erythropoiesis by activating erythropoietin (EPO) expression [19]. The distinct outcomes of HIF-1 and HIF-2 signaling arise from their distinct temporal activation patterns [12], specific DNA binding [21], and the expression of HIF-2 only in restricted cell-types and tissues versus ubiquitous expression of HIF-1.

Besides HIFs, many other molecular factors mediate cellular hypoxic responses [11]. Those include the aforementioned transcription factors Nrf2, which coordinates in particular protective adaptations against oxidative stress [22], and NF-κB, key regulator of immune responses [23]. Like PHDs, the catalytic activities of several other oxygen-dependent enzymes, including nicotinamide adenine dinucleotide phosphate (NADPH) oxidase (NOX), nitric oxide synthases (NOS), and heme oxygenase-1 (HO-1), contribute to biochemical changes in response to hypoxia. Numerous other mechanisms contribute to cellular consequences of adaptations to hypoxia, including remodeling of metabolism and ion homeostasis.

Signaling pathways related to AMP-activated protein kinase (AMPK) and mTOR are crucial to protect cells from hypoxia-provoked energy deficits. Activation by the ATP breakdown product AMP enables AMPK to sense ATP depletion (and likely also hypoxia directly [24]) and in response coordinate energy-generating and -conserving mechanisms, such as activation of phosphofructokinase, the key regulated step in glycolysis, and reduction of energy-intensive protein synthesis via inhibition of mTOR [25]. Both AMPK and HIFs also modulate mitochondrial biogenesis and mitophagy (mitochondrial degradation) pathways and thereby mitigate hypoxia-induced mitochondrial dysfunction [11].

In summary, cellular responses to mild hypoxic stress induce numerous protective adaptations, which may culminate in long-term increased resilience and metabolic efficiency, which may underlie the health benefits of hypoxia exposures.

2.3 Systemic responses to hypoxia

While many of the cellular responses to hypoxia described previously occur in most cells, there are also tissue- and organ-specific responses that elicit systemic adaptations. In some cases, these responses may be maladaptive, such as those associated with high altitude illnesses [26]. Here, we focus again on potentially beneficial responses to hypoxia that may underlie the positive health outcomes of controlled hypoxia exposures. Figure 2.3 summarizes cellular and systemic responses and adaptations to IH.

Acute systemic hypoxia is sensed by chemoreceptors, primarily the peripheral chemoreceptor neurons in the carotid bodies. Afferent signals from these chemoreceptors activate the sympathetic nervous system and/or suppress parasympathetic activity [27] and mediate ventilatory and cardiovascular responses directed toward improving oxygen uptake and distribution throughout the body. The hypoxic ventilatory response (HVR) is associated with ventilatory plasticity, that is, progressive augmentation of the HVR and ventilatory long-term facilitation, which could be particularly beneficial in respiratory diseases [28].

Cardiovascular responses to acute hypoxia include increased heart rate, cardiac output, and systemic arterial pressure, which collectively improve systemic oxygen provision [13]. Controlled hypoxia exposures, especially IH, may improve cardiovascular responses to hypoxia and attenuate hypoxic sympatho-excitation, which may ultimately lower systolic blood pressure and is therefore

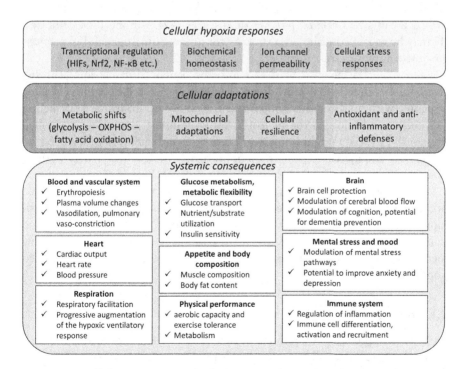

FIGURE 2.3 Cellular responses and adaptations to hypoxia and systemic outcomes.

a promising approach for treatment of hypertension [29–31] but may also have cardio- and vascular endothelium-protective properties benefiting many cardiovascular conditions [32–35]. Related mechanisms that possibly improve cardiovascular health through IH are augmentation of nitric oxide (NO) formation, vascular NO stores [33], and NO-mediated vasodilation, as well as metabolic, anti-oxidative, and anti-inflammatory consequences [13].

Hypoxia shifts blood distribution as a result of pulmonary hypoxic vaso-constriction combined with concomitant in most other tissues [22]. In addition, plasma volume and total hemoglobin mass are augmented by hypoxia [36]. Adaptations of the blood include increased erythropoiesis, which, by increasing oxygen-carrying capacity of the circulation, may increase physical performance [37] and protect the brain [38]. The hypoxic dose required to induce hematological changes, which may be modest or negligible in many protocols employing moderate IH [32], remains debated.

Hypoxia affects nutrient utilization and metabolism as well as appetite [39]. Particularly, consequences of hypoxia on systemic glucose homeostasis and lipid metabolism have raised interest in IH-based approaches to treat obesity and metabolic diseases, such as diabetes [40, 41].

The potential of applying IH to modulate psychological stress-related pathways (e.g., the hypothalamic-pituitary-adrenal axis and the sympatho-adrenomedullary axis) with hypoxia has resulted in suggestions to apply controlled IH in stress-related psychiatric diseases [42]. Among those illnesses, IH may be most promising as a strategy for anxiety disorders and in particular post-traumatic stress disorder.

Controlled IH has also been shown to be beneficial in neurological diseases: for example, it may slow down or temporarily reverse cognitive decline in people with mild cognitive impairment, a common prodrome of dementia [43, 44]. In addition to the neuroprotective cellular adaptations described previously, hypoxia might boost brain function via regulation of the cerebral blood flow and increased generation of protective molecules, such as erythropoietin and brain-derived neurotrophic factor (BDNF) [13].

Taken together, hypoxia substantially modulates the functioning of most organs and induces pronounced systemic changes. Understanding the physiological responses to hypoxia and accounting for hypoxic dose effects and individual differences will inform the development of hypoxia-based treatments to specifically improve dysfunctional organs in at-risk or diseased populations.

2.4 Conclusions

As hypoxia represents a vital threat to humans and other aerobic organisms, it demands appropriate cellular and systemic responses. Increasing understanding of the physiological consequences of hypoxia has informed the development and clinical application of IH, a new approach with great promise for treatment of diverse diseases. Many intermittent hypoxia conditioning/exposure/training protocols demonstrate the potential to increase physical and psychological functions, and their noninvasive character makes them highly facile interventions for numerous diseases. To fully exploit IH's potential, it is essential to clearly elucidate the underlying mechanisms, define the impact of the hypoxic dose, and optimize protocols for specific applications. This book summarizes and evaluates hypoxia-based strategies for different therapeutic purposes so as to provide the reader a broad overview of IH applications and lay the foundation for future research to optimize hypoxia treatments for health applications.

Abbreviations

BDNF	brain-derived neurotrophic factor
CBP	cyclic AMP response element-binding protein
EPO	erythropoietin
FIH1	factor inhibiting HIF-1
HIF	hypoxia-inducible transcription factor
HRE	hypoxia response element
IH	intermittent hypoxia
mTOR	mammalian target of rapamycin
NADPH	nicotinamide adenine dinucleotide phosphate
NF-κB	nuclear factor-κB
Nrf2	nuclear factor erythroid 2-related factor 2
PHD	prolyl hydroxylases
ROS	reactive oxygen species
SP1	specific protein 1

References

1. Jain, I.H., et al., *Leigh syndrome mouse model can be rescued by interventions that normalize brain hyperoxia, but not hif activation.* Cell Metab, 2019. 30(4): p. 824–832.
2. Jain, I.H., et al., *Hypoxia as a therapy for mitochondrial disease.* Science, 2016. 352(6281): p. 54–61.
3. Ast, T., et al., *Continuous, but not intermittent, regimens of hypoxia prevent and reverse ataxia in a murine model of Friedreich's ataxia.* Hum Mol Genet, 2023. 32(16): p. 2600–2610.
4. Ferrari, M., et al., *Hypoxia treatment reverses neurodegenerative disease in a mouse model of Leigh syndrome.* Proc Natl Acad Sci USA, 2017. 114(21): p. E4241–E4250.
5. Burtscher, M., *Lower mortality rates in those living at moderate altitude.* Aging, 2016. 8(10): p. 2603–2604.
6. Faeh, D., et al., *Lower mortality from coronary heart disease and stroke at higher altitudes in Switzerland.* Circulation, 2009. 120(6): p. 495.

7. Burtscher, J., G.P. Millet, and M. Burtscher, *Does living at moderate altitudes in Austria affect mortality rates of various causes? An ecological study.* BMJ Open, 2021. **11**(6): p. e048520.
8. Burtscher, J., et al., *Moderate altitude residence reduces male colorectal and female breast cancer mortality more than incidence: Therapeutic implications?* Cancers (Basel), 2021. **13**(17): p. 4420.
9. Stacey, B.S., et al., *Lifelong exposure to high-altitude hypoxia in humans is associated with improved redox homeostasis and structural-functional adaptations of the neurovascular unit.* J Physiol, 2023. **601**(6): p. 1095–1120.
10. Baik, A.H. and I.H. Jain, *Turning the oxygen dial: Balancing the highs and lows.* Trends Cell Biol, 2020. **30**(7): p. 516–536.
11. Lee, P., N.S. Chandel, and M.C. Simon, *Cellular adaptation to hypoxia through hypoxia inducible factors and beyond.* Nat Rev Mol Cell Biol, 2020. **21**(5): p. 268–283.
12. Lendahl, U., et al., *Generating specificity and diversity in the transcriptional response to hypoxia.* Nat Rev Genet, 2009. **10**(12): p. 821–832.
13. Burtscher, J., et al., *Mechanisms underlying the health benefits of intermittent hypoxia conditioning.* J Physiol, 2023. DOI: 10.1113/JP285230
14. Burtscher, J., et al., *A rationale for hypoxic and chemical conditioning in Huntington's disease.* Int J Mol Sci, 2021. **22**(2).
15. Ruas, J.L., L. Poellinger, and T. Pereira, *Role of CBP in regulating HIF-1-mediated activation of transcription.* J Cell Sci, 2005. **118**(2): p. 301–311.
16. Arany, Z., et al., *An essential role for p300/CBP in the cellular response to hypoxia.* Proc Natl Acad Sci USA, 1996. **93**(23): p. 12969–12973.
17. Xia, X., et al., *Integrative analysis of HIF binding and transactivation reveals its role in maintaining histone methylation homeostasis.* Proc Natl Acad Sci, 2009. **106**(11): p. 4260–4265.
18. Wenger, R.H., D.P. Stiehl, and G. Camenisch, *Integration of oxygen signaling at the consensus HRE.* Sci STKE, 2005. **2005**(306): p. re12–re12.
19. Burtscher, J., et al., *Environmental and behavioral regulation of HIF-mitochondria crosstalk.* Free Radic Biol Med, 2023. **206**: p. 63–73.
20. Mole, D.R., et al., *Genome-wide association of hypoxia-inducible factor (HIF)-1α and HIF-2α DNA binding with expression profiling of hypoxia-inducible transcripts.* J Biol Chem, 2009. **284**(25): p. 16767–16775.
21. Smythies, J.A., et al., *Inherent DNA-binding specificities of the HIF-1α and HIF-2α transcription factors in chromatin.* EMBO Rep, 2019. **20**(1).
22. Burtscher, J., et al., *Adaptive responses to hypoxia and/or hyperoxia in humans.* Antioxid Redox Signal, 2022. 37(13): p. 887–912.
23. Scholz, C.C., et al., *Regulation of IL-1β-induced NF-κB by hydroxylases links key hypoxic and inflammatory signaling pathways.* Proc Natl Acad Sci USA, 2013. **110**(46): p. 18490–18495.
24. Dengler, F., *Activation of AMPK under hypoxia: Many roads leading to Rome.* Int J Mol Sci, 2020. **21**(7).
25. Liu, L., et al., *Hypoxia-induced energy stress regulates mRNA translation and cell growth.* Mol Cell, 2006. **21**(4): p. 521–531.
26. Luks, A.M. and P.H. Hackett, *Medical conditions and high-altitude travel.* N Engl J Med, 2022. **386**(4): p. 364–373.
27. Meyer, M.J., et al., *Changes in heart rate and rhythm during a crossover study of simulated commercial flight in older and vulnerable participants.* Front Physiol, 2019. **10**: p. 1339.
28. Puri, S., G. Panza, and J.H. Mateika, *A comprehensive review of respiratory, autonomic and cardiovascular responses to intermittent hypoxia in humans.* Exp Neurol, 2021. **341**: p. 113709.

29. Chacaroun, S., et al., *Physiological responses to two hypoxic conditioning strategies in healthy subjects.* Front Physiol, 2016. **7**: p. 675.
30. Panza, G.S., et al., *Daily exposure to mild intermittent hypoxia reduces blood pressure in male OSA patients with hypertension.* Am J Respir Crit Care Med, 2022. **205**(8): p. 949–958.
31. Glazachev, O.S., et al., *Safety and efficacy of intermittent hypoxia conditioning as a new rehabilitation/ secondary prevention strategy for patients with cardiovascular diseases: A systematic review and meta-analysis.* Curr Cardiol Rev, 2021. **17**(6): p. e051121193317.
32. Mallet, R.T., et al., *Beta1-adrenergic receptor antagonism abrogates cardioprotective effects of intermittent hypoxia.* Basic Res Cardiol, 2006. **101**(5): p. 436–446.
33. Manukhina, E.B., et al., *Normobaric, intermittent hypoxia conditioning is cardio- and vasoprotective in rats.* Exp Biol Med (Maywood), 2013. **238**(12): p. 1413–1420.
34. Jarrard, C.P., et al., *Hypoxic preconditioning attenuates ischemia-reperfusion injury in young healthy adults.* J Appl Physiol (1985), 2021. **130**(3): p. 846–852.
35. Stray-Gundersen, S., et al., *Hypoxic preconditioning reduces endothelial ischemia-reperfusion injury in older adults.* Am J Phys Regul Integr Comp Phys, 2022. **323**(5): p. R832–R838.
36. Siebenmann, C., P. Robach, and C. Lundby, *Regulation of blood volume in lowlanders exposed to high altitude.* J Appl Physiol (1985), 2017. **123**(4): p. 957–966.
37. Rodriguez, F.A., et al., *Intermittent hypobaric hypoxia stimulates erythropoiesis and improves aerobic capacity.* Med Sci Sports Exer, 1999. **31**(2): p. 264–268.
38. Ehrenreich, H., et al., *Introducing the brain erythropoietin circle to explain adaptive brain hardware upgrade and improved performance.* Mol Psychiatry, 2022. **27**(5): p. 2372–2379.
39. Matu, J., et al., *The effects of hypoxia on hunger perceptions, appetite-related hormone concentrations and energy intake: A systematic review and meta-analysis.* Appetite, 2018. **125**: p. 98–108.
40. Kayser, B. and S. Verges, *Hypoxia, energy balance and obesity: From pathophysiological mechanisms to new treatment strategies.* Obes Rev, 2013. **14**(7): p. 579–592.
41. Netzer, N., et al., *Hypoxia, oxidative stress and fat.* Biomol, 2015. **5**(2): p. 1143–1150.
42. Burtscher, J., et al., *The interplay of hypoxic and mental stress: Implications for anxiety and depressive disorders.* Neurosci Biobehav Rev, 2022. **138**: p. 104718.
43. Bayer, U., et al., *Intermittent hypoxic-hyperoxic training on cognitive performance in geriatric patients.* Alzheimers Dement (N Y), 2017. **3**(1): p. 114–122.
44. Wang, H., et al., *Intermittent hypoxia training for treating mild cognitive impairment: A pilot study.* Am J Alzheimers Dis Other Dement, 2020. **35**: p. 1533317519896725.

3A

ISCHEMIC PRECONDITIONING

A practical tool for enhancing exercise performance

François Billaut and Gustavo R. Mota

3.1 Induction of an adaptive physiological cascade

Ischemic preconditioning (IPC) is an endogenous physiological phenomenon that has gained significant attention in the field of exercise and sport science due to its potent systemic physiological actions and practical field applications [1, 2]. IPC relies on the so-called and fascinating principle of conditioning. The famous Russian physiologist and Nobel prize laureate Ivan Pavlov first described the adaptive reactions of the organism to external factors as a "warning" signal, which in essence forms the basis for the universal phenomenon of anticipatory regulation [3]. According to modern concepts, an adaptogenic stimulus (i.e., the "warning" signal, which specifically represents injurious or stress factors of mild intensity) induces reorganization of the plasticity of the elements of all physiological systems. This reorganization prepares all cells and tissues to the expected deleterious exposures and is associated with an induction of evolutionarily acquired gene-determined protective mechanisms. This results in environmentally determined adaptive change in the phenotype, a process termed hormesis [4]. Hormesis is a basic principle of physiology which is generally defined as the integrated responses of cells or organisms to a factor which induces stimulatory or beneficial effects at low doses and inhibitory or adverse effects at high doses. In this context, a conditioning phenomenon aimed at enhancing adaptation to extreme factors represents one of the typical examples of the adaptogenic "warning" signaling and, therefore, of hormesis. It has been proposed that various (pre)conditioning modalities (e.g., via systemic hypoxia or local ischemia) share some common protective mechanisms that convey

DOI: 10.4324/9781003402879-4

immediate and long-term ergogenic effects conducive to improved health and performance [5, 6].

The term "ischemic preconditioning" was introduced at the end of the last century by Murry and colleagues demonstrating, in the canine model, that brief ischemic episodes could protect the myocardium from a subsequent sustained ischemic insult [7]. Then, a few years later, hypoxic/ischemic tolerance induced by pre-exposure to brief, sublethal preconditioning ischemic episodes was also demonstrated in the brain of rodents [8]. Importantly, this later study further reported that attention to the characteristics of the ischemic treatment (cycle duration and interval) was paramount to perturb cellular metabolism, cause protein synthesis, and exhibit tissue protection. IPC increases physiological stress on varied structures (e.g., muscle fiber, nociceptive fiber, endothelium) during both the ischemic and reperfusion phases, which combine to activate a variety of bioactive substances and induce ergogenic effects across multiple physiological functions. Athletes can thus momentarily subject themselves to safe doses of ischemia in order to activate their innate defenses and face the challenge of physical exercise insult.

3.2 Techniques of ischemic preconditioning

Current IPC applications involve subjecting one or multiple limb(s) to brief periods (e.g., 3 to 5 minutes) of complete occlusion of blood flow, followed by periods of reperfusion (e.g., 5 minutes), which are repeated three to five times. The pressure is applied using tourniquets or blood pressure cuffs and must be greater than the individual arterial occlusion pressure to induce limb ischemia (i.e., typical pressure range in scientific studies: 150–300 mmHg). IPC is applied at rest within ~5 to 90 min prior to exercise to initiate the physiological cascade of events that may acutely enhance performance. IPC may also be implemented chronically, where it is performed before exercise training sessions over a few weeks, to increase the training stimulus and optimize training-induced physiological adaptations [9, 10]. In both these acute and chronic scenarios, there are two main strategies to implement IPC, which makes this maneuver readily accessible to several populations and usable in varied athletic contexts.

Local IPC is the most extensively studied strategy. It involves targeting a specific muscle group, intended for exercise with ischemia/reperfusion stress (Figure 3A.1). In this scenario, a tourniquet or cuff is applied proximally to the muscles about to be engaged in the exercise. For example, a cyclist or runner would perform the IPC maneuver on their lower limbs just before a cycling or running test. The ischemic episode temporarily reduces blood flow to the target muscles, followed by the restoration of normal blood flow, which triggers a cascade of physiological responses within the muscles. These responses include increased blood vessel dilation, improved oxygen and

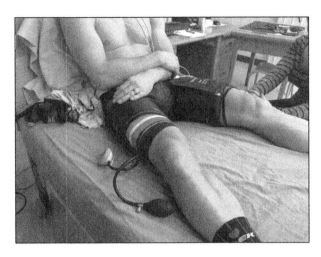

FIGURE 3A.1 Local application of a cuff to both upper thighs to induce ischemic preconditioning before cycling exercise.

nutrient delivery, and heightened metabolic activity. Such changes are believed to enhance the muscles' readiness and overall performance during subsequent exercise, making IPC a valuable strategy for optimizing exercise outcomes in numerous sports.

Remote IPC (RIPC) involves the application of an ischemia/reperfusion insult to a muscle group that is not actively engaged in the subsequent exercise. In that scenario, a blood pressure cuff would be alternatively inflated and deflated on the upper part of the arm(s) before embarking on an exercise that predominantly activates the lower limbs, such as running or cycling. Remarkably, while the blood flow occlusion and reperfusion occur remotely, this strategy capitalizes on the body's systemic physiological responses and adaptations to the temporary reduction in blood flow to any territory. Interestingly, both IPC and RIPC maneuvers have been shown to provide similar benefits [11], but RIPC applications may be less uncomfortable and trigger fewer nocebo effects than occluding blood flow directly to the muscles intended for use during exercise.

3.3 Potential mechanisms and effects on human performance

The preconditioning response confers protection that can last from minutes to days through manifold biological effects, including the immediate hypoxia-derived release of autacoids (e.g., adenosine, bradykinin, nitric oxide, opioids), ion channel permeability, posttranslational modification of proteins and upregulation of gene expression [2, 12]. These changes are induced via neuronal and humoral pathways and systemic protective

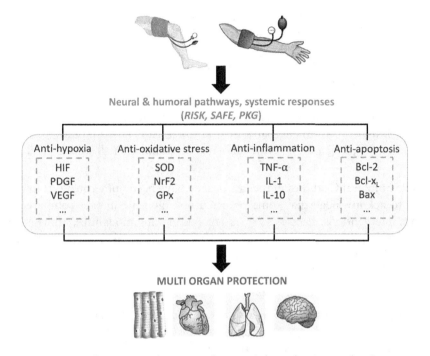

FIGURE 3A.2   Mechanistic pathways and potential mechanisms of ischemic pre-conditioning. Through the production of blood-borne factors and the stimulation of neural and humoral pathways and systemic responses, the protective signal is conveyed to multiple tissues and organs where pro-survival signalling pathways mediate protective effects. These salvage pathways include the reperfusion injury salvage kinase (RISK) pathway, the survivor activator factor enhancement (SAFE) pathway, and the cGMP–protein kinase G (PKG) pathway, to enhance gene expression and reduce oxidative stress, inflammation, and apoptosis.

HIF, hypoxia-inducible factor; PDGF, platelet-derived growth factor; VEGF, vascular endothelial growth factor; SOD, superoxide dismutase; Nrf2, nuclear factor erythroid-2 related factor 2; GPx, glutathione peroxidase; TNF-α, tumor necrosis factor; IL-1, interleukin 1; IL-10, interleukin 10; Bcl-2, B-cell lymphoma-2; Bcl-x_L, B-cell lymphoma-extra-large; Bax, Bcl-2-associated X. (personal source)

responses (Figure 3A.2). Although several physiological responses are still under investigation, human preconditioning studies on exercise performance have revealed the following mechanisms:

- Improved blood flow and muscle metabolism: the mechanical compression and reperfusion impact the endothelium and improve blood flow regulation (functional sympatholysis), resulting in increased delivery and extraction of oxygen by skeletal muscles during exercise [13, 14]. So far, these have been acknowledged to be the main mechanisms that underlmy the ergogenic effect of IPC.

- Reduction in muscle damage: IPC may reduce exercise-induced muscle damage by attenuating inflammation and oxidative stress, suggesting a quicker recovery and reduced muscle soreness [15].
- Neuromuscular adaptations: IPC may influence the nervous system, improving muscle recruitment patterns and enhancing neuromuscular coordination [16, 17], although this is not a robust finding in all studies [18].

While human IPC studies in the last decade have been numerous, it is important to acknowledge that some reported no ergogenic impact compared to sham interventions. Factors such as preconditioning modalities, athletes' fitness level, and the psychological placebo effect have all been incriminated when IPC failed to enhance performance [19, 20]. That said, the following ergogenic effects of IPC have been identified:

- Enhanced endurance: IPC may increase endurance capacity by optimizing oxygen utilization and delaying fatigue.
- Improved exercise tolerance: IPC may enhance the body's ability to tolerate high-intensity exercise.
- Increased muscle strength: IPC has been shown to improve muscle strength, potentially due to improved blood flow and neuromuscular function.
- Faster recovery: IPC may reduce muscle damage and inflammation, leading to quicker recovery between training sessions.

3.4 Future directions

Despite increasing evidence that IPC maneuvers enhance exercise performance, important questions remain regarding their practical application. A first and urgent concern to address is whether females can benefit as much as males do [21]. The effects of female ovarian hormones on the threshold required to elicit protection and/or an ergogenic effect should be investigated thoroughly with strong mechanistic research designs to promote efficient guidelines for both sexes. While it is refreshing to see more studies investigating the chronic impact of IPC associated to training, shorter-duration protocols than the classic 4×5-min ischemia/5-min reperfusion will certainly become more appealing to a greater number of athletes [22]. In this training perspective, the possibility that combining IPC with environmental stress, such as altitude or heat, might offer more rapid or robust physiological adaptations [1], thereby attaining training objectives in fewer sessions or with lower mechanical load, further merits attention.

3.5 Conclusion

Ischemic preconditioning has emerged as a promising technique to enhance physical performance through multifaceted mechanisms, relying on the body's endogenous defense systems to achieve ischemic and hypoxic tolerance. Although further research is essential to comprehensively unravel its intricate physiological foundations and refine its application protocols in diverse sport contexts, the phenomenon presents an exciting prospect for athletes and individuals aspiring to elevate their exercise performance.

Abbreviations

IPC   ischemic preconditioning
RIPC   remote ischemic preconditioning

References

1. Billaut, F., P. Paradis-Deschênes, and P.T. Richard, *Utilization of ischemic preconditioning for athletes competing and training at altitude: applications and perspectives.* J Sci Sport Exerc, 2022. **4**: p. 346–357.
2. Koch, S., et al., *Biomarkers for ischemic preconditioning: Finding the responders.* J Cereb Blood Flow Metab, 2014. **34**: p. 933–941.
3. Anokhin, P.K., *Biology and neurophysiology of the conditioned reflex and its role in adaptive behavior.* 3: Pergamon.
4. Calabrese, E.J. and M.P. Mattson, *Hormesis provides a generalized quantitative estimate of biological plasticity.* J Cell Commun Signal. 2011. **5**: p. 25–38.
5. Calabrese, E.J., et al., *Hormesis determines lifespan.* Ageing Res Rev, 2024. **94**: p. 102181.
6. Rybnikova, E. and M. Samoilov, *Current insights into the molecular mechanisms of hypoxic pre- and postconditioning using hypobaric hypoxia.* Front Neurosci-switz, 2015. **9**: p. 388.
7. Murry, C.E., R.B. Jennings, and K. Reimer, *Preconditioning with ischemia: A delay of lethal cell injury in ischemic myocardium.* Circulation 1986. **74**: p. 1124–1136.
8. Kitagawa, K., et al., *'Ischemic tolerance' phenomenon found in the brain.* Brain Res, 1990. **528**: p. 21–24.
9. Paradis-Deschênes, P., et al., *Ischemic preconditioning enhances aerobic adaptations to sprint-interval training in athletes without altering systemic hypoxic signaling and immune function.* Front Sports Act Liv, 2020. **2**: p. 41.
10. Slysz, J.T. and J.F. Burr, *Impact of 8 weeks of repeated ischemic preconditioning on running performance.* Eur J Appl Physiol, 2019. **119**: p. 1431–1437.
11. Ferreira, T., et al., *Ischemic preconditioning and repeated sprint swimming.* Med Sci Sports Ex, 2016. **48**: p. 1967–1975.
12. Mallet, R. T., et al., *Cardioprotection by intermittent hypoxia conditioning: Evidence, mechanisms, and therapeutic potential.* Am J Physiol Heart Circ, 2018. **315**: p. H216–H232.
13. Kido, K., et al., *Ischemic preconditioning accelerates muscle deoxygenation dynamics and enhances exercise endurance during the work-to-work test.* Physiol Reports, 2015. **3**: p. e12395.

14. Paradis-Deschênes, P., D.R. Joanisse, and F. Billaut, *Ischemic preconditioning increases muscle perfusion, oxygen uptake, and force in strength-trained athletes.* Appl Physiol Nutr Metab, 2016. **41**: p. 938–944.

15. Franz, A., et al., *Ischemic preconditioning blunts muscle damage responses induced by eccentric exercise.* Med Sci Sports Exer, 2018. **50**: p. 109–115.

16. Bouffard, S., P. Paradis-Deschênes, and F. Billaut, *Neuromuscular adjustments following sprint training with ischemic preconditioning in endurance athletes: Preliminary Data.* Sports, 2010. **9**: p. 124.

17. Wilk, M., et al., *Impact of ischemic intra-conditioning on power output and bar velocity of the upper limbs.* Front Physiol, 2021. **12**: p. 626915.

18. Halley, S.L., P. Marshall, and J.C. Siegler, *The effect of IPC on central and peripheral fatiguing mechanisms in humans following maximal single limb isokinetic exercise.* Physiol Reports, 2019. **7**: p. e14063–12.

19. Richard, P. and F. Billaut, *Time-trial performance in elite speed skaters after remote ischemic preconditioning.* Int J Sports Physiol Perform, 2018. **13**: p. 1308–1316.

20. Marocolo, M., et al., *Ischemic preconditioning and exercise performance: Are the psychophysiological responses underestimated?* Eur J Appl Physiol, 2023. **123**: p. 683–693.

21. Paradis-Deschênes, P., D.R. Joanisse, and F. Billaut, *Sex-specific impact of ischemic preconditioning on tissue oxygenation and maximal concentric force.* Front Physiol, 2017. **7**: p. 674.

22. Salagas, A., et al., *Effectiveness of either short-duration ischemic pre-conditioning, single-set high-resistance exercise, or their combination in potentiating bench press exercise performance.* Front Physiol, 2022. **13**: p. 1083299.

3B

THE VOLUNTARY HYPOVENTILATION AT LOW LUNG VOLUME (VHL) METHOD

Xavier Woorons

3.1 Introduction

The live low train high (LLTH) approach, when applied in certain conditions, seems beneficial for improving performance at sea level. Nonetheless, it is problematic to implement for many athletes due to difficulties in accessing sufficiently high altitudes (>2,500 m) in many countries. Furthermore, devices used to simulate altitude (hypoxic tents and chambers, apparatus for breathing O_2-depleted air) remain expensive and have practical drawbacks, as they do not allow athletes to train in the field.

Since the mid-2000s [1], numerous studies (around 20 to date) have shown that it is possible to simulate hypoxic training conditions without being at altitude and without using devices to create a hypoxic environment. This can be achieved through voluntary hypoventilation at low lung volume (VHL). The VHL technique involves repeating short periods of end-expiratory breath holding (EEBH) during exercise [2]. This "exhale–hold" technique significantly reduces O_2 concentrations throughout the body and therefore creates a state of hypoxia.

3.2 VHL exercise-induced hypoxia

Until the early 2020s, studies investigating the acute effects of VHL exercise had typically used EEBH durations of 4 to 6 s, resulting in mean minimal arterial oxygen saturation (SpO_2) values of 87–88%. However, in more recent times, a more ambitious approach to VHL was tested, consisting of performing EEBH for as long as possible, up to the breaking point [3–5]. This approach induced a much larger fall in SpO_2, with minimal values of

DOI: 10.4324/9781003402879-5

73–75% recorded during repetitions of running exercises performed between 80% and 125% of the maximal aerobic velocity [4, 5]. Such levels of hypoxaemia are comparable to what could be reached at altitudes of ~4,000 m according to a recently established mathematical model [6].

The marked arterial desaturation induced by VHL exercise has an impact on muscle tissue, causing tissue hypoxia. In the study by Woorons et al. [4, 5], it was showed that muscle oxygenation decreased very early (from the first repetition) and substantially compared with the same intermittent exercise performed under normal breathing conditions. The hypoxic effect of VHL exercise leads to greater stimulation of the anaerobic glycolysis, provoking a surge in blood lactate concentration [7, 8], which accentuates the level of acidosis.

Due to its hypoxic effect, the VHL approach has been recognized as a potentially beneficial training method for a wide range of sports [9, 10]. It has recently been included in the nomenclature of the hypoxic training methods [11] and more specifically within the LLTH paradigm [12]. It should be noted, however, that unlike an exercise performed in a hypoxic environment, the drop in both SpO_2 and muscle oxygenation only occurs for a few seconds during the EEBH. SpO_2 then rises sharply and rapidly during the recovery periods when breathing can resume (Figure 3B.1). The impact of this discontinuity of the hypoxic stimulus on the training adaptations could therefore be questioned.

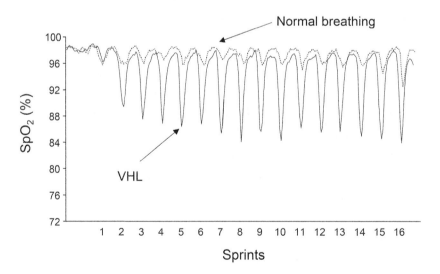

FIGURE 3B.1 Arterial oxygen saturation (SpO_2) measured continuously in swimmers during one set of 16 x 15-m crawl sprints (start/30 s) performed with normal breathing or with voluntary hypoventilation at low lung volume (VHL).

(Modified from Trincat R, Woorons X, and Millet GP, 2017).

3.3 Effects of training with VHL

In a pioneer study carried out on VHL training [13], only a moderate improvement in performance was observed after a 4-week training period in running at moderate intensity including EEBH of 4 s. However, since 2016, all the studies dealing with this topic have reported significant improvements in both anaerobic performance and repeated-sprint ability (RSA) after a period of 3–6 weeks of VHL training. These results are mainly attributed to the combination of the EEBH with exercises performed at high intensity or maximal velocity (RSH-VHL).

In a 2016 study, triathletes who performed VHL exercises at supramaximal intensity in swimming twice a week for 5 weeks improved their performance in the 100 m, 200 m, and 400 m freestyle by 4.4%, 3.6%, and 3.5%, respectively [14]. On the other hand, the control group of triathletes who performed the same exercises with unrestricted breathing showed no significant enhancement in performance (+0.4% on average). A 2017 study also reported an improvement in RSA in swimmers after six sessions of RSH-VHL over a 2-week period, while no change was observed in the control group [15]. In a group of highly trained rugby players, Fornasier Santos et al. [16] showed that seven sessions of RSH-VHL over a 4-week period largely improved RSA (Figure 3B.2). Once again, performance remained unchanged in the group that performed the same repeated-sprint training with unrestricted breathing. The effectiveness of RSH-VHL for improving RSA was confirmed in subsequent studies in cyclists [17], basketball players [18], ice hockey players [19], and soccer players [20].

RSH-VHL has demonstrated potential for improving anaerobic performance. After 3 weeks and six sessions of cycle repeated-sprint exercises with EEBH, highly trained cyclists exhibited an average 6% improvement in the Wingate test [17]. This improvement in performance was accompanied by a significant increase in the maximum blood lactate concentration (pre/post training: 13.9 vs. 16.2 mmol/L). In the Woorons et al. [14] study on triathletes, the improved performance in the 100-m and 200-m freestyle, primarily reliant on the anaerobic lactic component, coincided with higher maximum blood lactate levels. Furthermore, the rate of blood lactate accumulation soared by 48% and 29% in the 100 m and 200 m freestyle, respectively. These results suggest that VHL training, when performed at supramaximal intensity, could improve both the anaerobic lactic capacity and power.

While the improvement of anaerobic glycolysis is an important physiological adaptation induced by VHL training, a reduction in acidosis could also contribute to improved performance. As early as 2008, Woorons et al. [13] observed that at 90% of the maximal heart rate, runners who had trained with VHL exhibited higher blood pH (i.e., lower blood acidosis), higher blood bicarbonate concentration, and lower blood lactate concentration.

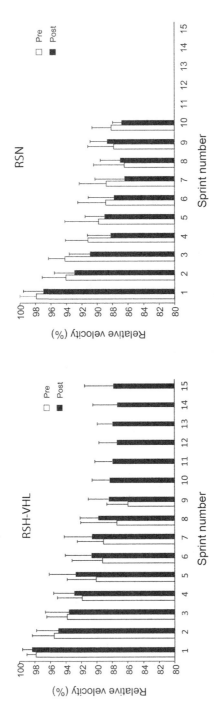

FIGURE 3B.2 40-m running sprints and relative velocity in rugby players before and after a 4-week hypoxic repeated-sprint training program.

(Modified from Fornasier Santos C, Millet GP, and Woorons X, 2018).

Therefore, it may be possible that VHL training could improve blood and/or muscle buffering capacity or enhance the efficiency of lactate transporters. Such adaptations could be pivotal in delaying fatigue onset during continuous or intermittent short high-intensity efforts. Recent findings by Lapointe et al. [18], showing a reduction in potassium ion concentration (associated with muscle fatigue) in basketball players who performed 4 weeks (eight sessions) of RSH-VHL, further support this hypothesis.

Regarding aerobic performance, no study to date has demonstrated an improvement in VO_2max or its associated velocity, lactic threshold, maximal ventilation or maximal heart rate after VHL training at either moderate or high intensity. However, recent studies suggest that aerobic metabolism may still contribute to improved performance, particularly during repeated-sprint exercises. For instance, Lapointe et al. [18] reported improved muscle reoxygenation during recovery periods following running repeated-sprint exercises in basketball players who performed 4 weeks of RSH-VHL. However, no enhancement in muscle O_2 utilization during the sprints was noted. Previously, Woorons et al. [17] recorded an increase in oxygen uptake during an RSA test including ten 6-s sprints (unrestricted breathing) in cyclists after completing six sessions of RSH-VHL. Nevertheless, in this study too, no improvement in muscle O_2 extraction was observed. These results suggest that a greater involvement of aerobic metabolism during a repeated-sprint exercise after RSH-VHL may be attributed to improved O_2 transport rather than muscle tissue adaptations.

A large increase in left ventricular stroke volume has been found during repetitions of supramaximal efforts with EEBH up to the breaking point [3]. The authors of this study hypothesized that after several weeks of such training, cardiac compliance could be improved, resulting in an augmented stroke volume, which plays a major role in O_2 transport. This hypothesis gains support from a recent study in which an improvement in performance on the yo-yo test (a predominantly aerobic shuttle running test) was found in team sports players after 3 weeks and six sessions of high-intensity VHL training in cycling [21]. The transfer of benefits from cycling to running in this specific test suggests that, for aerobic metabolism, unlike anaerobic metabolism, the physiological adaptations following VHL training may not occur specifically in the muscle but rather at the level of O_2 transport, possibly via a greater quantity of blood ejected by the heart during each contraction.

3.4 Conclusion

The new approach to VHL training, involving the repetition of supramaximal exercises with EEBH up the breaking point, appears promising. The first studies investigating the physiological adaptations resulting from this type of training and its effects on performance should be published in coming years.

Abbreviations

EEBH	end-expiratory breath holding
RSA	repeated-sprint ability
RSH-VHL	repeated-sprint training in hypoxia induced by voluntary hypo-ventilation at low lung volume
SpO_2	arterial oxygen saturation
VHL	voluntary hypoventilation at low lung volume.

References

1. Woorons, X., et al., *Prolonged expiration down to residual volume leads to severe arterial hypoxemia in athletes during submaximal exercise.* Respir Physiol Neurobiol, 2007. **15**: p. 75–82.

2. Woorons, X., *Hypoventilation training, push your limits!* Arpeh, ed., 2014. ISBN: 978-2-9546040-1-5.

3. Woorons, X., et al., *Exercise with end-expiratory breath holding induces large increase in stroke volume.* Int J Sports Med, 2021a. **42**: p. 56–65.

4. Woorons, X., F. Billaut, and C. Lamberto, *Running exercise with end-expiratory breath holding up to the breaking point induces large and early fall in muscle oxygenation.* Eur J Appl Physiol, 2021b. **121**: p. 3515–3525.

5. Woorons, X., et al., *Physiological responses to supramaximal running exercise with end-expiratory breath holding up to the breaking point.* J Hum Kinet, 2024. DOI: 10.5114/jhk/174465

6. Woorons, X., and J.P. Richalet, *Modelling the relationships between arterial oxygen saturation, exercise intensity and the level of aerobic performance in acute hypoxia.* Eur J Appl Physiol, 2021. **121**: p. 1993–2003.

7. Woorons, X., et al., *Exercise with hypoventilation induces lower muscle oxygenation and higher blood lactate concentration: Role of hypoxia and hypercapnia.* Eur J Appl Physiol, 2010. **110**: p. 367–377.

8. Woorons, X., et al., *Swimmers can train in hypoxia at sea level through voluntary hypoventilation.* Respir Physiol Neurobiol, 2014. **190**: p. 33–39.

9. Millet, G.P., et al., *Combining hypoxic methods for peak performance.* Sports Med, 2010. **40**: p. 1–25.

10. Millet G.P., et al., *Repeated sprint training in hypoxia—an innovative method.* Dtsch Z Sportmed, 2019. 2019: p. 115–122.

11. Girard, O., F. Brocherie, and G. Millet, *Effects of altitude/hypoxia on single- and multiple-sprint performance: a comprehensive review.* Sports Med, 2017. 47: p. 1931–1949.

12. Girard, O., et al., *An updated panorama of "living low-training high" altitude/hypoxic methods.* Front Sports Act Living, 2020. **31**: p. 2:26.

13. Woorons, X., et al., *Effects of a 4-week training with voluntary hypoventilation carried out at low pulmonary volumes.* Respir Physiol Neurobiol, 2008. **160**: p. 123–130.

14. Woorons, X., et al., *Hypoventilation training at supramaximal intensity improves swimming performance.* Med Sci Sports Exerc, 2016. **48**: p. 1119–1128.

15. Trincat, L., et al., *Repeated sprint training in hypoxia induced by voluntary hypoventilation in swimming.* Int J Sports Physiol Perform, 2017. **24**: p.1–24.

16. Fornasier-Santos, C., G. Millet, and X. Woorons, *Repeated-sprint training in hypoxia induced by voluntary hypoventilation improves running repeated-sprint ability in rugby players.* Eur J Sport Sci, 2018. **18**: p. 504–512.

17. Woorons, X., G. Millet, and P. Mucci, *Physiological adaptations to repeated sprint training in hypoxia induced by voluntary hypoventilation at low lung volume.* Eur J Appl Physiol, 2019. **119**: p. 1959–1970.

18. Lapointe, J., et al., *Impact of hypoventilation training on muscle oxygenation, myoelectrical changes, systemic [k+], and repeated-sprint ability in basketball players.* Front Sports Act Living, 2020. **3**: p. 2:29.

19. Brocherie, F., et al., *Effects of repeated-sprint training in hypoxia induced by voluntary hypoventilation on performance during ice hockey off-season.* Int J Sports Sci Coaching, 2022. **18**: p. 1–7.

20. Ait Ali Braham, M., et al., *Effects of a 6-week repeated-sprint training with voluntary hypoventilation at low and high lung volume on repeated-sprint ability in female soccer players.* Int J Sports Physiol Perform, 2024. **1**: p. 1–8.

21. Woorons, X., F. Billaut, and H. Vandewalle, *5 transferable benefits of cycle hypoventilation training for run-based performance in team-sport athletes.* Int J Sports Physiol Perform, 2020. **27**: p. 1–6.

4

HISTORICAL DEVELOPMENT OF ALTITUDE TRAINING AND HYPOXIC CONDITIONING

Randall L. Wilber

4.1 Decision at Baden-Baden: October 1963

The history of altitude training and hypoxic conditioning (ATHC) begins in 1946, shortly after the conclusion of World War II. A PubMed search using the term "altitude training" produced two publications from 1946, both dealing with high altitude training for pilots. From 1946 to 1963, a total of 15 scientific papers were published, mostly evaluating the effect of high altitude on fighter jet pilots or astronauts. There were no publications during this period that examined the effect of altitude training on athletic performance. A pivotal event took place in October 1963 when the International Olympic Committee (IOC) held its annual meeting in Baden-Baden, Germany that would change the way environmental physiologists and athletes viewed altitude training. The primary agenda item was the vote to determine the host city for the 1968 Olympic Games, with Buenos Aires (Argentina), Detroit (United States of America), Lyon (France), and Mexico City (Mexico) as the contenders [1]. Despite Detroit being considered the favorite, Mexico City's presentation emphasized the unique opportunity of hosting the Olympic Games in Latin America after Mexico City had successfully staged the 1955 Pan American Games. In addition, one member of the Mexico City delegation, Eduardo Hay, MD, argued that the city's altitude (2,239 m/7,349 ft) was well *below* the threshold elevation of 3,000 m (9,840 ft) at which point, he stated, physical performance begins to become impaired due to hypoxia [1]. The Mexico City presentation was impressive and convincing in front of the 58 IOC members present in Baden-Baden for the vote. Following presentations by Buenos Aires, Detroit, Lyon, and Mexico City, a one-hour deliberation preceded the announcement of the vote results: Mexico City 30, Detroit 14,

DOI: 10.4324/9781003402879-6

Lyon 12, Buenos Aires 2 [1]. Mexico City won on the first ballot, due in part to its own diligence and impressive final presentation, but also to the unanimous support from entire Soviet bloc of nations (n = 10), who voted for Mexico City [1] over other candidates, including their bitter Cold War opponent, the United States of America. Mexico City had met their goal of being the first city in Latin America to host the Olympic Games and simultaneously earned the distinction of being the first city located at moderate altitude to host the Olympics.

Despite Dr. Hay's assertion in Baden-Baden that the "threshold of impaired performance" occurs above 3,000 m (9,840 ft), concerns among athletes and environmental physiologists persisted about the potential negative impact on athletic performance at the 2,239 m (7,349 ft) elevation of Mexico City. As a result, formal research on altitude training began in the years immediately following the IOC's selection of Mexico City as host of the 1968 Olympic Games. The first paper dealing with altitude training and athletic performance, titled *Altitude and Maximum Performance in Work and Sports Activity*, was published in November 1965 in *the Journal of the American Medical Association* [2]. The authors stated,

> The decision to hold the Olympic Games of 1968 in Mexico City, a city with an elevation of around 2,250 meters (nearly one-half mile higher than Denver) has created a public interest in effects of higher altitudes on physical performance capabilities.
>
> *[2]*

In December 1965, *The Magglingen Symposium on Sports at Medium Altitude*, was held in Magglingen, Switzerland. Sponsored by the Research Committee of the International Council of Sports and Physical Education, Swiss Olympic Committee, and Swiss Medical Association, the Magglingen symposium concluded that "the Olympic athletes should train at altitude before going to Mexico City, and then have another short period of adaptation to the local environment prior to the competition." [3]. In March 1966, the United States Olympic Committee (USOC) along with the Lovelace Foundation for Medical Education and Research, and the University of New Mexico sponsored *The International Symposium on the Effects of Altitude on Physical Performance* held in Albuquerque, New Mexico, USA. Among the papers presented at that international conference were [4]:

- *Time Course of Acclimatization to Altitude*. Wolf H. Weihe (Switzerland)
- *Physiology and Performance of Track Athletes at Various Altitudes in the United States and Peru*. Elsworth Buskirk (United States)
- *The Effects of Altitude on Non-Acclimatized Athletes During Effort*. Jorge Soni (Mexico)

- *Training for Maximum Performance at Altitude.* John Faulkner (United States)
- *Aerobic and Anaerobic Work Capacity at an Altitude of 2,250 Meters.* Bengt Saltin (Sweden)
- *High Altitude Acclimatization in Women.* John Hannon (United States)

In 1966 and 1967, seven important papers were published on the topic of altitude training and athletic performance including five studies conducted at elevations similar to Mexico City. The authors of this cohort of papers include some of the most eminent scientists in the field of environmental physiology: Bruno Balke, Elsworth Buskirk, Frank Consolazio, Jack Daniels, John Faulkner, Griffith Pugh, and Bengt Saltin.

- Balke, B., J.A. Faulkner, and J.T. Daniels, *Maximum performance capacity at sea-level and at moderate altitude before and after altitude training.* Schweiz Z Sportmed, 1966. **14**: p. 106–116 [5].
- Buskirk, E.R., J. Kollias, R.F. Akers, E.K. Prokop, and E.P. Reategui, *Maximal performance at altitude and on return from altitude in conditioned runners.* J Appl Physiol, 1967. **23**: p. 259–266 [6].
- Evans, W.O., and C.F. Consolazio, *Effects of high altitude on performance of three different types of work.* Percept Mot Skills, 1967. **25**: p. 41–50 [7].
- Faulkner, J.A., J.T. Daniels, and B. Balke, *Effects of training at moderate altitude on physical performance capacity.* J Appl Physiol, 1967. **23**: p. 85–89 [8].
- Pugh, L.G.C.E., *Athletes at altitude.* J Physiol, 1967. **192**: p. 619–46 [9].
- Saltin, B, *Aerobic and anaerobic work capacity at 2300 meters.* Med Thorac, 1967. **24**: p. 205–10 [10].
- Scano, A., and G. Meineri, *Behavior of pulmonary ventilation and alveolar gas tension in athletes before, during and after 5 weeks of sojourn at an altitude of 2250 m.* Riv Med Aeronaut Spaz, 1967. **30**: p. 645–62 [11].

This trend would continue into the Olympic year 1968 when there appeared 11 publications related to altitude and athletic performance, equal to a two-fold increase versus 1967, and equal to 52% of the total number of papers published since 1946. One noteworthy paper from 1968 was titled, *Heart Frequencies and Substrate Concentrations in the Blood of Horses During Training in Mexico City (2250 m above sea level).* [12].

4.2 1968 Mexico City Olympics

The 1968 Mexico City Olympics were held from 12 to 27 October 1968. However, in October and November 1965, Mexico City hosted "International Sports Week," also known as the "Little Olympics," which served as a rehearsal competition staged approximately three years before the 1968

Mexico City Olympics. The 1965 Little Olympics were designed to allow probable 1968 Olympians to experience the physiological effects of competing at 2,239 m (7,349 ft). The competition drew 200 athletes from 17 nations and provided physicians and environmental physiologists with valuable data on athletes performing at maximal exercise capacity at moderate altitude [13]. Sir Roger Bannister, MD, widely known and respected for being the first runner to break four minutes in the mile run, was a member of the British medical team at the 1965 Little Olympics. Bannister presciently concluded,

> At 7,000 feet there is nearly 25 percent less oxygen in the atmosphere, and as we have seen, performance is limited by the transport of oxygen. I do not agree with the remark attributed to Finnish coach Onin Niakanen that 'there will be those that will die,' but altitude could be the critical additional factor leading to collapse under special circumstances.
>
> *[13]*

In March 1966, following the 1965 Little Olympics, the USOC produced the *Report of the Medical Section of the United States Team to the Games in Mexico City – October 1965*. Based on scientific observations made at the 1965 Little Olympics, this document reported on "the effects of altitude and other factors which might adversely influence the performance of the United States athletes in Mexico City" during the forthcoming 1968 Mexico City Olympics [14]. The American medical team evaluated probable 1968 Olympians from the sports of athletics, boxing, cycling, and swimming. In addition, the following papers were presented in March 1966 at *The International Symposium on the Effects of Altitude on Physical Performance* (Albuquerque, New Mexico, USA) based on data collected at the 1965 Little Olympics [4]:

- *A Study of the Acclimatization to Altitude in Japanese Athletes.* Kasuo Ikeda (Japan)
- *Experiences on Adaptations to Average Altitude for Subjects Trained to Cycling.* Antonio Venerando (Italy)
- *Observations on Cycling and Track Events in Mexico City at the Little Olympics of 1965.* Daniel Hanley (United States)
- *The Effect of Altitude Upon Swimming Performance.* James Counsilman (United States)
- *Physical Performance in Mexico City.* Roy Shephard (Canada)
- *United States Olympic Committee Swimming Team Performance in International Sports Week.* Roy Goddard (United States)
- *Comments on International Sports Week in Mexico City, October 1965.* Eduardo Hay (Mexico)
- *Interpretation of Performance Predictions for Tokyo Olympic Games, 1964, with Extrapolations for 1968.* Ernst Jokl (United States)

In April 1966, the British Olympic Association (BOA) produced the *Report of Medical Research Project into the Effects of Altitude in Mexico City in 1965*, based on their findings from the 1965 Little Olympics. Among the conclusions put forth by the BOA medical group [15] was, "it is estimated as a rough guide for those present in Mexico City for at least 4 weeks before competition that the times will be slower by approximately the following amounts:

- Events lasting 3–4 minutes ... 6–8 seconds
- Events lasting 4–8 minutes ... 8–20 seconds
- Events lasting 8–12 minutes ... 20–35 seconds"

Based on the scientific findings resulting from the 1965 Little Olympics, altitude preparation strategies and training bases were set up in several countries including the Soviet Union (Armenia, Kazakhstan), France (Font-Romeu), Switzerland (Magglingen, San Moritz), Japan (Mount Norikura), and the United States (Alamosa, Colorado; South Lake Tahoe, Nevada) [13].

The Games of the XIX Olympiad opened officially in Mexico City on 12 October 1968 with 5,516 athletes (4,735 men, 781 women) from 112 nations participating. This marked the first Olympic Games held in Latin America and introduced several technological advancements such as a synthetic athletics track, electronic timing system for athletics and swimming, and being the first Olympic Games at moderate altitude [16]. Based on the results of the 1965 Little Olympics, many environmental physiologists and coaches predicted that the elevation of Mexico City (2,239 m/7,349 ft) would favor performance in the sprint, jump, and throwing events in the sport of athletics but negatively affect long-distance running events. This prediction largely held true. Notably, Bob Beamon set a memorable world record in the long jump (8.90 m or 29 ft 2.5 in), breaking it by an incredible 56 cm (22.0 in) or approximately 6.6% [17]. Researchers later attributed part of Beamon's success to the lower barometric pressure in Mexico City, resulting in less aerodynamic resistance during the aerial phase of his jump [18]. In addition to Bob Beamon's groundbreaking long jump record, the 1968 Mexico City Olympics witnessed several world records in men's 100-m, 200-m, and 400-m sprints, as well as the 4 × 100-m relay and 4 × 400-m relay. World records were also established in the men's 110-m hurdles, 400-m hurdles, and triple jump. Among the 16 sprint, jump, and throwing events in the men's athletics competition, a total of nine world records and seven Olympic records were set [17] (Table 4.1). The women's sprint, jump, and throwing events in the 1968 Mexico City Olympics showed similar impressive results, although the women competed in fewer track and field events than their male counterparts (Table 4.1).

TABLE 4.1 Results of the high-altitude Olympic Games 1968 in Mexico City

EVENT	GOLD	SILVER	BRONZE	WORLD RECORD PRIOR TO 1968 MEXICO CITY OLYMPICS
100 m	Hines (USA) 9.95 **WR**	Miller (JAM) 10.04	Greene (USA) 10.07	10.03
4 x 100-m Relay	USA 38.24 **WR**	CUB 38.40	FRA 38.43	39.05
110 m Hurdles	Davenport (USA) 13.33 **WR**	Hall (USA) 13.42	Ottoz (ITA) 13.46	13.43
200 m	Smith (USA) 19.83 **WR**	Norman (AUS) 20.06	Carlos (USA) 20.10	19.92
400 m	Evans (USA) 43.86 **WR**	James (USA) 43.97	Freeman (USA) 44.41	44.19
4 x 400-m Relay	USA 2:56.16 **WR**	KEN 2:59.64	FRG 3:00.57	2:59.6
400 m Hurdles	Hemery (GBR) 48.12 **WR**	Hennige (FRG) 49.02	Sherwood (GBR) 49.03	48.94
800 m	Doubell (AUS) 1:44.30 =**WR**	Kiprugut (KEN) 1:44.57	Farrell (USA) 1:45.46	1:44.30
1,500 m	Keino (KEN) 3:34.91 **OR**	Ryun (USA) 3:37.89	Tummler (FRG) 3:39.08	3:31.1
3,000 m Steeplechase	Biwott (KEN) 8:51.02	Kogo (KEN) 8:51.56	Young (USA) 8:51.86	8:24.2
5,000 m	Gammoudi (TUN) 14:05.01	Keino (KEN) 14:05.16	Temu (KEN) 14:06.41	13:16.6
10,000 m	Temu (KEN) 29:27.40	Wolde (ETH) 29:27.75	Gammoudi (TUN) 29:34.20	27:39.4
Marathon	Wolde (ETH) 2:20:27	Kimihara (JPN) 2:23:31	Ryan (NZL) 2:23:45	2:09:36
20 km Racewalk	Holubnychy (URS) 1:33:58	Pedraza (MEX) 1:34:00	Smaga (URS) 1:34:03	1:25:22
50 km Racewalk	Hohne (GDR) 4:20:14	Kiss (HUN) 4:30:17	Young (USA) 4:31:55	3:55:36
Long Jump	Beamon (USA) 8.90 m **WR**	Beer (GDR) 8.19 m	Boston (USA) 8.16 m	8.35 m
Triple Jump	Saneyev (URS) 17.39 m **WR**	Prudencion (BRZ) 17.27 m	Gentile (ITA) 17.22 m	17.03 m
High Jump	Fosbury (USA) 2.24 m **OR**	Caruthers (USA) 2.22 m	Gavrilov (URS) 2.20 m	2.28 m
Pole Vault	Seagren (USA) 5.40 m **OR**	Schiprowski (FRG) 5.40 m	Nordwig (GDR) 5.40 m	5.41 m
Shot Put	Matson (USA) 20.54 **OR**	Woods (USA) 20.12 m	Gushchin (URS) 20.09 m	21.78 m
Discus	Oerter (USA) 64.78 **OR**	Milde (GDR) 63.08 m	Danek (CZK) 62.92 m	68.40 m

(Continued)

TABLE 4.1 (Continued)

EVENT	GOLD	SILVER	BRONZE	WORLD RECORD PRIOR TO 1968 MEXICO CITY OLYMPICS
Javelin	Lusis (URS) 90.10 m **OR**	Kinnunen (FIN) 88.58 m	Kulcsar (HUN) 87.06 m	91.98 m
Hammer Throw	Zsivotzky (HUN) 73.36 m **OR**	Klim (URS) 73.28 m	Lovasz (HUN) 69.78 m	73.76 m
Decathlon	Toomey (USA) 8193 **OR**	Walde (FRG) 8111	Bendlin (USA) 8064	8319
80 m Hurdles	Caird (AUS) 10.39 **OR**	Kilborn (AUS)	Cheng (TPE)	10.41
100 m	Tyus (USA) 11.08 **WR**	Ferrell (USA) 11.15	Szewinska (POL) 11.19	11.12
4 x 100-m Relay	USA 42.88 **WR**	CUB 43.36	URS 43.41	43.49
200 m	Szewinska (POL) 22.58 **WR**	Boyle (AUS) 22.74	Lamy (AUS) 22.88	22.86
400 m	Besson (FRA) 52.03	Board (GBR) 52.12	Pechonkina (URS) 52.25	52.01
800 m	Manning (USA) 2:00.92 **OR**	Silai (ROM) 2:02.58	Gommers (NED) 2:02.63	2:00.5
Long Jump	Viscopoleanu (ROM) 6.82 m **WR**	Sherwood (GBR) 6.68 m	Talysheva (URS) 6.66 m	6.76 m
High Jump	Rezkova (CZK) 1.82 m	Okorokova (URS) 1.80 m	Kozyr (URS) 1.80 m	1.91 m
Shot Put	Gummel (GDR) 19.61 m **WR**	Lange (GDR) 18.78 m	Chizhova (URS) 18.19 m	18.87 m
Discus	Manoliu (ROM) 58.18 m **OR**	Westermann (FRG) 57.76 m	Kleiber-Kontsek (HUN) 54.90 m	62.54 m
Javelin	Nemeth (HUN) 60.36 m	Penes (ROM) 59.92 m	Janko (AUT) 58.04 m	62.40 m
Pentathlon	Becker (FRG) 5098	Prokop (AUT) 4966	Toth (HUN) 4959	5246

WR: World Record; OR: Olympic Record.

Conversely, no world records were set in the men's middle-distance or long-distance events during the 1968 Mexico City Olympics, except for Australia's Ralph Doubell, who tied the world record in the 800-m run. Gold medalists in the men's 1,500-m, 3,000-m steeplechase, 5,000-m, 10,000-m, and marathon ran slower by ~0.8, 5.3, 6.1, 6.5, and 8.4%, respectively, compared to the world records in place at the time of the event [17] (Table 4.1). Mexico City's altitude negatively impacted performance in long-distance events, as evident by the performance of Ron Clarke of Australia, who was the world record holder in the 5,000-m and 10,000-m. Clarke finished fifth in the 5,000-m race, running about 1 minute slower than his world record, and sixth in the 10,000-m race, running more than 2 minutes slower than his world record [17]. Interestingly, several medalists in men's middle-distance and long-distance events came from the altitude-based nations of Ethiopia and Kenya, where the athletes were born and raised in highlands very similar in elevation to Mexico City. The 1968 Mexico City Olympics marked the beginning of a trend where Ethiopian and Kenyan distance runners dominated several subsequent Olympic Games [19]. In Mexico City, Kenyan athletes won 39% (7 of 18) of the medals, including three gold medals, in events ranging from 800-m to the marathon (Table 4.1).

4.3 The early years of altitude training

The 1968 Mexico City Olympics made it obvious that in order to compete successfully at *altitude* in endurance events, it was advantageous either to be a native of an altitude-based country such as Ethiopia or Kenya or to have completed extensive altitude training beforehand. Logically, the next question that many athletes, coaches, and environmental physiologists began asking was, "What effect does living and/or training at altitude have on *sea level* performance?" Thus, the post–Mexico City Olympics period, spanning from 1968 until the mid-1990s, witnessed a significant surge in research devoted to the effect of altitude training on the enhancement of sea level performance. During this era, the focus of research was on the efficacy of traditional "live high and train high" (LH + TH) altitude training (Figure 4.1). Early studies primarily measured *sea level performance*, with less emphasis on delving into specific physiological mechanisms and adaptations. Several investigations during this time were characterized by inherent design flaws, such as the lack of a sea level control group, inadequate pre-altitude iron normalization, and altitude training blocks carried out above 4,000 m (13,120 ft) causing insufficient training stimulus [17]. Despite these limitations, the heightened interest following the 1968 Mexico City Olympics played a crucial role in advancing altitude training

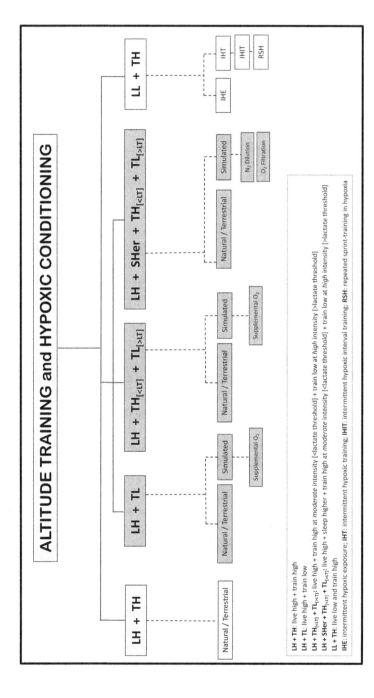

FIGURE 4.1 Altitude training and hypoxic conditioning (ATHC) strategies.

research and laying the foundation for years to come. Key questions addressed during the early years of altitude training research included:

- How many days does an athlete need to train at altitude in order to improve sea level performance?
- How many days after the athlete returns to sea level is the best time to compete?
- How long does the "altitude effect" last after an athlete returns to sea level?

During the early period of research on LH + TH altitude training, the results were equivocal regarding its effect on sea level performance. For example, a classic study by Adams et al. [20] involved 12 trained male distance runners divided into two training groups: one (SL-to-ALT) trained at 16 m (52 ft) at the University of California–Davis (Davis, California, USA), and the other (ALT-to-SL) trained simultaneously at 2,300 m (7,544 ft) at the United States Air Force Academy (Colorado Springs, Colorado, USA). Both groups followed the same 20 km (12.4 miles) per day running regimen at 75% maximal oxygen uptake (VO_2max) for 20 days at their respective locations, then moved directly to the opposite training location for an additional 20 days. Compared with baseline values, 2-mile run time was 7 seconds slower following the ALT-to-SL blocks, suggesting that 20 days of moderate-intensity training at 2,300 m and living at the same elevation for 24 hours per day did not improve sea-level endurance performance in the first three days post-altitude. In contrast, Daniels and Oldridge [21] found positive effects of LH + TH altitude training. Six male elite distance runners from the United States National Team lived and trained for periods of 14, 14, 7, and 7 days at 2,300 m (7,544 ft) in Alamosa, Colorado, USA. The athletes returned to sea level for five days (SL2) after the first 14-day altitude training block and returned to sea level again for five days (SL3) after the second 14-day altitude training block. During SL2 and SL3, the runners competed in sanctioned national or international competitions. The runners completed the study after the final seven-day altitude block and were evaluated within five days after returning to sea level (SLPost). Compared with pre-altitude baseline values, 3-mile run time measured at SLPost improved by 3%, with five of the six runners establishing 14 personal bests in sanctioned 1-mile and 3-mile races when competing during SL2, SL3, and SLPost. One runner broke the world record for the 1-mile during SL2 and lowered it again during SL3. The authors concluded that "there is an indication that this type of training is beneficial in improving performance at altitude and shows considerable promise of benefitting sea-level running performance." [21]. This study is considered by some as the first "live high and train low" (LH + TL)

(Figure 4.1) study done almost 30 years ahead of the first recognized LH + TL study by Levine and Stray-Gundersen [22], based on its design of four successive altitude blocks (7-14 days) followed by sea level blocks (5 days) during which the runners competed in elite-level competition. In addition, this period saw initial studies on Kenyan distance runners, exploring physical and physiological characteristics that might explain their success in athletics endurance events, particularly after their notable performance in the 1968 Mexico City Olympics [23, 24].

4.4 Living high and training low

In 1997, a paper appeared in the *Journal of Applied Physiology* titled, "Living High–Training Low: Effect of Moderate-Altitude Acclimatization with Low-Altitude Training on Performance." In that paper, the authors speculated that "if athletes could live at moderate altitude, above 2,500 m, but train at low altitude, below 1,500 m, they could acquire the physiological advantages of altitude acclimatization for maximizing oxygen transport, without the detraining associated with hypoxic exercise" [22]. Results showed that living for four weeks at a relatively high altitude (2,500 m / 8,200 ft) resulted in a significant increase in red blood cell (RBC) mass (5%) and hemoglobin concentration (9%). Simultaneous training at a lower elevation (1,250 m/4,100 ft) on select days during the 4-week LH + TL block allowed the runners to achieve running velocities similar to their sea level running velocities, thereby purportedly inducing beneficial cardiopulmonary and neuromuscular adaptations. Upon returning to sea level, significant improvements in VO_2max (5%) and 5,000-m run performance (1%) were observed three days post-LH + TL. In addition, performance in the 5,000-m run was similar on days 7, 14, and 21 post-LH + TL compared with day 3 post-LH + TL, suggesting that the benefits of a 4-week LH + TL block may last for up to 3 weeks upon return to sea level. The authors concluded that

> four weeks of living high and training low improves sea-level running performance in trained runners due to altitude acclimatization (increase in red cell mass volume and VO_2max) and maintenance of sea-level training velocities, most likely accounting for the increase in velocity at VO_2max and maximal steady state.
>
> *[22]*

Beginning in the early 2000s, LH + TL altitude training underwent several iterations (Figure 4.1). For example, "live high" (and potentially "sleep higher" via natural altitude or simulated altitude) plus "train high at *moderate* intensity," with moderate intensity defined as *below* lactate threshold

(LT) plus "train low at *high* intensity," with high intensity defined as *above* lactate threshold. The goal of living high, and potentially sleeping higher via natural or simulated altitude, is to stimulate a robust erythropoietic response and an increase of 2% to 3% in total hemoglobin mass [25, 26]. By remaining high when conducting *moderate*-intensity training sessions, the hypoxia-induced erythropoietic response is maintained [27]. In addition, the overall efficiency of the cardiopulmonary system is maintained or improved [27]. Conversely, conducting *high*-intensity training sessions at significantly lower elevations induces peripheral and nonhematological adaptations, including improved mitochondrial efficiency, increased oxidative and nonoxidative enzymatic activity, and augmentation of skeletal muscle capillarity [28]. The 2000s also saw the practical application of LH + TL by elite athletes, coaches, and environmental physiologists in natural environments such as Park City, Utah, USA (2,500 m/8,200 ft) and Salt Lake City, Utah, USA (1,250 m/4,100 ft), as well as simulated altitude environments such as nitrogen apartments, hypoxic tents, and the use of supplemental oxygen. The decade also witnessed advancements in LH + TL research, including the evaluation of hematological and nonhematological factors contributing to enhanced sea level performance post-altitude. Research designs became more rigorous, incorporating control groups, iron supplementation, and elite athletes into studies [29]. The widespread interest in LH + TL research during the 2000s led to the initiation and growth of international conferences organized around the theme of "altitude training" held in Colorado Springs, USA; Takayama City, Japan; Font-Romeu, France; Beijing, China; and Jyvaskyla, Finland. Two of these international forums continue to the present day.

In the 2000s, the use of simulated altitude in conjunction with LH + TL altitude training prompted discussions on ethical issues, particularly regarding the use of simulated altitude modalities (nitrogen apartment, hypoxic tent) at the Olympic level. During the 2000 Sydney Olympics, athletes living in the Olympic Athlete Village were prohibited from using simulated altitude devices, and this prohibition has persisted to the present day [29]. In addition, there was significant public opposition in Norway regarding the use of simulated altitude apartments by the country's Olympic athletes. In July 2001, the Norwegian Winter Olympic Team vacated the nitrogen house they had constructed in Heber City, Utah, USA for use in preparation for the 2002 Salt Lake City Winter Olympics [17]. In September 2006, the World Anti-Doping Agency (WADA) released an official statement regarding the use of simulated altitude modalities. WADA Chairman Richard Pound stated,

> In response to our stakeholders who requested that there be full consideration of hypoxic conditions in the context of the prohibited list, WADA performed a scientific and ethical review of the matter and engaged in a thorough consultation with experts and stakeholders. While we do *not*

deem this method appropriate for inclusion on the Prohibited List at this time, we still wish to express the concern that, in addition to the results varying individually from case to case, use of this method may pose health risks if not properly implemented and under medical supervision.

[29]

4.5 Living low and training high

In the mid-2000s, "live low and train high" (LL + TH) altitude training emerged as an alternative to LH + TH and LH + TL (Figure 4.1). LL + TH altitude training involves athletes living in a natural, normobaric normoxic environment while being exposed to discrete and relatively short intervals of simulated normobaric hypoxia or hypobaric hypoxia [30, 31]. LL + TH via normobaric hypoxia can be achieved through devices like commercial nitrogen-dilution and oxygen-filtration devices, hypoxic training rooms, or via inspiration of hypoxic gas. LL + TH via hypobaric hypoxia is typically done in a barometric pressure chamber. LL + TH can be used by athletes in the resting state (intermittent hypoxic exposure, IHE) or during formal training sessions (intermittent hypoxic training, IHT; intermittent hypoxic interval training, IHIT). An additional iteration of IHIT is "repeated sprint-training in hypoxia" (RSH), which differs slightly from IHT and IHIT in that it involves *maximal* or near-maximal sprints, purportedly achieving greater recruitment of type II-X fast glycolytic fibers [30]. It is speculated that IHT, IHIT, and RSH can augment skeletal muscle mitochondrial density, myoglobin content, capillary-to-fiber ratio, and fiber cross-sectional area, particularly in type II-X fast glycolytic fibers [32, 33] via upregulation of hypoxia-inducible factor 1a (HIF-1a) [30, 31]. In the mid-2000s, LL + TH altitude training became popular due to its reduced cost, travel requirements, and time away from home compared to mountain-based altitude training blocks. While research supporting LL + TH for the enhancement of endurance performance in elite athletes has been limited [29], there is strong support for its use (particularly IHIT and RSH) in nonendurance sport at sea level [34]. Indeed, LL + TH altitude training has been credited with expanding the application of ATHC for athletes in team sports, sprint-based sports, combat sports, and individual sports [30, 34], broadening its use beyond the traditional focus on endurance athletes.

During this time, the concept of the "optimal hypoxic dose" (OHD) became a topic of debate [35]. This debate emerged due to the contrast between the acute nature of LL + TH hypoxic exposure *versus* the chronic nature of LH + TH and LH + TL hypoxic exposure. This debate extended to the physiological differences between normobaric hypoxia (e.g., LL + TH) and hypobaric hypoxia (e.g., LH + TH & LH + TL), and the effect of each ATHC strategy on inducing beneficial physiological adaptations for enhanced performance [36, 37]. This period witnessed a more sophisticated and detailed approach to altitude training, considering factors such as the duration, intensity, and specific physiological demands of a particular sport. Researchers and practitioners started examining cellular and molecular mechanisms driving enhanced performance in conjunction with ATHC in more detail. For example, Zoll et al. [38] found significant increases in mRNA concentrations of various factors related to hypoxia adaptation in the vastus lateralis muscle of a hypoxia-trained group after 6 weeks of LH + TL training. This included hypoxia-inducible factor 1 (104%), glucose transporter-4 (32%), phosphofructokinase (32%), peroxisome proliferator-activated receptor gamma coactivator 1 (60%), citrate synthase (28%), cytochrome oxidase 1 (74%) and 4 (36%), carbonic anhydrase-3 (74%), and manganese superoxide dismutase (44%). These findings marked a shift toward a deeper understanding of the molecular and cellular responses to altitude training.

4.6 Current issues and trends

Over the past decade, the number of publications listed in PubMed under the search term "altitude training" has increased exponentially: 2013 (120 publications), 2014 (155), 2015 (176), 2016 (222), 2017 (234), 2018 (254), 2019 (287), 2020 (306), 2021 (400), 2022 (428), 2023 (476). This growth demonstrates a robust and expanding interest in understanding and implementing altitude-training related strategies. *Combining* different ATHC strategies has become a popular concept among environmental physiologists and elite athletes. Millet et al. [39] first introduced the idea of

> a new combination of hypoxic method (which we suggest naming Living High-Training Low and High, interspersed; LHTLHi) combining LH + TL (five nights at 3000 m and two nights at sea level) with training at sea level except for a few (2-3 per week) IHT sessions of supra-threshold training.

This approach was suggested as an effective way to prepare athletes for competition at both sea level and competition at altitude when periodized systematically over several weeks. Mujika et al. [40] expanded on this concept, advocating that

> published and field-based data strongly suggest that altitude training in elite endurance athletes should follow a long- and short-term *periodized* approach, integrating exercise training and recovery manipulation, performance peaking, adaptation monitoring, nutritional approaches, and the use of normobaric hypoxia in conjunction with terrestrial altitude.

Figure 4.2 ref. [40] shows the critical performance components of terrestrial altitude, normobaric hypoxia, and sea level training, along with the ancillary components of nutritional intervention, blood chemistry, and heat/humidity

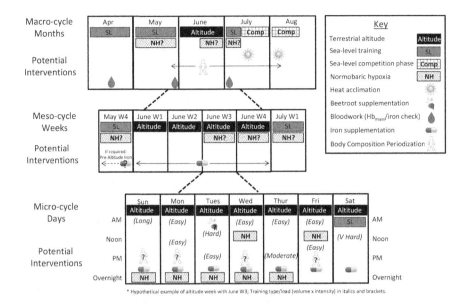

FIGURE 4.2 Potential macro-, meso-, and micro-periodization and integration of nutrition, heat, and artificial altitude with terrestrial altitude. The hypothetical proposal features a 4-week terrestrial altitude block in June to set up a competition phase from mid-July into August indicates hypothetical interventions that require further scientific validation.

Reprinted with permission from Mujika, I., A.P. Sharma, and T. Stellingwerff, *Contemporary periodization of altitude training for elite endurance athletes: A narrative review.* Sports Med, 2019. 49: 1651–1669.

acclimation or acclimatization. Mujika et al. [40] have provided a comprehensive framework for the proper integration of critical performance components within the construct of training cycles to achieve optimal results in ATHC. This integration extends across macro-cycles, meso-cycles, and micro-cycles emphasizing a periodized and systematic approach. Other recommendations include the use of normobaric hypoxia (IHE, IHT, IHIT) as a pre-acclimation strategy in preparation for LH + TH or LH + TL altitude training blocks. Additionally, normobaric hypoxia (IHE; hypoxic apartment) is suggested for use at sea level post-altitude to mitigate neocytolysis, thereby slowing the decrease in altitude-induced hemoglobin mass. In line with this periodized and integrated ATHC approach, recent nutritional strategies recommended by Stellingwerff et al. [41] focus on altered energy availability, iron, carbohydrate, hydration, antioxidant requirements, and various performance supplements. Particular attention is paid to the importance of blood testing prior to, during, and after an altitude training block to monitor serum ferritin levels and introduce iron supplementation as needed.

The concept of OHD has been revisited in recent studies [42], acknowledging a wide range of OHD recommendations using *number of days* and *elevation* as the defining parameters. Recommendations for OHD have ranged from 2 weeks of natural altitude at 2,500 m (8,200 ft) [43] to over 17 days of natural altitude at 4,000+ m (13,120+ ft) [44] for the specific purpose of stimulating a robust increase in hemoglobin mass. A question arises, "Would a longer stay at a lower altitude elicit the same hemoglobin mass response as a shorter stay at a higher altitude if the same overall 'dose' of altitude was provided?" [42]. Accordingly, it has been proposed that OHD be expressed as *kilometer hours*, defined as $km \cdot h = (m/1,000) \times h$, where m indicates elevation of exposure in meters and h indicates total duration of exposure in hours [42]. This conceptualization of OHD in kilometer hours may provide athletes and coaches with more options in terms of where they can effectively conduct altitude training blocks based on what natural highlands may be realistically available to them.

Over the past 10 years, there has been a notable increase in the number of professional-level altitude training facilities around the world. For example, the United States Olympic and Paralympic Committee (USOPC) has established the Team USA Altitude Training Network. This network comprises 14 altitude training sites located in the Rocky Mountains and Sierra Nevada Mountains of the western United States. The elevations of these sites range from 1,525 m (5,002 ft) to 2,780 m (9,118 ft) [45, 46]. This altitude training network is accessible to U.S. National Team athletes from summer and winter Olympic sports, providing convenient access to many sites suitable for both LH + TL and LH + TH altitude training. In addition, Team USA has developed an international altitude training network in the Engadin region of Switzerland (1,829–2,439 m/6,000–8,000 ft) and in Nagano Prefecture in Japan (1,750–2,569 m/5,740–8,425 ft) to facilitate altitude training for Team USA athletes in conjunction with major international competitions held in Europe and Asia [46].

4.7 Into the future

The future of ATHC holds several intriguing possibilities, both in terms of research and practical application by athletes and coaches. Following are some key areas that might be explored in the near future:

- Further evaluation of nonhematological physiological responses that could enhance performance not only in endurance sport but also in non-endurance sport. There is a need for increased knowledge regarding OHD as it relates specifically to nonhematological effects. In addition, there is a need for investigation into the timeline of decay of nonhematological effects upon return to sea level.

- Advances in technology and innovation may lead to increased interest in exploring epigenomic processes related to ATHC. These processes involve non-sequence-based features of the human genome and could provide insights into how altitude training impacts gene expression and adaptation [47].
- Further evaluation of the concept of "cross acclimation" or "cross tolerance," which suggests that heat pre-acclimation/acclimatization might simultaneously enhance altitude tolerance via similar mechanistic pathways (i.e., HIF).
- With climate change and global warming, there is a possibility that future Olympic Games, both Summer and Winter, will be held at higher elevations [48]. This shift may be driven by the need for better environmental and competition conditions, for example, reduced hyperthermia in the Summer Olympics and more robust snow conditions in the Winter Olympics. Research will be needed to understand the effects of moderate altitude on various sports including those that have traditionally been contested at low altitude or sea level. It will also require increased knowledge regarding the physiological preparation needed for optimal performance at higher elevations.

Abbreviations

ATHC	altitude training and hypoxic conditioning
IHE	intermittent hypoxic exposure
IHT	intermittent hypoxic training
IHIT	intermittent hypoxic interval training
IOC	International Olympic Committee
LH + TH	live high and train high
LH + TL	live high and train low
LL + TH	live low and train high
OHD	optimal hypoxic dose
RSH	repeated sprint-training in hypoxia
USOC	United States Olympic Committee.

References

1. Maraniss, D., *Once in a great city: A Detroit story*. New York, Simon & Schuster, 2015.
2. Balke, B., F.J. Nagle, and J. Daniels, *Altitude and maximum performance in work and sports activity*. JAMA, 1965. **194**: p. 646–649.
3. Proceedings of *The Magglingen Symposium on Sports at Medium Altitude. Research Committee of the International Council of Sports and Physical Education, Swiss Olympic Committee, and Swiss Medical Association. Magglingen*, Switzerland, 1966.

4. Proceedings of *The International Symposium on the Effects of Altitude on Physical Performance. United States Olympic Committee, Lovelace Foundation for Medical Education and Research, and the University of New Mexico.* Albuquerque, New Mexico, USA, 1967.

5. Balke, B., J.A. Faulkner, and J.T. Daniels, *Maximum performance capacity at sea-level and at moderate altitude before and after altitude training.* Schweiz Z Sportmed, 1966. **14:** p. 106–116.

6. Buskirk, E.R., et al., *Maximal performance at altitude and on return from altitude in conditioned runners.* J Appl Physiol, 1967. **23:** p. 259–266.

7. Evans, W.O., and C.F. Consolazio, *Effects of high altitude on performance of three different types of work.* Percept Mot Skills, 1967. **25:** p. 41–50.

8. Faulkner, J.A., J.T. Daniels, and B. Balke, *Effects of training at moderate altitude on physical performance capacity.* J Appl Physiol, 1967. **23:** p. 85–89.

9. Pugh, L.G.C.E., *Athletes at altitude.* J Physiol, 1967. **192:** p. 619–646.

10. Saltin, B. *Aerobic and anaerobic work capacity at 2300 meters.* Med Thorac, 1967. **24:** p. 205–210.

11. Scano, A., and G. Meineri, *Behavior of pulmonary ventilation and alveolar gas tension in athletes before, during and after 5 weeks of sojourn at an altitude of 2250 m.* Riv Med Aeronaut Spaz, 1967. **30:** p. 645–662.

12. Keul, J., et al, *Heart frequencies and substrate concentrations in the blood of horses during training in Mexico City (2,250 m above sea level).* Pflugers Arch Gesamte Physiol Menschen Tiere, 1968. **301:** p. 358–367.

13. Burns, B., *The track in the forest: The creation of a legendary 1968 U.S. Olympic Team.* Chicago, Chicago Review Press, 2019.

14. *Report of the Medical Section of the United States Team to the Games in Mexico City–October 1965.* United States Olympic Committee. Colorado Springs, Colorado, USA, 1966.

15. *Report of Medical Research Project into the Effects of Altitude in Mexico City in 1965.* British Olympic Association. London, England, 1966.

16. Hoffer, R., *Something in the air: American passion and defiance in the 1968 Mexico City Olympics.* New York, Free Press, 2009.

17. Wilber, R.L., *Altitude training and athletic performance.* Champaign-Urbana, Human Kinetics, 2004.

18. Ward-Smith, A. J., *Altitude and wind effects on long jump performance with particular reference to the world record established by Bob Beamon.* J Sports Sci, 1986. **4:** p. 89–99.

19. Wilber, R.L., and Y.P. Pitsiladis, *Kenyan and Ethiopian distance runners: What makes them so good?* Int J Sports Physiol Perf, 2012. **7:** p. 92–102.

20. Adams, W.C., et al., *Effects of equivalent sea-level and altitude training on VO$_2$max and running performance.* J Appl Physiol, 1975. **39:** p. 262–266.

21. Daniels, J., and N. Oldridge, *The effects of alternate exposure to altitude and sea level on world-class middle-distance runners.* Med Sci Sports Exerc, 1970. **2:** p. 107–112.

22. Levine, B.D., and J. Stray-Gundersen, *"Living high-training low": Effect of moderate-altitude acclimatization with low-altitude training on performance.* J Appl Physiol, 1997. **83:** p. 102–112.

23. Saltin, B., et al., *Morphology, enzyme activities and buffer capacity in leg muscles of Kenyan and Scandinavian runners.* Scand J Med Sci Sports, 1995. **5:** p. 222–230.

24. Saltin, B., et al., *Aerobic exercise capacity at sea level and at altitude in Kenyan boys, junior and senior runners compared with Scandinavian runners.* Scand J Med Sci Sports, 1995. **5**: p. 209–221.

25. Chapman, R.F., et al., *Defining the "dose" of altitude training: How high to live for optimal sea level performance enhancement.* J Appl Physiolc, 2014. **116**: p. 595–603.

26. Levine, B.D., and J. Stray-Gundersen, *Point: Positive effects of intermittent hypoxia (live high: train low) on exercise performance are mediated primarily by augmented red cell volume.* J Appl Physiol, 2005. **99**: p. 2053–2055.

27. Stray-Gundersen, J., R.F. Chapman, and B.D. Levine, *"Living high-training low" altitude training improves sea level performance in male and female elite runners.* J Appl Physiol, 2001. **91**: p. 1113–1120.

28. Gore, C.J., and W.G. Hopkins, (2005). *Counterpoint: Positive effects of intermittent hypoxia (live high: train low) on exercise performance are not mediated primarily by augmented red cell volume.* J Appl Physiol, 2005. **99**: p. 2055–2057.

29. Wilber, R.L., *Application of altitude/hypoxic training by elite athletes.* Med Sci Sports Exerc, 2007. **39**: p. 1610–1624.

30. Brocherie, F., et al., *Effects of repeated-sprint training in hypoxia on sea-level performance: A meta-analysis.* Sports Med, 2017. **47**: p. 1651–1660.

31. Girard, O., et al., *An updated panorama of "living low-training high" altitude/hypoxic methods.* Front Sports Act Living, 2020. **2**: p. 26.

32. Desplanches, D., et al., *Effects of training in normoxia and normobaric hypoxia on human muscle ultrastructure.* Pflügers Archiv, 1993. **425**: p. 263–267.

33. Vogt, M., et al., *Molecular adaptations in human skeletal muscle to endurance training under simulated hypoxic conditions.* J Appl Physiol, 2001. **91**: p. 173–182.

34. Millet, G.P., and F. Brocherie, *Hypoxic training is beneficial in elite athletes.* Med Sci Sports Exerc, 2020. **52**: p. 515–518.

35. Wilber, R.L., J. Stray-Gundersen, and B.D. Levine, *Effect of hypoxic "dose" on physiological responses and sea-level performance.* Med Sci Sports Exerc, 2007. **39**: p. 1590–1599.

36. Millet, G.P., R. Faiss, and V. Pialoux, *Point: Counterpoint: Hypobaric hypoxia induces/does not induce different responses from normobaric hypoxia.* J Appl Physiol, 2012. **112**: p. 1783–1784.

37. Mounier, R., and J.V. Brugniaux, *Counterpoint: Hypobaric hypoxia does not induce different responses from normobaric hypoxia.* J Appl Physiol, 2012. **112**: p. 1784–1786.

38. Zoll, J., et al., *Exercise training in normobaric hypoxia in endurance runners. III. Muscular adjustments of selected gene transcripts.* J Appl Physiol, 2006. **100**: p. 1258–1266.

39. Millet, G.P., et al., *Combining hypoxic methods for peak performance.* Sports Med, 2010. **40**: p. 1–25.

40. Mujika, I., A.P. Sharma, and T. Stellingwerff, *Contemporary periodization of altitude training for elite endurance athletes: A narrative review.* Sports Med, 2019. **49**, p. 1651–1669.

41. Stellingwerff, T., et al., *Nutrition and altitude: Strategies to enhance adaptation, improve performance and maintain health: A narrative review.* Sports Med, 2019. **49**: p. 169–184.

42. Garvican-Lewis, L.A., K. Sharpe, and C.J. Gore, *Time for a new metric for hypoxic dose?* J Appl Physiol, 2016. **121**: p. 352–355.

43. Gore C.J., et al., *Altitude training and haemoglobin mass from the optimised carbon monoxide rebreathing method determined by a meta-analysis.* Br J Sports Med, 2013. **47 Suppl 1**: p. i31–i39.
44. Rasmussen, P., et al. *Red cell volume expansion at altitude: A meta-analysis and Monte Carlo simulation.* Med Sci Sports Exerc, 2013. **45**: p. 1767–1772.
45. Girard, O., et al., *"Living high-training low" for Olympic medal performance: what have we learned 25 years after implementation?* Int J Sports Physiol Perf, 2023. **18**: p. 563–572.
46. Wilber, R.L., *Practical application of altitude/hypoxic training for Olympic medal performance: The team USA experience.* J Sci Sport Exerc, 2022. **4**: p. 358–370.
47. Julian, C.G., *Epigenomics and human adaptation to high altitude.* J Appl Physiol, 2017. **123**: p. 1362–1370.
48. Watts, N., *The 2020 report of The Lancet Countdown on health and climate change: Responding to converging crises.* The Lancet, 2020. **397**: p. 129–170.

SECTION 2

5

NEURODEGENERATIVE DISEASES

Johannes Burtscher

5.1 Background

Neurodegenerative diseases include rare and common neurological diseases, such as dementias like Alzheimer's disease (AD), motor diseases like Parkinson's disease (PD) or Huntington's disease (HD), and inflammatory diseases like multiple sclerosis (MS). Most cases of AD and PD are idiopathic, meaning that no clear (genetic) cause is known. In these cases, age is the most important risk factor [1]. Around 5–10% of AD and PD are caused by genetic mutations, while for example HD is always caused by an extension of the *Huntingtin (Htt)* gene. Idiopathic cases usually still have genetic risk factors that in conjunction with environmental risk factors can trigger pathogenic disease processes. MS is a chronic inflammatory disease with neurodegeneration in the spinal cord and brain, and both genetic and environmental factors play important roles in its development [2, 3]. Since neurodegenerative diseases are characterized by the death of neurons, which can usually not be replaced, once initiated, the disease processes inexorably continue.

Local hypoxia in the brain is thought to be a crucial factor in the development and progression of neurodegenerative disorders and is tightly linked to mitochondrial dysfunctions, protein-aggregation pathologies, and brain lesions, which frequently represent major neuropathological characteristics. While protective mechanisms are in place to counteract hypoxic injury, revolving notably around hypoxia inducible factors (HIFs), these mechanisms may be dysfunctional in neurodegenerative diseases.

The pathology of most neurodegenerative diseases overlaps, for example regarding mitochondrial dysfunctions, oxidative stress, neuroinflammation, protein aggregation, and neuronal death. The diverse symptoms are owed to

DOI: 10.4324/9781003402879-8

different affected brain regions, differential compositions/toxicity of the protein aggregations/lesion sites, specific mitochondrial dysfunctions, and other characteristics. The classical view of differences between AD, PD, and HD is depicted in Figure 5.1. Importantly, however, a much greater complexity is becoming increasingly recognized. This includes a great heterogeneity of pathology and symptomatology also within disease categories. Different proteins are today known to contribute to the formation of disease-specific protein inclusions, and the differentiation of affected mitochondrial components is less clearcut than previously assumed and not restricted to the vulnerability of elements of the mitochondrial electron transport system.

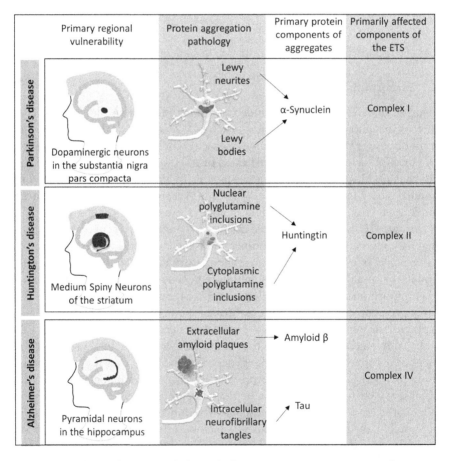

FIGURE 5.1   Classical neuropathological characteristics in major neurodegenerative diseases. ETS, electron transport system.

Adapted from [4].

Before summarizing the specific evidence on hypoxia and hypoxia conditioning in these neurodegenerative diseases, a short overview will be provided on neurological conditions, which are very obviously linked to hypoxia/ischemia (stroke) and for which the understanding of hypoxia conditioning as clinical application is already better understood: stroke and spinal cord injury.

5.2 Spinal cord injury and stroke

Early experiments demonstrated that exposure to sub-harmful hypoxia (hypoxia conditioning) protected the brain from subsequent severe hypoxia in rodents by triggering neuroprotective adaptations [5, 6]. These findings paved the way for later insights in the potential of hypoxia conditioning for neuroprotection. Specifically, hypoxia conditioning proved effective in animal models of spinal cord injury by improving respiratory and nonrespiratory plasticity and in humans with incomplete spinal cord injury by improving symptoms such as walking capacity, functional hand movement, and respiration (see Chapter 6). Short intermittent hypoxia conditioning, when related to spinal cord injury, is usually termed (therapeutic) acute intermittent hypoxia (tAIH). The field on clinical applications of hypoxia conditioning in spinal cord injury is more advanced than research in neurodegenerative diseases, although large-scale clinical trials have yet to be performed and increasing numbers of clinical trials are performed for all kinds of other neurological diseases as well [7, 8].

Stroke is probably the best example for the dual role of hypoxia; hypoxia/ischemia in stroke is responsible for subsequent brain damage, but cellular and tissue adaptations induced by exposures to hypoxia or ischemia can partially prevent this [9]. The term *pre*-conditioning has frequently been used in this field to indicate that the ischemia/hypoxia exposures took place before the stroke event, which is informative in animal models but usually not practical in humans, who had already experienced stroke when they need treatment. However, *post*-conditioning was also shown to be effective, even if performed remotely, for example by transiently blocking the blood flow (thereby inducing peripheral ischemia) by cuff inflation on the upper arm [10].

In animal stroke models, for example nine exposures of 2–4 h to 8% or 11% oxygen for 2 weeks, improved inflammation, stroke volume, and blood–brain-barrier integrity [11]. Daily cycles of 5 min exposures of mice to 13% ambient hypoxia, separated by 5 min normoxia, for two weeks improved microvascular angiogenesis and cerebral microcirculation, thereby protecting from stroke [12]. However, the therapeutic window for intermittent hypoxia treatments appears to be narrow: A fraction of inspired oxygen (FiO_2)>15% is likely not sufficient to induce brain benefits, and FiO_2<10% can result in neurologic deficits [13]. The efficacy of hypoxia conditioning is further determined by other factors of the "hypoxic dose" (duration, frequency, and pattern of application).

5.3 Hypoxia and neurodegenerative disorders

The systemic benefits of hypoxia conditioning include the reduction of cardiovascular risk factors for many neurological diseases, such as obesity, hypertension or metabolic deficits. Intermittent hypoxia can also be harnessed to modulate cerebral blood flow [14], which can be generally beneficial in neurodegenerative conditions by preventing ischemia and by boosting clearance of potentially harmful molecules, like for example pro-inflammatory molecules. In the following chapters, the specific role of hypoxia—and the corresponding potential of hypoxia conditioning—in some neurodegenerative diseases will be discussed.

5.3.1 Mild cognitive impairment, Alzheimer's disease, and other dementias

Severe hypoxia leads to cognitive deficits both in ambient hypoxia or in chronic diseases in which oxygen supply is reduced, such as chronic obstructive pulmonary disease (COPD) or obstructive sleep apnea (OSA) syndrome, which are associated with cognitive impairment. Hypoxia therefore may play a role in the cognitive decline that occurs in dementias and specifically in AD and its prodrome, mild cognitive impairment (MCI) [15]. This hypothesis is supported by the occurrence of molecular markers of hypoxia in brains of AD patients [16]. AD is the most common neurodegenerative disease and is characterized by protein aggregation pathology (amyloid-β protein-containing extracellular plaques and tau protein-containing intracellular neurofibrillary tangles), neuroinflammation, and mitochondrial dysfunction. The hippocampus, a brain structure importantly involved in learning and memory formation, is especially vulnerable to neurodegeneration in AD, which is related to cognitive deficits in patients.

Animal models suggest that hypoxia conditioning can attenuate pathological processes in AD. For example, hypoxia conditioning (2 h of 10% oxygen per day during three consecutive days) in AD-model rats attenuated astrogliosis, energy deficits, and oxidation and prevented cognitive deficits [17]. While no results of clinical trials in AD patients are yet available, several studies suggest that hypoxia conditioning is beneficial in MCI, as summarized in Table 5.1. Importantly, in these studies protocols consisting of short cycles of intermittent hypoxia (several minutes of hypoxia, separated by similarly long intervals of normoxia or hyperoxia) were applied on several days per week and for 3–8 weeks. While these protocols are probably not yet

TABLE 5.1 Hypoxia conditioning in mild cognitive impairment (MCI)

Study population	Experimental groups (number)	Hypoxia conditions	Main results	Ref.
Patients with MCI	Healthy + sham (7), MCI + sham (6), Healthy + IHHC (6), MCI + IHHC (10)	4 cycles/session of 5 min FIO_2 12%, interspersed with 3 min hyperoxia FIO_2 33%, 5 sessions/week for 3 weeks	• Slight cognitive improvement (MoCA) in MCI+IHHC only directly after IHHC • Latency of cognitive evoked potentials improved in MCI+IHHC • Decreased neutrophil extracellular trap formation and amyloid β expression in MCI+IHHT	[18]
Patients with MCI	IHC (7)	8 cycles/session of 5 min FIO_2 10%, interspersed with 5 min normoxia, 3 sessions/week for 8 weeks	• Resting arterial pressures reduced by 5–7 mm Hg • Cerebral oxygen saturation increased • Hypoxemia-induced cerebral vasodilation improved • Higher scores in mini-mental status exam and digit span test	[19]
Patients with MCI	Healthy (7), MCI + sham (6), MCI + IHHC (8)	4 cycles/session of 5 min FIO_2 12%, interspersed with 5 min hyperoxia F_1O_2 33%, 5 sessions/week for 3 weeks	• Slight cognitive improvement immediately post-IHHC • Event related potentials unchanged • Amyloid precursor protein ratio improved • Amyloid β and neutrophil extracellular traps improved	[20]
Multi-morbidity due to advanced age	IHHC (18) + multimodal rehabilitation, Sham (16) + multimodal rehabilitation	4–8 cycles/session of 4–6 min FIO2 12%, interspersed with 1–2 min hyperoxia FIO2 35%, total 16–20 session in 5–6 weeks	• Cognitive performance improved: dementia and clock drawing test • Walking capacity improved in both groups but more in IHHC group	[21]

Source: Adapted from [22].

Abbreviations: FIO_2: fraction of inspired oxygen; IHC: intermittent hypoxia conditioning; IHHC: intermittent hypoxia hyperoxia conditioning; MoCA: Montreal Cognitive Assessment test.

completely optimized, they do provide an important signpost for future studies, in particular for neurological diseases, for which no clinical trials on hypoxia conditioning have yet been performed.

5.3.2 Parkinson's disease and synucleinopathies

PD is the second most common neurodegenerative disorder, and its global prevalence is increasing more rapidly than any other neurological disease [23]. The cardinal symptoms are motor symptoms, including bradykinesia (slowness of movement), muscle rigidity, resting tremor, and impairments of posture and gait, but nonmotor symptoms are common, too, and can precede the diagnosis by decades [24]. Among these symptoms are autonomic and cognitive deficits, hyposmia, sleep disturbances, apathy, anxiety, and depression (for relevance of hypoxia conditioning, see Chapter 7). Motor symptoms follow the loss of dopaminergic neurons in the *substantia nigra, pars compacta*, which leads to an insufficient dopaminergic innervation of basal ganglia, cortical regions, and other brain areas. Pathological protein aggregation, mitochondrial dysfunction, and perturbed homeostasis of calcium and iron are thought to play important roles in disease progression. Lewy bodies and Lewy neurites are the characteristic protein aggregation pathology in PD, and its main proteinaceous component is the protein α-synuclein. Various mutations in the gene encoding for α-synuclein, *SNCA*, are established genetic causes of PD [25]. α-synuclein is also importantly involved in other neurodegenerative diseases that together with PD have been classified as α-synucleinopathies and include PD with dementia, dementia with Lewy bodies (DLB), and multiple system atrophy (MSA). Instead of Lewy pathology, MSA is characterized by glial cytoplasmic inclusions (also containing α-synuclein) and can be further subclassified in MSA with (1) predominant cerebellar ataxia or (2) predominant parkinsonism.

Severe hypoxia is a risk factor for PD, PD-related symptoms, and α-synucleinopathies. Several case studies report the occurrence of parkinsonism [26–28] or the development of PD in people with genetic risk factors [29] following high altitude sojourns. In addition, patients with PD and other synucleinopathies frequently suffer from ventilatory dysfunction [30]. They are also characterized by an impaired chemosensitivity and hypoxic ventilatory response [31, 32]. In line with a role of hypoxia in PD pathogenesis, polymorphisms in HIF-1 may represent risk factors to develop PD, aberrant HIF-activities have been reported in animal models of synucleinopathies, and modulation of HIFs was protective [33]. Moreover, increased HIF-levels were observed in MSA and in PD brains [34]. Mechanistically, prolonged tissue hypoxia may promote pathology by impairing mitochondrial functions or aggravating α-synuclein pathology and conditioning-induced adaptations may mitigate these effects. Hypoxia exposure further modulates the dopaminergic systems, likely by changing dopamine synthesis, reuptake, or receptor-sensitivity [35]. This effect could be controlled in a rat model of PD (5×15 min exposures to 12% oxygen, interspersed with 15 min normoxia, daily for two weeks) to increase dopamine availability [36].

Although the theoretical promise of hypoxia conditioning in PD is high, little information is yet available on its application in patients. Clinical trials are however ongoing, and the design and rational for one was recently published [37]. In this study PD patients will be subjected to only one session of hypoxia exposure: continuous hypoxia for 45 min or 5×5 min hypoxia interspersed with 5 min normoxia, both protocols at 12.7% or 16.3% oxygen. This study will be important for future research, but a single exposure might not be enough to induce lasting benefits like the longer protocols used for MCI (see previous discussion).

5.3.3 Huntington's disease, multiple sclerosis, and amyotrophic lateral sclerosis

HD is a rare dominantly inherited neurodegenerative disease, characterized by motor and cognitive symptoms. *Htt* mutation leads to the expression of an expanded polyglutamine stretch in the Htt protein, which damages mitochondria and cells, especially in the striatum. Although there is very limited direct evidence showing efficacy of hypoxia conditioning in HD, such approaches appear to be particularly promising for HD [38]. First, the striatum is highly vulnerable to hypoxia [39]. Second, in HD model mice an increased sensitivity to hypoxia at young age and an increasing resistance at older age have been observed [40], suggesting intrinsic hypoxic conditioning processes due to repeated tissue hypoxia. And third, the stabilization of HIFs has been shown to be beneficial in several cell and animal models (see Table 5.2).

The chronic inflammatory and neurodegenerative disease MS is the most common neurological disease in young adults. In animal models of MS, both moderate chronic and intermittent hypoxia exposures were beneficial. Chronic hypoxia exposure (10% oxygen) preserved vascular integrity and excessive immune cell activity in MS model mice [45]. An intermittent hypoxia conditioning protocol (10 cycles per day of 5 min at 11% oxygen, alternating with 5 min normoxia for seven days) protected axons and myelination, reduced inflammation, and improved clinical scores in a mouse model of MS [46]. Not much information on the efficiency of hypoxia conditioning is yet available in MS patients. One study tested a hypoxic training protocol (12 brisk walking sessions within 4 weeks at 15% oxygen) in MS patients and found improvements in physical performance and mood that were, however, similar to the normoxic training group [47].

Amyloid lateral sclerosis (ALS) is a neuromuscular disease characterized by degeneration of motor neurons and eventual failure of breathing. Hypoxia

TABLE 5.2 Hypoxia inducible factor (HIF) stabilization in Huntington's disease models

Model	HIF-stabilization	Main results	Ref.
Human fetal striatal neuroblasts	HIF-1 inducer cobalt chloride	• Modulation of proliferation and differentiation • Increased VEGF	[41]
Mouse striatal and cortical neurons, 3-NP toxicity	HIF-1 inducer DFO	• Attenuated cytotoxicity • Increased VEGF • No rescue of complex II deficits	[42]
Caenorhabditis elegans with mutated Htt	HIF-1 stabilization by knockdown of egl-9 or vhl-1	• Reduced paralysis • Increased lifespan	[43]
C6 astroglial cells, 3-NP toxicity	HIF-1 inducers cobalt chloride, mimosine, and DFO	• Reduced cytotoxicity	[44]

Source: Adapted from [38].

Abbreviations: 3-NP, 3-nitropropionic acid (toxin that is used to trigger cell death to model HD); DFO, desferrioxamine; VEGF, vascular endothelial growth factor.

conditioning in a rat model of ALS preserved phrenic long-term facilitation and breathing capacity [48] and thus represents a promising approach also for this disease.

Overall, hypoxia conditioning is a promising approach for HD, MS, and ALS, but scientific evidence is very scarce still. More animal studies to delineate the mechanisms of beneficial hypoxia in these diseases and clinical trials to clearly establish safety and efficacy (depending on the hypoxic dose) are needed.

5.3.4 Leigh disease and Friedreich's ataxia

Recently, spectacular results have been obtained in models of Leigh disease and Friedreich's ataxia in the group of Vamsi Mootha when mice were exposed to hypoxia. Leigh syndrome is a mitochondrial disease, and patients develop neurodegeneration early in life. In a Leigh syndrome mouse model, chronic exposure to continuous hypoxia (11% oxygen) prevented the development of the disease and extended survival [49].

Friedreich's ataxia is a rare, multisystemic, neurodegenerative disease leading to severe motor symptoms (ataxia) with a usual onset between childhood and adolescence. Chronic continuous hypoxia (11% oxygen) was shown to prevent and even reverse the development of ataxia in Friedreich's ataxia model mice [50]. Conversely, chronic intermittent hypoxia (11% oxygen for 16 h per day) was harmful both in Leigh syndrome [51] and Friedreich's ataxia [50] models. It is important to point out that this kind of intermittent hypoxia is used as a model for OSA, and the hypoxic dose is too high to be beneficial like hypoxia conditioning protocols presented previously that usually involve exposure of only several minutes hypoxia per day for no longer than a few weeks.

5.4 Conclusions

Uncontrolled, severe hypoxia and ischemia are dangerous for cells and tissues and in particular in the brain, which strongly depends on oxygen to satisfy its high energy demand. In addition, neurons are vulnerable to oxidative stress, a prominent consequence of hypoxia–reperfusion sequences. Unsurprisingly, hypoxia is involved in neurodegeneration and closely associated with neuropathological processes involving mitochondrial dysfunction, oxidative stress, (neuro)inflammation, and protein aggregation.

Emerging evidence suggests that the controlled exposure to hypoxia induces protective cellular and systemic adaptations that may be protective in many neurogenerative diseases both by reducing systemic (e.g., cardiovascular and respiratory) risk factors and by increasing brain function (vascular remodeling, control of brain blood flow and mitochondrial capacities) and resilience (management of oxidative stress, inflammation, and protein aggregation) [4].

Recent promising results in animal models for rare, early onset neurodegenerative disease (Leigh syndrome and Friedreich's ataxia) suggest great potential for permanent hypoxic environments to attenuate disease progression in such conditions. However, studies to confirm these results in different models and in patients are needed. The permanent exposure to hypoxia is also not very practical to apply, therefore new ideas and solutions are necessary.

Many of the more common age-related neurodegenerative diseases appear to be amenable to mild intermittent hypoxia conditioning protocols (often 15–20 cycles of around 30 min of mild hypoxia $FiO_2 \geq 10\%$ distributed over several weeks), alleviating notably cognitive and motor symptoms. Importantly these protocols must be clearly distinguished from models of chronic intermittent hypoxia, in which hypoxia episodes are often longer than 8 h per day, with FiO_2 sometimes <10%. While some clinical data on these strategies are already available, optimization of them is necessary. Several clinical trials are currently ongoing or are expected to start soon for hypoxia conditioning in neurodegenerative diseases, so we will soon see if the high expectations are justified.

Abbreviations

3-NP	3-nitropropionic acid
AD	Alzheimer's disease
ALS	amyloid lateral sclerosis
DFO	desferrioxamine
DLB	dementia with Lewy bodies
COPD	chronic obstructive pulmonary disease
FiO_2	Fraction of inspired oxygen
HD	Huntington's disease
HIF	hypoxia inducible factors
IHC	intermittent hypoxia conditioning
IHHC	intermittent hypoxia hyperoxia conditioning
MCI	mild cognitive impairment
MoCA	Montreal Cognitive Assessment test
MS	multiple sclerosis
MSA	multiple system atrophy
OSA	obstructive sleep apnea
PD	Parkinson's disease
SNCA	gene encoding for α-synuclein
tAIH	therapeutic Acute Intermittent Hypoxia
VEGF	vascular endothelial growth factor

References

1. Hou, Y., et al., *Ageing as a risk factor for neurodegenerative disease*. Nat Rev Neurol, 2019. **15**(10): p. 565–581.
2. Dyment, D.A., G.C. Ebers, and A.D. Sadovnick, *Genetics of multiple sclerosis*. Lancet Neurol, 2004. **3**(2): p. 104–110.
3. Ebers, G.C., *Environmental factors and multiple sclerosis*. Lancet Neurol, 2008. **7**(3): p. 268–277.
4. Burtscher, J., et al., *Boosting mitochondrial health to counteract neurodegeneration*. Prog Neurobiol, 2022. **215**: p. 102289.
5. Dahl, N.A. and W.M. Balfour, *Prolonged anoxic survival due to anoxia preexposure: Brain ATP, lactate, and pyruvate*. Am J Physiol, 1964. **207**(2): p. 452–456.
6. Noble, R.L., *The development of resistance by rats and guinea pigs to amounts of trauma usually fatal*. Am J Physiol, 1943. **138**: p. 346–351.
7. Burtscher, J., et al., *Hypoxia and brain aging: Neurodegeneration or neuroprotection?* Ageing Res Rev, 2021. **68**: p. 101343.
8. Vose, A.K., et al., *Therapeutic acute intermittent hypoxia: A translational roadmap for spinal cord injury and neuromuscular disease*. Exp Neurol, 2022. **347**: p. 113891.
9. Dirnagl, U., K. Becker, and A. Meisel, *Preconditioning and tolerance against cerebral ischaemia: From experimental strategies to clinical use*. Lancet Neurol, 2009. **8**(4): p. 398–412.

10. An, J.Q., et al., *Safety and efficacy of remote ischemic postconditioning after thrombolysis in patients with stroke.* Neurology, 2020. **95**(24): p. e3355–e3363.

11. Stowe, A.M., et al., *Repetitive hypoxia extends endogenous neurovascular protection for stroke.* Annals Neurol, 2011. **69**(6): p. 975–985.

12. Guan, Y., et al., *Intermittent hypoxia protects against hypoxic-ischemic brain damage by inducing functional angiogenesis.* J Cereb Blood Flow Metab, 2023. **43**: p. 1656–1671.

13. Guan, Y., et al., *Effects of Hypoxia on cerebral microvascular angiogenesis: Benefits or damages?* Aging Dis, 2023. **14**(2): p. 370–385.

14. Iwamoto, E., et al., *Intermittent hypoxia enhances shear-mediated dilation of the internal carotid artery in young adults.* J Appl Physiol, 2020. **129**(3): p. 603–611.

15. Daulatzai, M.A., *Death by a thousand cuts in Alzheimer's disease: Hypoxia—the prodrome.* Neurotoxicity Res, 2013. **24**(2): p. 216–243.

16. March-Diaz, R., et al., *Hypoxia compromises the mitochondrial metabolism of Alzheimer's disease microglia via HIF1.* Nature Aging, 2021. **1**(4): p. 385–399.

17. Correia, S.C., et al., *Hypoxic preconditioning averts sporadic Alzheimer's disease-like phenotype in rats: A focus on mitochondria.* Antioxid Redox Signal, 2022. **37**(10–12): p. 739–757.

18. Serebrovska, Z.O., et al., *Response of circulating inflammatory markers to intermittent hypoxia-hyperoxia training in healthy elderly people and patients with mild cognitive impairment.* Life (Basel), 2022. **12**(3): 1533317519896725.

19. Wang, H., et al., *Intermittent hypoxia training for treating mild cognitive impairment: A pilot study.* Am J Alzheimers Dis Other Demen, 2020. **35**: p. 1533317519896725.

20. Serebrovska, Z.O., et al., *Intermittent hypoxia-hyperoxia training improves cognitive function and decreases circulating biomarkers of Alzheimer's disease in patients with mild cognitive impairment: A pilot study.* Int J Mol Sci, 2019. **20**(21): p. 5405.

21. Bayer, U., et al., *Intermittent hypoxic–hyperoxic training on cognitive performance in geriatric patients.* Alzheimer's & Dementia: Translational Research & Clinical Interventions, 2017. **3**(1): p. 114–122.

22. Burtscher, J., et al., *Hypoxia and brain aging: Neurodegeneration or neuroprotection?* Ageing Res Rev, 2021. **68**: p. 101343.

23. Dorsey, E.R., et al., *The emerging evidence of the Parkinson pandemic.* J Parkinsons Dis, 2018. **8**(s1): p. S3–s8.

24. Kalia, L.V. and A.E. Lang, *Parkinson's disease.* Lancet, 2015. **386**(9996): p. 896–912.

25. Lashuel, H.A., et al., *The many faces of alpha-synuclein: From structure and toxicity to therapeutic target.* Nat Rev Neurosci, 2013. **14**(1): p. 38–48.

26. Hur, T., *Parkinsonism after climbing high amplitude mountain: A case report.* J Neurol Sci, 2015. **357**: p. e270.

27. Park, K. and K.I. Yang, *Delayed parkinsonism following high mountain climbing: A case report.* Neurology Asia, 2013. **18**(1): p. 99–101.

28. Swaminath, P.V., et al., *Parkinsonism and personality changes following an acute hypoxic insult during mountaineering.* Mov Disord, 2006. **21**(8): p. 1296–1297.

29. Tang, Y., et al., *Parkinson's disease in a patient with GBA and LRRK2 covariants after acute hypoxic insult: A case report.* BMC Neurol, 2023. **23**(1): p. 226.

30. Vijayan, S., et al., *Brainstem ventilatory dysfunction: A plausible mechanism for dyspnea in Parkinson's disease? Move Disord Offic J Move Disord Soc*, 2020: 10.1002/mds.27932
31. Serebrovskaya, T., et al., *Hypoxic ventilatory responses and gas exchange in patients with Parkinson's disease.* Respiration; J Thorac Dis, 1998. **65**(1): p. 28–33.
32. Onodera, H., et al., *Impaired chemosensitivity and perception of dyspnoea in Parkinson's disease.* Lancet, 2000. **356**(9231): p. 739–740.
33. Burtscher, J., et al., *Hypoxia conditioning as a promising therapeutic target in Parkinsons disease?* Mov Disord, 2021. **35**(12): p. 2333–2338.
34. Heras-Garvin, A., et al., *Signs of chronic hypoxia suggest a novel pathophysiological event in α-synucleinopathies.* Mov Disord, 2020. 35: p. 2333–2338.
35. Serebrovskaya, T., et al., *Geriatric men at altitude: Hypoxic ventilatory sensitivity and blood dopamine changes.* Respiration, 2000. **67**(3): p. 253–260.
36. Belikova, M.V., E.E. Kolesnikova, and T.V. Serebrovskaya, *Intermittent hypoxia and experimental Parkinson's disease*, in *Intermittent Hypoxia and Human Diseases*. 2012, Springer. p. 147–153.
37. Janssen Daalen, J.M., et al., *Multiple N-of-1 trials to investigate hypoxia therapy in Parkinson's disease: Study rationale and protocol.* BMC Neurol, 2022. **22**(1): p. 262.
38. Burtscher, J., et al., *A rationale for hypoxic and chemical conditioning in Huntington's disease.* Int J Mol Sci, 2021. **22**(2): p. 582.
39. Calabresi, P., et al., *Synaptic transmission in the striatum: From plasticity to neurodegeneration.* Prog Neurobiol, 2000. **61**(3): p. 231–265.
40. Klapstein, G.J. and M.S. Levine, *Age-dependent biphasic changes in ischemic sensitivity in the striatum of Huntington's disease R6/2 transgenic mice.* J Neurophysiol, 2005. **93**(2): p. 758–765.
41. Ambrosini, S., et al., *Fibroblast growth factor and endothelin-1 receptors mediate the response of human striatal precursor cells to hypoxia.* Neuroscience, 2015. **289**: p. 123–133.
42. Niatsetskaya, Z., et al., *HIF prolyl hydroxylase inhibitors prevent neuronal death induced by mitochondrial toxins: Therapeutic implications for Huntington's disease and Alzheimer's disease.* Antioxid Redox Sign, 2010. **12**(4): p. 435–443.
43. Mehta, R., et al., *Proteasomal regulation of the hypoxic response modulates aging in C. elegans.* Science (New York, N.Y.), 2009. **324**(5931): p. 1196–1198.
44. Yang, Y.T., T.C. Ju, and D.I. Yang, *Induction of hypoxia inducible factor-1 attenuates metabolic insults induced by 3-nitropropionic acid in rat C6 glioma cells.* J Neurochem, 2005. **93**(3): p. 513–525.
45. Halder, S.K. and R. Milner, *Chronic mild hypoxia accelerates recovery from pre-existing EAE by enhancing vascular integrity and apoptosis of infiltrated monocytes.* Proc Natl Acad Sci U S A, 2020. **117**(20): p. 11126–11135.
46. Tokarska, N., et al., *Acute intermittent hypoxia alters disease course and promotes CNS repair including resolution of inflammation and remyelination in the experimental autoimmune encephalomyelitis model of MS.* Glia, 2023. **71**(8): p. 2045–2066.
47. Mähler, A., et al., *Metabolic, mental and immunological effects of normoxic and hypoxic training in multiple sclerosis patients: A pilot study.* Front Immunol, 2018. **9**: p. 2819–2819.

48. Nichols, N.L., et al., *Mechanisms of enhanced phrenic long-term facilitation in SOD1(G93A) rats.* J Neurosci, 2017. **37**(24): p. 5834–5845.

49. Jain, I.H., et al., *Hypoxia as a therapy for mitochondrial disease.* Sci, 2016. **352**(6281): p. 54–61.

50. Ast, T., et al., *Continuous, but not intermittent, regimens of hypoxia prevent and reverse ataxia in a murine model of Friedreich's ataxia.* Hum Mol Genet, 2023. **32**(16): p. 2600–2610.

51. Ferrari, M., et al., *Hypoxia treatment reverses neurodegenerative disease in a mouse model of Leigh syndrome.* Proc Natl Acad Sci U S A, 2017. **114**(21): p. E4241–E4250.

6

SPINAL CORD INJURY

Gino Panza and Fei Zhao

6.1 Introduction

Spinal cord injury (SCI) results in significant impairments of the autonomic and cardiovascular systems [1], sleep [2], and motor control [3]. Ultimately, these impairments contribute to reduced physical function, deconditioning, and disability (Figure 6.1). As an individual becomes forced into inactivity, as a constraint on a healthy lifestyle, inactivity further impairs each physiological system creating a perpetual loop of worsening limitations that increase disability and mortality. Therefore, identifying new interventions to promote health and physical function is imperative.

Over the last few decades, there have been improvements in physical rehabilitation for individuals living with SCI [4], but due to the lack of somatic muscle activation, many therapies utilize robotics or various forms of electrical simulation to improve autonomic and functional capacity [5]. However, mild intermittent hypoxia (MIH) is a therapy that shows promise in amplifying neural plasticity in individuals with SCI and may be additive to various rehabilitation approaches [6]. The purpose of this chapter is to highlight when MIH is beneficial or detrimental, and when these protocols may facilitate improvements in sleep, autonomic, and motor function for individuals with SCI.

6.2 Sleep and chronic intermittent hypoxia

Individuals with high-level SCI commonly experience impaired pulmonary and upper airway function [7] contributing to an increased prevalence of sleep apnea (SA) compared to the general population [8]. SA leads to nocturnal

DOI: 10.4324/9781003402879-9

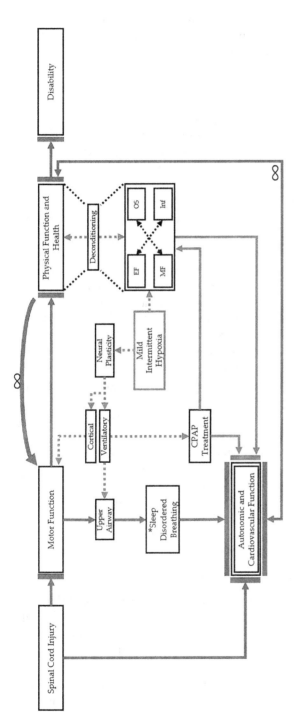

FIGURE 6.1 Red end-caps indicate negative consequences of spinal chord injury (SCI) as the green lines and end-caps indicate positive adaptations following intervention. The positive adaptations following mild intermittent hypoxia or continuous positive airway pressure (CPAP) can be linked to several other boxes in the schematic, but only a few are provided for clarity. Black short-dashed lines with arrows indicate potential mediators between or within boxes. Dashed green arrows indicate suggested hypotheses or preliminary data in humans and the suggested relationship. Solid green arrows indicate stronger evidence for the relationships. Positive adaptations from interventions, in theory, mitigate or reverse the red lines between associated variables. Please note that the peripheral adaptations associated with mitochondrial function, inflammation and oxidative stress are found in all cells. Thus, the schematic does not imply these potential mediators are only found in skeletal muscle.

Adapted from [2]. ∞ = perpetual loop, EF = endothelial function, Inf = inflammation, MF = mitochondrial function, OS = oxidative stress.

chronic intermittent hypoxia (CIH) and intermittent hypercapnia during sleep, which is thought to further impair autonomic function [9] and potentially mitigate physical rehabilitation efforts in those with SCI [2]. An important detail about MIH protocols delivered in controlled laboratory settings is the timing of delivery relative to sleep, as this can yield beneficial or detrimental effects on SA severity.

When administered during morning hours, MIH induces ventilatory plasticity that may improve upper airway function [10, 11], and when administered during sleep with continuous positive airway pressure, elicit reductions in airway resistance and therapeutic pressure to treat SA [12]. However, if administered immediately before sleep, MIH can worsen SA [13]. This is likely due to changes in peripheral chemoreceptor sensitivity, or the hypoxic ventilatory response (HVR) in humans. HVR contributes to SA severity [9] since disturbances in blood gas concentrations lead to hyperventilation following breathing events, ultimately resulting in hypocapnia and decreased stimulation to the upper airway muscles, which perpetuate apneic events [14]. Thus, if peripheral chemoreceptor sensitivity is increased, individuals will have a greater degree of hyperventilation subsequently resulting in another apneic event yielding a MIH-induced increase in SA severity when administered immediately prior to sleep [13, 15].

Considering that the increased prevalence of SA in those with SCI [8] is coupled with increased HVR during non–rapid eye movement sleep [16], and that repeated exposure to MIH can increase HVR [17], suggests MIH preceding sleep has the potential to worsen SA severity in persons with SCI. Conversely, when administered in the morning, MIH resulted in improved upper airway function during sleep in those with SA and no SCI [10]. Thus, MIH holds promise for improving upper airway function during sleep, which may benefit individuals with SCI and SA. It is critical to point out, however, that optimal timing of MIH (morning versus evening [11, 18]) will need to be established in those with SCI. Thus, experimentally delivered MIH, as opposed to nocturnal CIH experienced from SA [19], holds promise for improving upper airway function during sleep for those with SCI and SA.

6.3 Autonomic and cardiovascular function

There remains ambiguity in the terminology used surrounding MIH [19]. Some investigators study the pathophysiology of SA and recruit healthy individuals and expose them to longer duration MIH protocols as a model of SA (i.e., CIH, 180 minutes) [20]. Others study the potential benefit of IH and recruit various healthy and patient populations, and expose them to shorter bouts of IH (i.e. MIH, 24 minutes [19]) while measuring other clinically important outcomes like blood pressure (BP). For example, significant improvements in BP and other measures of autonomic function (heart rate and BP variability) were found when hypertensive individuals were exposed to a 24-minute MIH protocol (morning) for 15 days [10] with some studies suggesting improvements in nitric oxide as the mechanism of action [21]. Conversely, six hours of IH (i.e., simulating CIH from SA) has been shown to increase resting BP in healthy individuals [17], highlighting the importance of the study populations and dose of hypoxia [19]. The current evidence surrounding MIH in noninjured individuals with altered cardiovascular function indicates its efficacy in improving autonomic and cardiovascular control. Thus, there is potential for MIH to provide benefits to individuals with SCI and autonomic dysfunction, but these are not typically investigated in studies involving MIH and SCI.

Individuals with SCI commonly experience altered autonomic and cardiovascular function [22, 23]. This dysfunction may result in two distinct BP responses termed autonomic dysreflexia and orthostatic hypotension. Autonomic dysreflexia is a sudden rise in BP following a noxious or non-noxious stimulus (+20/10 mmHg), while orthostatic hypotension is a drop in BP during position movements (–20/–10 mmHg) [24]. These are intriguing autonomic responses since autonomic dysreflexia is the result of an overactive sympathetic spinal reflex initiated below the level of injury that cannot be inhibited by supraspinal input, and orthostatic hypotension is the inability to quickly activate sympathetic fibers. Managing these responses in individuals with SCI presents a unique challenge since treatment for one may augment the other [25, 26]. Thus, interventions with several mechanisms may improve cardiovascular care for individuals with SCI.

While MIH has shown efficacy in improving hypertension in individuals without SCI [17], the impact of MIH on BP and autonomic dysfunction in those with SCI has yet to be studied. Most studies measure BP for safety but have not directly investigated the impact of MIH on BP. Typically, resting BP does not change following repeated daily MIH [27–30], but one study did report a significant decrease in systolic BP after 5 days of MIH [31], suggesting no maladaptive changes in cardiovascular control following several days of MIH. Acute exposure to MIH also does not seem to elevate BP [27, 29, 32, 33], although one study reported a significant decrease following MIH when supplemented with ibuprofen [34]. Likewise, no changes in BP are typically found following the hypoxic exposure on the final day of repeated daily MIH protocols [27, 29, 31, 33].

These findings are intriguing considering MIH, as well as CIH from SA, is thought to increase muscle sympathetic nerve activity [9, 17] potentially explaining the sustained increases in BP following MIH [17] and hypertension for those with SA and no SCI [9]. For those with SCI and impaired supraspinal input, it may not be surprising that sustained increases in BP are not found following MIH, but this does not mean that autonomic dysreflexia is not worsened with acute MIH exposure since these studies do not perturb the sympathetic reflex below the lesion. Conversely, a heightened sympathetic system may mitigate orthostatic hypotension for these individuals, but orthostatic challenges have not been investigated following MIH to date. Unfortunately, despite the importance of treating autonomic dysreflexia and orthostatic hypotension in those with SCI, most studies on MIH are focused on its potential impact on motor function and do not test for autonomic dysreflexia or orthostatic hypotension. However, no changes in resting BP for these individuals does suggest there is no maladaptive resting cardiovascular plasticity following MIH.

6.4 Motor function

MIH induces a form of plasticity termed ventilatory long-term facilitation (vLTF), which is a sustained increase in minute ventilation following MIH and has been studied heavily in animals and humans [17]. Recently, studies have shown more robust neuroplastic changes in animals and humans following MIH [17, 35], and that the plasticity following MIH may be leveraged to improve motor function for individuals with SCI. Improvements in motor function following MIH include limb-specific tasks and functional tasks for the muscles of breathing, and upper and lower limb function. Improvements have been found after acute MIH alone, repeated daily MIH, and repeated MIH with concurrent task-specific training.

When MIH is accompanied by slight, sustained, hypercapnia, vLTF has been consistently shown in humans [17, 36]. Importantly, vLTF is not found after MIH in noninjured persons when hypercapnia is only administered during the hypoxic episodes [37], suggesting sustained hypercapnia may be critical for manifestation of vLTF. Despite limited human data, it appears the expression of vLTF is present in those with motor incomplete SCI when CO_2 is maintained throughout the entire protocol [38]. However, the expression of vLTF by itself may not be clinically important considering that multiple aspects of pulmonary function are impaired following SCI [39], and MIH can affect multiple aspects of breathing besides minute ventilation. For example, in those without SCI, improvements in the neural drive to breath were found following hypoxia in the absence of vLTF [37]. This could explain why improvements in maximum inspiratory pressure, but no change in maximum expiratory pressure or forced vital capacity, have been found in individuals with SCI following acute MIH [40]. However, it remains unknown if protocols that consistently elicit vLTF in those with SCI would lead to improvements in maximum expiratory pressure or forced vital capacity, as this remains to be tested.

The strength of the available evidence of MIH in humans with SCI resides in studies investigating some measure of hand or leg function. Exposure to acute MIH has been shown to increase grip strength with concurrent improvements in functional hand tests 1 hour, and up to 24 hours, following MIH exposure [41]. Likewise, acute improvements in ankle torque have been reported [33, 34], which coincide with increases in electromyography [33, 42]. MIH in conjunction with task-specific training has also shown improvements in hand function in those with SCI. MIH plus hand-opening exercises resulted in significant increases in box-and-block tests and the Jebsen-Taylor hand function tests when compared to sham plus hand-opening exercises, and these outcomes were concomitant with significant increases in maximal aperture and electromyography following MIH [30].

Improvements in lower body motor function have been found following repeated daily MIH, with positive effects on the 10 m and 6 min walk tests lasting at least one week [27]. Moreover, studies indicate further improvements in motor function when MIH is combined with some form of locomotor training [27, 31]. Four weeks of MIH *plus* body weight-supported treadmill training showed improvements in the 10 m walk test compared to sham and body weight supported-treadmill training for the initial 3 weeks. Conversely, improvements in the timed up and go test were found after the fourth week of training. The improvements in the 10 m walk test were concurrent with significant improvements in the 6 min walk test after the first 5 days and each week of training (4 weeks), including follow-up testing, when compared to only body weight–supported treadmill training [43]. This combined training also improved dynamic, but not static, balance [44]. Currently, the hypothesis is that MIH leads to plasticity within the corticospinal tract as evidenced by increased motor evoked potentials in those with and without SCI [32, 45]. However, this was not replicated in individuals without SCI from another laboratory [46]. Currently, there is only one large-scale study completed using MIH with individuals with SCI [43, 44], but there are a growing number of studies showing promising efficacy in improving various forms of motor function for these individuals. However, there remains a great deal of heterogeneity in the MIH protocols and methods employed in these studies; effective doses, minimum effective doses, and other parameters surrounding the specific protocols remain to be systematically investigated.

6.5 Conclusion

The current literature on MIH designed for beneficial effects has shown convincing efficacy in improving motor function for individuals with motor incomplete SCI, but evidence on the autonomic and cardiovascular impact is sparse, and findings involving sleep are nonexistent. Seemingly, effective MIH protocols are of short duration and mild intensity. The potency of MIH as a potentially beneficial or adjunctive therapy is remarkable due to the continued benefits reported despite heterogeneous research designs. There remains much to be learned regarding the mechanisms and most effective protocols of MIH for individuals with SCI; however, the current evidence remains promising.

Abbreviations

BP   blood pressure
CIH   chronic intermittent hypoxia
HVR   hypoxic ventilatory response
IH   Intermittent hypoxia
vLTF   ventilatory long-term facilitation
MIH   mild intermittent hypoxia
SA   Sleep apnea
SCI   Spinal cord injury

References

[1] Wecht, J.M. and Bauman, W.A. 2018. Implication of altered autonomic control for orthostatic tolerance in SCI. *Auton Neurosci Basic Clin.* **209**, 51–58. https://doi.org/10.1016/j.autneu.2017.04.004

[2] Panza, G.S. et al. 2021. Is sleep disordered breathing confounding rehabilitation outcomes in spinal cord injury research? *ArchPhys Med Rehab.* https://doi.org/10.1016/j.apmr.2021.08.015

[3] Kern, H. et al. 2005. Motor control in the human spinal cord and the repair of cord function. *Curr Pharmaceut Design.* **11**, 11, 1429–1439. https://doi.org/10.2174/1381612053507882

[4] Sandrow-Feinberg, H.R. and Houlé, J.D. 2015. Exercise after spinal cord injury as an agent for neuroprotection, regeneration and rehabilitation. *Brain Res.* **1619**, 12–21. https://doi.org/10.1016/j.brainres.2015.03.052

[5] Karamian, B.A. et al. 2022. The role of electrical stimulation for rehabilitation and regeneration after spinal cord injury. *J Orthopaed Traumatol: Offic J Ital Soc Orthopaed Traumatol.* **23**, 1, 2. https://doi.org/10.1186/s10195-021-00623-6

[6] Welch, J.F. et al. 2020. Synergy between acute intermittent hypoxia and task-specific training. *Exer Sport Sci Revs.* **48**, 3, 125–132. https://doi.org/10.1249/JES.0000000000000222

[7] Sankari, A. et al. 2019. Sleep-disordered breathing and spinal cord injury: A state-of-the-art review. *Chest.* **155**, 2, 438–445. https://doi.org/10.1016/j.chest.2018.10.002

[8] Graco, M. et al. 2021. Prevalence of sleep-disordered breathing in people with tetraplegia: A systematic review and meta-analysis. *Spinal Cord.* https://doi.org/10.1038/s41393-020-00595-0

[9] Dempsey, J.A. et al. 2010. Pathophysiology of sleep apnea. *Physiol Rev.* **90**, 1, 47–112. https://doi.org/10.1152/physrev.00043.2008

[10] Panza, G.S. et al. 2022. Daily exposure to mild intermittent hypoxia reduces blood pressure in male patients with obstructive sleep apnea and hypertension. *Am J Resp Crit Care Med* **205**, 8, 949–958. https://doi.org/10.1164/rccm.202108-1808OC

[11] Panza, G.S. et al. 2022. Divergent ventilatory and blood pressure responses are evident following repeated daily exposure to mild intermittent hypoxia in males with OSA and hypertension. *Front Physiol.* **13**, 897978. https://doi.org/10.3389/fphys.2022.897978

[12] El-Chami, M. et al. 2017. Exposure to intermittent hypoxia and sustained hypercapnia reduces therapeutic CPAP in participants with obstructive sleep apnea. *J Appl Physiol (Bethesda, Md.: 1985).* jap.00204.2017. https://doi.org/10.1152/japplphysiol.00204.2017

[13] Yokhana, S.S. et al. 2012. Impact of repeated daily exposure to intermittent hypoxia and mild sustained hypercapnia on apnea severity. *J Appl Physiol (Bethesda, Md.: 1985).* **112**, 3, 367–377. https://doi.org/10.1152/japplphysiol.00702.2011

[14] Mateika, J.H. et al. 2017. The impact of intermittent or sustained carbon dioxide on intermittent hypoxia initiated respiratory plasticity. What is the effect of these combined stimuli on apnea severity? *Resp Physiol Neurobiol.* https://doi.org/10.1016/j.resp.2017.10.008

[15] Alex, R.M. et al. 2019. Exposure to mild intermittent hypoxia increases loop gain and the arousal threshold in participants with obstructive sleep apnoea. *J Physiol.* (Apr. 2019). https://doi.org/10.1113/JP277711

[16] Vaughan, S. et al. 2022. Tetraplegia is associated with increased hypoxic ventilatory response during nonrapid eye movement sleep. *Physiol Rep.* **10**, 17, e15455. https://doi.org/10.14814/phy2.15455

[17] Puri, S. et al. 2021. A comprehensive review of respiratory, autonomic and cardiovascular responses to intermittent hypoxia in humans. *Exper Neurol.* 113709. https://doi.org/10.1016/j.expneurol.2021.113709

[18] Gerst, D.G. et al. 2011. The hypoxic ventilatory response and ventilatory long-term facilitation are altered by time of day and repeated daily exposure to intermittent hypoxia. *J Appl Physiol.* **110**, 1, 15–28. https://doi.org/10.1152/japplphysiol.00524.2010

[19] Panza, G.S. et al. 2023. Intermittent hypoxia: a call for harmonization in terminology. *J Appl Physiol (Bethesda, Md.: 1985).* **135**, 4, 886–890. https://doi.org/10.1152/japplphysiol.00458.2023

[20] Mateika, J.H. 2019. A reminder that experimentally induced intermittent hypoxia is an incomplete model of obstructive sleep apnea and its outcome measures. *J Appl Physiol (Bethesda, Md.: 1985).* **127**, 6, 1620–1621. https://doi.org/10.1152/japplphysiol.00549.2019

[21] Lyamina, N.P. et al. 2011. Normobaric hypoxia conditioning reduces blood pressure and normalizes nitric oxide synthesis in patients with arterial hypertension. *J Hypertens.* **29**, 11, 2265–2272. https://doi.org/10.1097/HJH.0b013e32834b5846

[22] Eldahan, K.C. and Rabchevsky, A.G. 2018. Autonomic dysreflexia after spinal cord injury: Systemic pathophysiology and methods of management. *Autonom Neurosci Basic Clin.* **209**, 59–70. https://doi.org/10.1016/j.autneu.2017.05.002

[23] Katzelnick, C.G. et al. 2019. Blood pressure instability in persons with SCI: Evidence from a 30-day home monitoring observation. *Am J Hypertens.* **32**, 10, 938–944. https://doi.org/10.1093/ajh/hpz089

[24] Wecht, J.M. et al. 2021. International standards to document autonomic function following SCI (ISAFSCI): Second edition. *Topics Spinal Cord Inj Rehab.* **27**, 2, 23–49. https://doi.org/10.46292/sci2702-23

[25] Chobanian, A.V. et al. 2003. Seventh report of the joint national committee on prevention, detection, evaluation, and treatment of high blood pressure. *Hypertens (Dallas, Tex.: 1979).* **42**, 6 (Dec. 2003), 1206–1252. https://doi.org/10.1161/01.HYP.0000107251.49515.c2

[26] Wecht, J.M. et al. 2023. Clinical trial of home blood pressure monitoring following midodrine administration in hypotensive individuals with spinal cord injury. *J Spinal Cord Med.* **46**, 4, 531–539. https://doi.org/10.1080/10790268.2021.1977904

[27] Hayes, H.B. et al. 2014. Daily intermittent hypoxia enhances walking after chronic spinal cord injury: A randomized trial. *Neurology.* **82**, 2, 104–113. https://doi.org/10.1212/01.WNL.0000437416.34298.43

[28] Navarrete-Opazo, A. et al. 2016. Intermittent hypoxia does not elicit memory impairment in spinal cord injury patients. *Arch Clin Neuropsychol Off J Nat AcadNeuropsychol.* **31**, 4, 332–342. https://doi.org/10.1093/arclin/acw012

[29] Trumbower, R.D. et al. 2022. Caffeine enhances intermittent hypoxia-induced gains in walking function for people with chronic spinal cord injury. *J Neurotraum.* **39**, 23–24, 1756–1763. https://doi.org/10.1089/neu.2022.0120

[30] Trumbower, R.D. et al. 2017. Effects of acute intermittent hypoxia on hand use after spinal cord trauma: A preliminary study. *Neurol.* **89**, 18, 1904–1907. https://doi.org/10.1212/WNL.0000000000004596

[31] Tan, A.Q. et al. 2021. Daily acute intermittent hypoxia combined with walking practice enhances walking performance but not intralimb motor coordination in persons with chronic incomplete spinal cord injury. *Exper Neurol.* **340**, 113669. https://doi.org/10.1016/j.expneurol.2021.113669

[32] Christiansen, L. et al. 2020. Acute intermittent hypoxia boosts spinal plasticity in humans with tetraplegia. *Exper Neurol.* (Sep. 2020), 113483. https://doi.org/10.1016/j.expneurol.2020.113483

[33] Trumbower, R.D. et al. 2012. Exposure to acute intermittent hypoxia augments somatic motor function in humans with incomplete spinal cord injury. *Neurorehab Neur Repair.* **26**, 2, 163–172. https://doi.org/10.1177/1545968311412055

[34] Lynch, M. et al. 2017. Effect of acute intermittent hypoxia on motor function in individuals with chronic spinal cord injury following ibuprofen pretreatment: A pilot study. *J Spinal Cord Med.* **40**, 3, 295–303. https://doi.org/10.1080/10790268.2016.1142137

[35] Vose, A.K. et al. 2022. Therapeutic acute intermittent hypoxia: A translational roadmap for spinal cord injury and neuromuscular disease. *Exper Neurol.* **347**, 113891. https://doi.org/10.1016/j.expneurol.2021.113891

[36] Panza, G.S. et al. 2023. The hypoxic ventilatory response and hypoxic burden are predictors of the magnitude of ventilatory long-term facilitation in humans. *J Physiol.* **601**, 20, 4611–4623. https://doi.org/10.1113/JP285192

[37] Welch, J.F. et al. 2022. Acute intermittent hypercapnic-hypoxia elicits central neural respiratory motor plasticity in humans. *J Physiol.* **600**, 10, 2515–2533. https://doi.org/10.1113/JP282822

[38] Tester, N.J. et al. 2014. Long-term facilitation of ventilation in humans with chronic spinal cord injury. *Am J Respir Crit Care Med.* **189**, 1, 57–65. https://doi.org/10.1164/rccm.201305-0848OC

[39] Schilero, G.J. et al. 2018. Traumatic spinal cord injury: Pulmonary physiologic principles and management. *Clin Chest Med.* **39**, 2, 411–425. https://doi.org/10.1016/j.ccm.2018.02.002

[40] Sutor, T. et al. 2021. Single-session effects of acute intermittent hypoxia on breathing function after human spinal cord injury. *Exper Neurol.* **342**, 113735. https://doi.org/10.1016/j.expneurol.2021.113735

[41] Sandhu, M.S. et al. 2021. Efficacy and time course of acute intermittent hypoxia effects in the upper extremities of people with cervical spinal cord injury. *Exper Neurol.* **342**, 113722. https://doi.org/10.1016/j.expneurol.2021.113722

[42] Sandhu, M.S. et al. 2019. Prednisolone pretreatment enhances intermittent hypoxia-induced plasticity in persons with chronic incomplete spinal cord injury. *Neurorehab Neur Repair.* **33**, 11, 911–921. https://doi.org/10.1177/1545968319872992

[43] Navarrete-Opazo, A. et al. 2017. Repetitive intermittent hypoxia and locomotor training enhances walking function in incomplete spinal cord injury subjects: A randomized, triple-blind, placebo-controlled clinical trial. *J Neurotraum.* **34**, 9, 1803–1812. https://doi.org/10.1089/neu.2016.4478

[44] Navarrete-Opazo, A. et al. 2017. Intermittent hypoxia and locomotor training enhances dynamic but not standing balance in patients with incomplete spinal cord injury. *Arch Phys MedRehab.* **98**, 3, 415–424. https://doi.org/10.1016/j.apmr.2016.09.114

[45] Christiansen, L. et al. 2018. Acute intermittent hypoxia enhances corticospinal synaptic plasticity in humans. *eLife.* **7**, (Apr. 2018). https://doi.org/10.7554/eLife.34304

[46] Finn, H.T. et al. 2022. The effect of acute intermittent hypoxia on human limb motoneurone output. *Exper Physiol.* **107**, 6, 615–630. https://doi.org/10.1113/EP090099

7

PSYCHIATRIC DISEASES

Eugenia Manukhina, H. Fred Downey,
Vadim E. Tseilikman and Johannes Burtscher

7.1 Oxygen and psychiatric diseases

Psychiatric illnesses encompass a wide array of mental disorders that are clas-sified in the WHO's *International Classification of Diseases* (ICD) and the *Diagnostic and Statistical Manual of Mental Disorders* (DSM). The categori-zations are not always clear, but the use of the term *mental disorders* accord-ing to the ICD usually implies "the existence of a clinically recognizable set of symptoms or behaviors associated in most cases with distress and with interference with personal functions" [1]. Among the many mental disorders are several that are clearly linked to hypoxia, and some for which hypoxia conditioning has been suggested as a novel treatment strategy—and in some cases this potential has already been demonstrated in animal models. While uncontrolled hypoxia can contribute to the development or progression of many neurological and psychiatric diseases [2], exposure to mild ambient hypoxic conditions is emerging as important strategy to treat some of these diseases. The reason for such diverging effects are different cellular and sys-temic consequences of hypoxia, depending on individual vulnerabilities to hypoxia and the hypoxic dose, namely the extent of oxygen availability reduction, the duration of it, and the frequency at which hypoxia occurs [3].

This chapter will discuss psychiatric diseases that have been linked to hypoxia. The main focus will be stress-related psychiatric diseases, including anxiety and depressive disorders and especially post-traumatic stress disorder (PTSD). To this end, the current knowledge of the impact of hypoxia on men-tal stress responses and under which circumstances hypoxia may increase the risk to develop stress-related psychiatric diseases, or conversely may be uti-lized as a therapeutic strategy, is elaborated. A short outlook on the potential

DOI: 10.4324/9781003402879-10

role of hypoxia in the etiology and disease progression of schizophrenia and other psychoses will then be provided, although the evidence of hypoxia as a potential therapeutic tool is much weaker for this group of disorders.

7.2 Overlaps in mental and hypoxic stress responses

Exposure to hypoxia and the experience of mental stress cause physiological responses that partly overlap [3]. The mental stress response is importantly mediated by the sympatho-adrenomedullary (SAM) axis and the hypothalamic-pituitary-adrenal (HPA) axis. The SAM axis consists of the sympathetic nervous system and the adrenal medulla and rapidly regulates metabolic and cardiovascular responses to acute stress, enabling quick reaction to a threat (fight or flight response), via regulation of adrenaline and noradrenaline [4]. The HPA axis complements SAM activation during stress via the regulation of glucocorticoids, such as cortisol [5]. Interestingly, both axes are also activated by hypoxia and contribute to physiological responses to hypoxia (Figure 7.1). Hypoxia sensing by peripheral chemosensors (carotid bodies) activates the sympathetic nervous system [6] and induces a ventilatory (including increased minute ventilation) and cardiovascular response (increased heart rate and blood pressure), resembling a mental stress response [7]. Similarly, the HPA axis is activated by hypoxia, resulting in a glucocorticoid response that depends on the severity and duration of the hypoxia exposure [8].

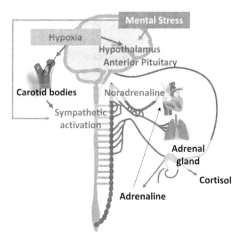

FIGURE 7.1 Physiological consequences of mental stress and hypoxia. Both types of stressors activate the sympatho-adrenal medullary- and the hypothalamic-pituitary adrenal-axis and induce overlapping responses, including cardiovascular and ventilatory effects.

7.3 Hypoxia in anxiety and depression

High-altitude exposure—and thus likely the associated hypobaric hypoxia—can elicit irreversible neuronal damage and negatively impact cognition and mood [9] and trigger anxiety symptoms (Table 7.1), such as panic attacks [8].

In addition, residence at high altitude has been linked to an increased prevalence of depressive disorders, although this effect is debated and may be confounded by various other factors (e.g., socioeconomic factors, including reduced social contacts) [8]. On the other hand, the controlled application of hypoxia (hypoxia conditioning) may reduce such symptoms, as shown in animal models for anxiety- and depressive-like symptoms, suggesting beneficial effects of intermittent hypoxia (IH) conditioning [16–18]. IH protocols of 4 h/day at 5,000 m simulated altitude for 2 weeks reduced anxiety and depressive-like behaviors in a chronic unpredictable mild stress model in rats [16] and daily 2 h/day exposure of rats to 5,000 m prevented the development of anxiety and depressive-like behaviors after unavoidable psychoemotional stress induced through electroshocks ("learned helplessness" paradigm) [18]. Mild IH exposure is thought to improve the regulation of the HPA axis and thereby may be beneficial in stress-related diseases, as demonstrated in rodent models of depressive- and anxiety-like

TABLE 7.1 Changes in anxiety after ascending to high or very high altitude

Study population	Main results	Ref.
40 healthy adults, ascent to 5,100 m over 14 days	– Significantly increased anxiety scores at higher altitudes	[10]
668 healthy males: ascent to 3,700 m after 24, 72, and 168 h	– Significantly increased anxiety scores after 24 h at 3,700 m – Thereafter decrease, but anxiety scores remained above baseline levels	[11]
80 healthy adults: progressive trek to 5,140 m	– Anxiety scores decreased until 3,619 m – Significant increase of anxiety scores above 4,072 m	[12]
850 young men: ascent by plane to 3,700 m over 2 h	– Significant increase in anxiety scores	[13]
426 young men: ascent from low altitude to 4,400 m over 40 days	– Increasing anxiety scores at higher altitudes	[14]
44 healthy adults: 19-day expedition to 5,372 m	– Anxiety symptoms increased significantly with altitude – 98% experienced anxiety symptoms at some point during the expedition	[15]

pathologies [17]. The efficiency of IH conditioning for stress-related disorders is best established in animal models for PTSD.

7.4 Hypoxia and PTSD

PTSD is caused by severe stress that follows a life-threatening experience, such as a natural disaster, military combat, traffic accident, incurable disease, or personal tragedy. In the general population the rate of PTSD reaches 6% to 12%. In veterans and survivors of natural disasters, the PTSD prevalence is considerably higher, up to 10–30% [19, 20].

The most common pharmaceutical treatments for PTSD often do not cure the condition completely, and they are frequently associated with serious side effects [21]. Thus, nonpharmacological treatment, or even prevention, of PTSD must be considered.

Anxiety shares with PTSD behavioral and neural elements, and anxiety disorders are among the most common PTSD comorbidities [22]. Predator stress, produced by exposure of rodents to cat urine scent or a live cat, is a well-validated model of PTSD [23, 24]. Using measurements from an elevated X-maze test, anxiety can be quantified with an anxiety index, which allows segregation of rats into PTSD-resistant and PTSD-vulnerable rats for studying mechanisms of stress resilience [25–28].

In studies of IH protection against PTSD, normobaric or hypobaric IH conditioning was used according to protocols that have demonstrated its high anti-stress and neuroprotective efficacy with no significant side effects [16, 29–32]. The anti-anxiety effect of IH was evident from a significant decrease in the anxiety index and the number or freezing reactions in predator stress-exposed rats [31, 33]. In a stress-restress model of PTSD, Rybnikova et al. [18, 32] showed that pre- and post-conditioning of rats with moderate hypobaric IH prevented development of anxiety and depression. These effects of IH were comparable with the effects of tetracyclic antidepressants but without any side effects.

PTSD induces high concentrations of catecholamines that may damage the prefrontal cortex and hippocampus by causing loss of dendritic spines and gray matter [34] (Figure 7.2). The PTSD-induced increased norepinephrine signaling results in part from suppressed activity and expression of monoaminoxidase A (MAO-A), a key mediator of biogenic amine metabolism [35]. The suppression of MAO-A activity in PTSD, in turn, is caused by the PTSD-associated decrease in glucocorticoids released from adrenal glands, which normally trigger the activation of MAO-A expression [36]. IH was shown to increase MAO-A activity and prevent its suppression in PTSD rats [25]. Thus, the IH protection may be due, at least partially, to prevention of PTSD-induced adrenal gland dystrophy and normalization of corticosteroid production [25, 33].

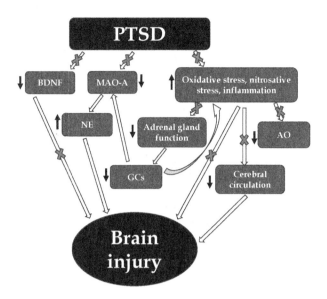

FIGURE 7.2 Protective mechanisms of IH conditioning in PTSD.

PTSD, post-traumatic stress disorder; BDNF, brain-derived neurotrophic factor; MAO-A, monoaminoxidase A; NE, norepinephrine; AO, antioxidants; GCs, glucocorticoids. White arrows, effects of PTSD; black arrows, direction of changes; red crosses, blocking effects of intermittent hypoxia (IH).

Another central protective mechanism of IH in PTSD may be related to prevention of stress-induced decrease in the hippocampal expression of brain-derived neurotrophic factor (BDNF), the major neuroplasticity factor that participates in regulation of the anxiety response to stress, prevents damage and death of hippocampal neurons, and stimulates neuronal regeneration [37]. BDNF expression was shown to be higher in PTSD-resilient rats than in PTSD-vulnerable rats, and apparently, it is an important factor of PTSD resilience [27]. Adaptation to IH was associated with increase in BDNF in the cerebral cortex [38].

Oxidative stress is an essential molecular mechanism widely implicated in the development of PTSD [39] (Figure 7.2). Normally, endogenous antioxidants increase in response to moderate levels of reactive oxygen species (ROS); however, PTSD is often associated with depletion of antioxidants [32, 40]. Both PTSD and anxiety disorders are typically associated with mitochondrial dysfunction that leads to dysregulation of oxidative pathways, generation of ROS, intensive lipid peroxidation and suppressed antioxidant activity, and oxidative damage to DNA, proteins, and lipids [39, 41]. Increased lipid peroxidation and protein oxidation in the brain of PTSD rats were evident from elevated concentrations of ketodienes, conjugated dienes and trienes, Schiff bases, and carbonylated proteins [25].

IH potentiates antioxidant defense by increasing activities and expression of antioxidant enzymes, including superoxide dismutase, catalase and glutathione peroxidase [42]. In PTSD rats, IH protection considerably reduced lipid peroxidation and protein oxidation in the brain and internal organs [25] (Figure 7.2). Although IH itself caused a moderate oxidative stress, this was much less pronounced than that induced by PTSD [25]. The ROS generation that follows each hypoxic exposure activates various defense mechanisms, including nuclear factor erythroid 2-related factor 2, a transcriptional factor for the expression of antioxidant and anti-inflammatory enzymes [32, 43].

Increased ROS generation and systemic inflammation in PTSD lead to expression and activation of all nitric oxide (NO) synthase isoforms and may result in toxic NO overproduction [44–46]. This nitrosative stress, together with oxidative stress, exacerbates PTSD by damaging brain cells, particularly in the hippocampus [45] and in the prefrontal cortex [46]. Normally, glucocorticoids suppress systemic inflammation and thereby limit NO overproduction [47, 48]. However, in PTSD, reduced glucocorticoids may not provide this protection.

IH can alleviate NO overproduction in brain by at least two ways [30, 49]. First, mild IH itself induces an increase in NO synthesis, and this NO restricts further NO production by a negative feedback mechanism. Second, IH facilitates NO storage in stable complexes, which is an adaptive mechanism to protect cells from the toxic effects of excessive NO. Also, the IH prevention of the PTSD-related decrease in glucocorticoids [33] may reduce systemic inflammation and thus reduce nitrosative stress.

Another important mechanism of IH protection of the brain in PTSD is improvement of cerebral blood flow [30, 50] (Figure 7.2). Susceptibility to experimental PTSD is associated with reduced basal cerebral blood flow, endothelial dysfunction, and depressed endothelial NO synthase mRNA expression in the cerebral cortex [28]. A negative correlation was found between cerebral blood flow and the anxiety index in PTSD rats [28]. The ability of IH to prevent endothelial dysfunction in the cerebral circulation [30] suggests that this is one of IH's protective mechanisms against PTSD-induced brain damage. Another protective mechanism of IH is stimulation of cerebral angiogenesis. Oxidative stress in microvessels is the major cause for rarefaction of cerebral microvasculature due to apoptosis of smooth muscle cells [51]. IH can effectively prevent this rarefaction of cerebral vasculature [52, 53]. A likely candidate for initiating angiogenesis is hypoxia-inducible factor 1 (HIF-1), a transcription factor that activates many downstream genes with hypoxia responsive elements, including vascular endothelial growth factor, a key mediator of angiogenesis [54].

Thus, IH conditioning is very promising as an alternative and/or supplementary therapy for PTSD since it targets multiple, nonspecific detrimental factors that are universally involved in PTSD. Future clinical studies should not only evaluate IH as a therapy to lessen or prevent PTSD and PTSD-induced comorbidities, but they should also strive to define optimal treatment regimens.

7.5 Hypoxia in schizophrenia and psychosis

Schizophrenia is a complex psychiatric disease, thought to be caused by a combination of genetic and environmental risk factors [55], with a prevalence of about 1% and frequently characterized by psychosis, disorganized motor behavior, and cognitive dysfunction. Among the environmental risk factors is hypoxia, particularly hypoxia during early neurodevelopment [56]. Accordingly, HIFs as major transcriptional regulators of cellular responses to hypoxia are associated with neurodevelopmental changes leading to schizophrenia [57]. Genetic links between schizophrenia and cellular responses to hypoxia have been established; for example, single-nucleotide polymorphisms in hypoxia response elements may represent a risk for schizophrenia [58–60]. Severe hypoxia exposure further can be associated with psychotic episodes even in adults, as observed for example in mountaineers at high altitudes [61, 62].

Notable cellular benefits of mild hypoxia are improved bioenergetics and increased flexibility in substrate utilization for energy production, enhanced oxidative stress defense, reduced inflammation and protein aggregation, as well as higher resilience to disturbances in calcium homeostasis, for example via regulation of N-methyl-D-aspartate receptors [3, 63]. Inter-dependent disturbances of mitochondrial functions, N-methyl-D-aspartate receptor, redox, and neuroinflammation regulation are also major factors in schizophrenia pathogenesis [64], possibly linking the outcomes of various genetic and environmental risk factors. Cuenod et al. [64] suggest pharmacological approaches to break resulting feed-forward interactions likely driving symptom manifestations. These factors are modulated by changes in oxygen availability as well [63, 65], rendering hypoxia-based interventions an interesting, hitherto unexplored, strategy for schizophrenia. In summary, a combination of genetic vulnerabilities and brain insults (e.g., severe hypoxia) likely cause schizophrenia and other types of psychosis. This leads to the disturbance of delicate cellular balances, including redox regulation, bioenergetics, and immune responses. Controlled mild hypoxia may improve cellular homeostasis and protect from future insults that can otherwise trigger psychotic episodes.

7.6 Conclusion

The strongest evidence for the potential of hypoxia conditioning to be beneficial in the treatment of psychiatric diseases currently comes from animal experiments suggesting hypoxia to be beneficial in PTSD [25, 66, 67], but hypoxia may also improve other stress-related diseases, including anxiety and depression disorders. In the applied hypoxia-based approaches, major mechanisms leading to benefits appear to be beneficial adaptations, partially mediated by HIFs, that render the brain more resilient to future insults (e.g., severe hypoxia, oxidative damage) and may have the potential to restore delicate physiological balances that were disrupted in psychiatric diseases [3].

Acknowledgments

This publication was a part of the State Assignment of the Institute of General Pathology and Pathophysiology # FGFU-2022-0011, "Identification of significant bio-indicators for various disorders of body function."

Abbreviations

BDNF	brain-derived neurotrophic factor
DSM	*Diagnostic and Statistical Manual of Mental Disorders*
HIF1	hypoxia-inducible factor 1
HPA	hypothalamic-pituitary-adrenal
ICD	*International Classification of Diseases*
IH	intermittent hypoxia
MAO-A	monoaminoxidase A
NO	nitric oxide
PTSD	post-traumatic stress-disorder
ROS	reactive oxygen species
SAM	sympatho-adrenomedullary

References

1. WHO, *The ICD-10 classification of mental and behavioural disorders: Clinical descriptions and diagnostic guidelines.* Vol. 1. 1992: WHO.
2. Burtscher, J., et al., *Hypoxia and brain aging: Neurodegeneration or neuroprotection?* Age Res Rev, 2021. **68**: p. 101343.
3. Burtscher, J., et al., *Boosting mitochondrial health to counteract neurodegeneration.* Prog Neurobiol, 2022. **215**: p. 102289.
4. Godoy, L.D., et al., *A comprehensive overview on stress neurobiology: Basic concepts and clinical implications.* Front Behav Neurosci, 2018. **12**: p. 127.
5. de Kloet, E.R., *Functional profile of the binary brain corticosteroid receptor system: mediating, multitasking, coordinating, integrating.* Eur J Pharmacol, 2013. **719**(1–3): p. 53–62.
6. Iturriaga, R., et al., *Carotid body chemoreceptors: physiology, pathology, and implications for health and disease.* Physiol Rev, 2021. **101**(3): p. 1177–1235.
7. Tank, A.W. and D. Lee Wong, *Peripheral and central effects of circulating catecholamines.* Compr Physiol, 2015. **5**(1): p. 1–15.
8. Burtscher, J., et al., *The interplay of hypoxic and mental stress: Implications for anxiety and depressive disorders.* Neurosci Biobehav Rev, 2022. **138**: p. 104718.

9. de Aquino Lemos, V., et al., *High altitude exposure impairs sleep patterns, mood, and cognitive functions.* Psychophysiol, 2012. **49**(9): p. 1298–1306.

10. Shah, N., et al., *The effects of apnea training, using voluntary breath holds, on high altitude acclimation: Breathe-high altitude study.* High Alt Med Biol, 2020. **21**(2): p. 152–159.

11. Bian, S.Z., et al., *The onset of sleep disturbances and their associations with anxiety after acute high-altitude exposure at 3700 m.* Transl Psychiatry, 2019. **9**(1): p. 175.

12. Boos, C.J., et al., *The relationship between anxiety and acute mountain sickness.* PloS One, 2018. **13**(6): p. e0197147–e0197147.

13. Bian, S.Z., et al., *Risk factors for high-altitude headache upon acute high-altitude exposure at 3700 m in young Chinese men: A cohort study.* J Headache Pain, 2013. **14**(1): p. 35.

14. Dong, J.Q., et al., *Anxiety correlates with somatic symptoms and sleep status at high altitudes.* Physiol Behav, 2013. **112–113**: p. 23–31.

15. Oliver, S.J., et al., *Physiological and psychological illness symptoms at high altitude and their relationship with acute mountain sickness: A prospective cohort study.* J Travel Med, 2012. **19**(4): p. 210–219.

16. Kushwah, N., et al., *Neuroprotective role of intermittent hypobaric hypoxia in unpredictable chronic mild stress induced depression in rats.* PLoS One, 2016. **11**(2): p. e0149309.

17. Rybnikova, E., et al., *Involvement of the hypothalamic-pituitary-adrenal axis in the antidepressant-like effects of mild hypoxic preconditioning in rats.* Psychoneuroendocrinol, 2007. **32**(7): p. 813–823.

18. Rybnikova, E.A., et al., *The possible use of hypoxic preconditioning for the prophylaxis of post-stress depressive episodes.* Neurosci Behav Physiol, 2008. **38**(7): p. 721–726.

19. Kessler, R.C., et al., *Lifetime prevalence and age-of-onset distributions of DSM-IV disorders in the National Comorbidity Survey Replication.* Arch Gen Psychiatry, 2005. **62**(6): p. 593–602.

20. Ryder, A.L., P.M. Azcarate, and B.E. Cohen, *PTSD and physical health.* Curr Psychiatry Rep, 2018. **20**(12): p. 116.

21. Katzman, M.A., et al., *Canadian clinical practice guidelines for the management of anxiety, posttraumatic stress and obsessive-compulsive disorders.* BMC Psychiatry, 2014. **14**(Suppl 1): p. S1.

22. Baltjes, F., et al., *Psychiatric comorbidities in older adults with posttraumatic stress disorder: A systematic review.* Int J Geriatr Psychiatry, 2023. **38**(6): p. e5947.

23. Cohen, H., M.A. Matar, and Z. Joseph, *Animal models of post-traumatic stress disorder.* Curr Protoc Neurosci, 2013. 64: p. 9–45.

24. Flandreau, E.I. and M. Toth, *Animal models of PTSD: A critical review.* Curr Top Behav Neurosci, 2018. **38**: p. 47–68.

25. Manukhina, E.B., et al., *Intermittent hypoxic conditioning alleviates posttraumatic stress disorder-induced damage and dysfunction of rat visceral organs and brain.* Int J Mol Sci, 2020. **21**(1): p. 345.

26. Tseilikman, V., et al., *A rat model of post-traumatic stress syndrome causes phenotype-associated morphological changes and hypofunction of the adrenal gland.* Int J Mol Sci, 2021. **22**(24): p. 13235.

27. Tseilikman, V.E., et al., *Mechanisms of susceptibility and resilience to PTSD: Role of dopamine metabolism and BDNF expression in the hippocampus.* Int J Mol Sci, 2022. **23**(23): p. 14575.

28. Kondashevskaya, M.V., et al., *Cerebral blood flow in predator stress-resilient and -susceptible rats and mechanisms of resilience.* Int J Mol Sci, 2022. **23**(23).

29. Meerson, F.Z., *Essentials of adaptive medicine: Protective effects of adaptation.* 1994, Moscow: Hypoxia Medical Ltd., p. 417.

30. Manukhina, E.B., et al., *Intermittent hypoxia training protects cerebrovascular function in Alzheimer's disease.* Exp Biol Med (Maywood), 2016. **241**(12): p. 1351–1363.

31. Ding, F.-S., et al., *Intermittent hypoxic preconditioning relieves fear and anxiety behavior in post-traumatic stress model mice.* Sheng Li Xue Bao [Acta physiologica Sinica], 2019. **71**(4): p. 537–546.

32. Rybnikova, E.A., et al., *Intermittent hypoxic training as an effective tool for increasing the adaptive potential, endurance and working capacity of the brain.* Front Neurosci, 2022. **16**: p. 941740.

33. Manukhina, E.B., et al., *Intermittent hypoxia improves behavioral and adrenal gland dysfunction induced by post-traumatic stress disorder in rats.* J Appl Physiol (1985), 2018. **125**(3): p. 931–937.

34. Datta, D. and A.F.T. Arnsten, *Loss of prefrontal cortical higher cognition with uncontrollable stress: Molecular mechanisms, changes with age, and relevance to treatment.* Brain Sci, 2019. **9**(5): p. 113.

35. Tseilikman, V., et al., *Post-traumatic stress disorder chronification via monoaminooxidase and cortisol metabolism.* Horm Metab Res, 2019. **51**(9): p. 618–622.

36. Grunewald, M., et al., *Mechanistic role for a novel glucocorticoid-KLF11 (TIEG2) protein pathway in stress-induced monoamine oxidase A expression.* J Biol Chem, 2012. **287**(29): p. 24195–24206.

37. Colucci-D'Amato, L., L. Speranza, and F. Volpicelli, *Neurotrophic factor BDNF, physiological functions and therapeutic potential in depression, neurodegeneration and brain cancer.* Int J Mol Sci, 2020. **21**(20): p. 7777.

38. Ryou, M.G., et al., *Intermittent hypoxia training prevents deficient learning-memory behavior in mice modeling Alzheimer's disease: A pilot study.* Front Aging Neurosci, 2021. **13**: p. 674688.

39. Miller, M.W., et al., *Oxidative stress, inflammation, and neuroprogression in chronic PTSD.* Harv Rev Psychiatry, 2018. **26**(2): p. 57–69.

40. Atli, A., et al., *Altered lipid peroxidation markers are related to post-traumatic stress disorder (PTSD) and not trauma itself in earthquake survivors.* Eur Arch Psychiatry Clin Neurosci, 2016. **266**(4): p. 329–336.

41. Kaplan, G.B., N.A. Dadhi, and C.S. Whitaker, *Mitochondrial dysfunction in animal models of PTSD: Relationships between behavioral models, neural regions, and cellular maladaptation.* Front Physiol, 2023. **14**: p. 1105839.

42. Gonchar, O. and I. Mankovska, *Moderate hypoxia/hyperoxia attenuates acute hypoxia-induced oxidative damage and improves antioxidant defense in lung mitochondria.* Acta Physiol Hung, 2012. **99**(4): p. 436–446.

43. Mallet, R.T., et al., *Cardioprotection by intermittent hypoxia conditioning: Evidence, mechanisms, and therapeutic potential.* Am J Physiol Heart Circ Physiol, 2018. **315**(2): p. H216–H232.

44. Harvey, B.H., et al., *Stress-restress evokes sustained iNOS activity and altered GABA levels and NMDA receptors in rat hippocampus.* Psychopharmacology (Berl), 2004. **175**(4): p. 494–502.

45. Oosthuizen, F., G. Wegener, and B.H. Harvey, *Nitric oxide as inflammatory mediator in post-traumatic stress disorder (PTSD): Evidence from an animal model.* Neuropsychiatr Dis Treat, 2005. **1**(2): p. 109–123.

46. Campos, F.L., et al., *Rodent models of Parkinson's disease: Beyond the motor symptomatology.* Front Behav Neurosci, 2013. **7**: p. 175.

47. Sapolsky, R.M., L.M. Romero, and A.U. Munck, *How do glucocorticoids influence stress responses? Integrating permissive, suppressive, stimulatory, and preparative actions.* Endocr Rev, 2000. **21**(1): p. 55–89.

48. Szabó, C., et al., *Attenuation of the induction of nitric oxide synthase by endogenous glucocorticoids accounts for endotoxin tolerance in vivo.* Proc Natl Acad Sci U S A, 1994. **91**(1): p. 271–275.

49. Manukhina, E.B., et al., *Formation and role of nitric oxide stores in adaptation to hypoxia.* Adv Exp Med Biol, 2006. **578**: p. 35–40.

50. Steinback, C.D. and M.J. Poulin, *Influence of hypoxia on cerebral blood flow regulation in humans.* Adv Exp Med Biol, 2016. **903**: p. 131–144.

51. Kobayashi, N., F.A. DeLano, and G.W. Schmid-Schönbein, *Oxidative stress promotes endothelial cell apoptosis and loss of microvessels in the spontaneously hypertensive rats.* Arterioscler Thromb Vasc Biol, 2005. **25**(10): p. 2114–2121.

52. Sokolova, I.A., et al., *Rarefication of the arterioles and capillary network in the brain of rats with different forms of hypertension.* Microvasc Res, 1985. **30**(1): p. 1–9.

53. Goryacheva, A.V., et al., *Adaptation to intermittent hypoxia prevents rarefaction of the brain vascular net in rats with experimental Alzheimer's disease.* FASEB J, 2011. **25**(1_supplement): p. 669.3.

54. Ran, R., et al., *Hypoxia preconditioning in the brain.* Dev Neurosci, 2005. **27**(2–4): p. 87–92.

55. Brown, A.S., *Epidemiologic studies of exposure to prenatal infection and risk of schizophrenia and autism.* Dev Neurobiol, 2012. **72**(10): p. 1272–1276.

56. Davies, C., et al., *Prenatal and perinatal risk and protective factors for psychosis: A systematic review and meta-analysis.* Lancet Psychiat, 2020. **7**(5): p. 399–410.

57. Schmidt-Kastner, R., et al., *Gene regulation by hypoxia and the neurodevelopmental origin of schizophrenia.* Schizophr Res, 2006. **84**(2–3): p. 253–271.

58. Okazaki, S., et al., *Polymorphisms in the hypoxia inducible factor binding site of the macrophage migration inhibitory factor gene promoter in schizophrenia.* PLoS One, 2022. **17**(3): p. e0265738.

59. Schmidt-Kastner, R., et al., *Analysis of GWAS-derived schizophrenia genes for links to ischemia-hypoxia response of the brain.* Front Psychiatry, 2020. **11**: p. 393.

60. Schmidt-Kastner, R., et al., *An environmental analysis of genes associated with schizophrenia: Hypoxia and vascular factors as interacting elements in the neurodevelopmental model.* Mol Psychiatry, 2012. **17**(12): p. 1194–1205.

61. Hüfner, K., et al., *Isolated psychosis during exposure to very high and extreme altitude - characterisation of a new medical entity.* Psychol Med, 2018. **48**(11): p. 1872–1879.

62. Hüfner, K., et al., *Assessment of psychotic symptoms in individuals exposed to very high or extreme altitude: A field study*. High Alt Med Biol, 2021. **22**(4): p. 369–378.
63. Burtscher, J., et al., *A rationale for hypoxic and chemical conditioning in Huntington's disease*. Int J Mol Sci, 2021. **22**(2).
64. Cuenod, M., et al., *Caught in vicious circles: A perspective on dynamic feed-forward loops driving oxidative stress in schizophrenia*. Mol Psychiatry, 2022. **27**(4): p. 1886–1897.
65. Burtscher, J., et al., *Adaptive responses to hypoxia and/or hyperoxia in humans*. Antioxid Redox Signal, 2022. **37**: p. 887–912.
66. Lin, C.C., et al., *Hyperbaric oxygen therapy restored traumatic stress-induced dysregulation of fear memory and related neurochemical abnormalities*. Behav Brain Res, 2019. **359**: p. 861–870.
67. Manukhina, E.B., et al., *Intermittent hypoxia improves behavioral and adrenal gland dysfunction induced by posttraumatic stress disorder in rats*. J Appl Physiol (1985), 2018. **125**(3): p. 931–937.

SECTION 3

8

HYPOXEMIA, PULMONARY DISORDERS, AND HYPOXIA CONDITIONING

Annalisa Cogo and Martin Burtscher

8.1 Introduction

The two most frequent chronic respiratory diseases are asthma and chronic obstructive pulmonary disease (COPD), and for this reason, most of the information available on exposure to environmental hypoxia (i.e., high altitude) and hypoxia conditioning (HC) effects concerns these two pathologies. The tolerance of hypoxia and effectiveness of HC in patients suffering from asthma or COPD depends on the disease severity and potential comorbidities, the level and duration of the hypoxia exposures, and in the case of intermittent HC (IHC), the interspersed reoxygenation periods, the number of hypoxia–reoxygenation cycles per session, and the number of sessions per week.

8.2 Hypoxemia

Hypoxemia is a low level of oxygen in the blood. A normal level of arterial oxygen at sea level is about 75–80 to 100 mm Hg or 10–13 kPa. Hypoxemia is any value under 60 mm Hg (8 kPa) or below 90% of oxygen saturation measured by pulse oximeter. Hypoxemia is not an illness, but it is a sign of a problem tied to breathing or blood flow. Hypoxemia is usually due to respiratory problems, except in situations of low inspired oxygen content (as at high altitude) or due to a right-to-left shunt as a consequence of heart disease. The first step of the oxygen cascade from the ambient air to the mitochondria is the respiratory system, mainly the lungs.

For optimal oxygen passage, every part of the respiratory system involved must function perfectly: ventilatory drive, respiratory muscles, rib cage

DOI: 10.4324/9781003402879-12

movements, airway caliber, lung elasticity, diffusion capacity, and ventilation/ perfusion ratio (VA/Qc).

The lung can be divided into two functional units: an air transport unit and a gas exchange unit. The two units act in synergy, and many respiratory pathologies can compromise one or both of them.

8.2.1 How hypoxemia occurs in different lung diseases

Whichever is the first impairment (ventilatory constraints, restrictive or obstructive airway defect, emphysema, or fibrosis—both affecting the alveolar diffusion and the VA/Qc), the outcome is reduced alveolar ventilation with gas exchange impairment. Concerning VA/Qc, we must highlight that there will always be some mismatch between blood flow and ventilation as one moves through different lung zones, but this is normal physiology and consistent with normal oxygenation. However, pathological conditions create extreme amounts of VA/Qc mismatching which are no longer consistent with proper oxygenation.

8.2.2 Notes on high altitude

The study of the human body at high altitudes can provide information on the response to hypoxia at sea level of subjects with chronic pathologies that can alter gas exchange. Exposure to hypoxia induces a series of physiological responses aiming to restore the oxygen content in the body and oxygen delivery to the tissues. These responses have different timing, with heart rate, ventilation, and pulmonary artery vasoconstriction increasing within minutes, whereas hematological changes occur after a minimum of one or two days [1]. Noteworthily, the magnitude of the responses can vary among persons, due to interindividual differences in the sensitivity to hypoxia.

The lung plays a pivotal role in the acclimatization process, but it may also be involved in maladaptive responses [2]. Two important physiological responses are the hypoxic ventilatory response and hypoxic pulmonary vasoconstriction leading to an increase in pulmonary artery pressure. A maladaptive response can lead to the development of high-altitude pulmonary edema [3].

8.2.3 Hypoxemia and respiratory disease

The next sections are primarily about hypoxia-related consequences of asthma and COPD.

8.3 Responses and adaptations to environmental hypoxia

Adaptation to hypoxia mainly concerns COPD patients. For asthmatics, climbing to high altitudes is linked to problems of bronchial reactivity and exercise-induced bronchospasm (EIB), which can be elicited by inhalation of cold and dry air.

For many years, information on environmental hypoxia exposure for COPD patients has been derived from research that investigated the safety of air travel for patients [4–6]. In recent years, however, interesting results have also been published on the exposure of COPD patients to environmental hypoxia both at rest and during exercise [7–9].

8.3.1 What happens to asthmatics exposed to high altitude?

First, we must emphasize again that it's not the elevation change (i.e., hypoxia) that can trigger asthma symptoms but the change in air temperature and humidity. Even if in animal models (awake sheep) exposure to severe and acute hypoxia (13% O_2) increased the hyperresponsiveness to methacholine [10], an analogous result was not reported in asthmatic humans exposed in the laboratory to hypoxia with peripheral oxygen saturation (SpO_2) maintained at 90% [11]. There is not much research on asthmatic subjects at high altitudes; what we know is that bronchial hyperresponsiveness is significantly reduced in mild asthma between 3,500 and 5,000 m [12, 13], and many asthmatic climbers have been able to reach high altitudes with no differences compared to non-asthmatics [14, 15].

Moreover, asthmatics engaged in the construction of the Qinghai–Tibet railroad reported less frequent and less severe symptoms, necessitating less medication to control the disease [16]. A conflicting result was reported during the ascent on Mt. Aconcagua. In this case, the exposure to environmental conditions as high as 6,000 m was associated with a moderate loss of asthma control, probably due to the extremely cold temperature. A similar 24-hour cold exposure at sea level induced similar effects [17].

In summary, there are no particular contraindications to altitude exposure for asthmatics as long as asthma is well controlled, appropriate pretravel assessment and planning is performed, and precautions regarding exercise and exposure to cold are taken [18]. Two independent risk factors for asthma attacks during altitude travel have been recognized: frequent use (>3 times weekly) of inhaled bronchodilators before travel, which means a poor control of asthma, and participation in intense physical exertion during treks [19].

8.3.2 What happens to COPD exposed to mild and high altitude?

Firstly, we have to highlight that some patients are very sensitive to hypoxia and develop symptoms requiring either descent or oxygen and medical treatment even at moderate altitude [20, 21]. It would be important to identify and advise such susceptible patients before they are exposed to hypoxia. Unfortunately, so far, no test or algorithm has been found that can predict the response to hypoxia. Generally speaking, it can be stated that in COPD patients already at 1,650 m the exercise capacity is significantly reduced due to respiratory constraints, while at 2,500 m oxygen desaturation is significantly reduced even at rest, as is the distance covered at 6-min walking test (6MWT) [7]. About 25% of the patients enrolled in the previously mentioned study needed O_2 therapy or descent due to the presence of symptoms [7].

In summary, people with COPD at altitude (mainly above 2,000 m) have exaggerated hypoxemia with possible excessive increase in blood pressure, electrocardiographic changes, impaired exercise capacity, and sleep disturbances. All these symptoms are reduced or disappear with the administration of oxygen [20, 22, 23]. Given these premises, at first glance it would seem difficult to imagine the usefulness and feasibility of IHC for COPD. However, we must consider that all the problems relating to exposure to altitude (including the various forms of acute altitude sickness) appear after a few hours of stay [24], especially if the subject spends the night at altitude. IHC instead is based on repeated short hypoxia exposures [25, 26].

In this way adverse events should be avoided, favouring beneficial stimuli. In fact, in a review published some years ago it has been emphasized that the type of hypoxia exposure is crucial in discriminating the positive effects for health from the harmful ones [27]. In fact, biological responses to intermittent hypoxia can be either adaptive or maladaptive, depending on the severity, frequency, and duration of hypoxemia [27, 28]. As outlined previously, the different detrimental versus beneficial effects of intermittent hypoxia may depend on the different number of hypoxia episodes, severity, and total exposure duration of hypoxia, which may mobilize the body's adaptive mechanisms or cause dangerous pathological processes in more severe or prolonged hypoxia events [28, 29].

8.4 Hypoxia conditioning as a treatment for respiratory diseases

Most investigated beneficial effects of HC pertain to the cardiovascular system, such as myocardial protection [30] and antihypertensive effects [31], but also neuroprotection has recently attained specific consideration [32–35]. Several authors suggest that rather moderate hypoxia (inspiratory fraction of oxygen, FiO_2: 9–16% with a SpO_2 of 75–80%) and low cycle numbers (10–15 episodes per day, lasting 1–2 min alternating with an equal duration of normoxia) are mostly associated with beneficial effects, while severe hypoxia (FiO_2: 2–8%) and higher numbers of episodes (>48 per day) are associated with an increased risk for pathology-promoting consequences [27]. A few studies have evaluated the therapeutic use of HC, specifically of IHC, in asthma and COPD [25, 36–38].

8.4.1 Hypoxia conditioning in bronchial asthma

A few early studies evaluated IHC effects on bronchial asthma [39–41]. Those studies, for instance when applying alternating 5-min hypoxic (12–15% O_2) and normoxic breathing intervals, demonstrated improvements in lung function (tests for vital capacity, maximal ventilation, and forced expired volume in 1 s) as well as in the regulation of respiration and alveolar ventilation in asthmatic patients. Beneficial effects have been attributed at least partially to the normalization of initially elevated oxidative stress and positive impact on specific and nonspecific immunological status [40]. It is therefore supposed that especially in severe asthmatics, IHC can be a therapeutic strategy leading to more efficient ventilation, especially for patients who fail or cannot follow the exercise-based rehabilitation protocols. Importantly, potentially harmful consequences versus benefits of therapeutic HC use, particularly in children, have been critically reviewed [36].

It should also be added that the only paper (to our knowledge) concerning the effect of intermittent hypoxia (10% O_2) in an animal model of asthma shows an altered immune response to allergens toward a more TH-1-predominant cellular phenotype with collagen deposition and matrix degradation, leading to airflow limitation [42].

8.4.2 Hypoxia conditioning in COPD

As is true for bronchial asthma, early and newer trials have reported beneficial effects of IHC in COPD patients [25, 38]. Findings derived from randomized, controlled clinical trials applying mild repetitive hypoxia exposures (12–15% O_2 for 3–5 min, followed by intervals of 3–5 min of normoxia, five to nine episodes per day, for 15 days) suggested the following potential health benefits in patients suffering from mild COPD: improved exercise tolerance and lung function (forced vital capacity and forced expiratory volume in 1 s), increases in total hemoglobin mass, arterial oxygen content and oxygen delivery, baroreflex sensitivity, and hypercapnic ventilatory response [37, 43, 44].

One interventional study (15 hypoxia sessions, 15–12% FiO_2 or normoxia), including 18 patients (10 males, 8 females; 33–72 years) suffering from mild COPD, demonstrated a 9.7% increase of total exercise time and a 13% increase in exercise time to the anaerobic threshold (incremental cycle spiro-ergometry) in the IHC group versus 0.0 and –7.8% in the control group ($p < 0.05$) [43]. Improvement in the total exercise time were positively related with increases in total hemoglobin ($r = 0.59$, $p < 0.05$), while the time to the anaerobic threshold was associated with improved lung diffusion capacity for carbon monoxide ($r = 0.48$, $p < 0.05$) [43]. These findings indicate that oxygen delivery to exercising muscles contributes to improved maximal and submaximal exercise performance after HC. Peripheral adaptations (oxygen extraction in the working muscles) due to mitochondrial remodeling in hypoxia, including improvements in oxidative phosphorylation efficiency and flexibility in substrate utilization, may be consequences of HC interventions [45]. Potential HC effects on aerobic exercise capacity related to changes of oxygen delivery and/or oxygen extraction in patients suffering from mild COPD are depicted in Figure 8.1. Furthermore, cardiovascular autonomic abnormalities at baseline, which had normalized with hypoxic training, may also contribute to those benefits [44], for example by favorably impacting blood flow distribution, namely vasoconstriction in inactive muscle and vasodilation in working muscles ("functional sympatholysis") [46].

In contrast to placebo, IHC interventions significantly increased baroreflex sensitivity (up to healthy levels), with no changes in the hypoxic ventilatory response but increased hypercapnic ventilatory response [47]. Importantly, elevated vagal and reduced sympathetic tone after IHC may be associated with lower lactate production and decreased ventilatory requirements during exercise [48], which is of particular benefit for COPD patients. It is well known that patients with autonomic dysfunction have low levels of fitness, which can be improved with exercise training [46] and likely also with IHC

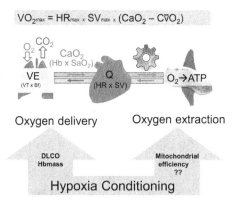

FIGURE 8.1   Potential hypoxia conditioning effects on exercise tolerance (maximal oxygen uptake, VO_2max) by improving oxygen delivery and/or oxygen extraction in patients suffering from mild chronic obstructive pulmonary disease.

ATP, adenosine triphosphate; Bf, breathing frequency; CaO_2, arterial oxygen content; $C\bar{v}O_2$, mixed venous oxygen content; DLCO, lung diffusion capacity for carbon monoxide; HR, heart rate; Q, cardiac output; SV, stroke volume; VE, pulmonary ventilation; VT, tidal volume.

interventions. Thus, IHC may represent a valuable tool to support the well-known benefits from exercise training in COPD on cardiorespiratory fitness [37]. This is particularly relevant since better cardiorespiratory fitness, i.e., VO$_2$max, is closely associated with reduced all-cause mortality even after adjusting for relevant confounders [49, 50].

Besides systemic physiological responses, molecular mechanisms, especially those related to the oxidant-antioxidant system, might play important roles in therapeutic IHC effects. It is undisputed that oxidative stress and oxidative damage, such as that associated with smoking, are important components in the pathogenesis of COPD [51]. Thus, improving the oxidant–antioxidant balance by IHC may contribute to the discussed beneficial effects [45]. Hypoxia exposure in combination with reoxygenation periods provokes the production of reactive oxygen species (ROS), which in turn activate nuclear factor erythroid 2-related factor 2 (Nrf2), a transcriptional regulator of antioxidant and anti-inflammatory gene products [45]. Antioxidant and anti-inflammatory effects potentially triggered by IHC are depicted in Figure 8.2. While chronic

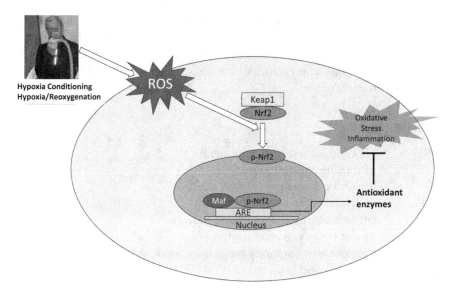

FIGURE 8.2   Schematic presentation of Nrf2-Keap1 signaling in oxidative stress. Hypoxia exposure and following reoxygenation may generate reactive oxygen species (ROS) leading to Nrf2 stabilization (which is inactivated when bound to Keap1 under basal conditions). Nrf2 accumulates and is translocated to the nucleus where Nrf2 heterodimerizes with small Maf protein and binds to the antioxidant responsive element (ARE) to activate the transcription of antioxidant genes. Antioxidants may then counteract oxidative stress and related inflammatory processes. Keap1, Kelch-like ECH-associated protein 1; Nrf2, nuclear factor-erythroid 2-related factor 2.

high-frequency intermittent hypoxia, as occurring in obstructive sleep apnea patients, produced oxidative stress without antioxidant compensation in healthy men [52], decreased oxidative stress markers were demonstrated in cardiac tissue (animal study) after IHC [53]. However, such mechanisms have to be confirmed in COPD by well-controlled studies.

8.5 Conclusions

IHC is currently evaluated as a nonpharmacological treatment in patients suffering from respiratory diseases, such as COPD, if appropriate protocols and an appropriate hypoxic dose are applied. The existing literature reports that exposure to a mild level of hypoxia for few, short episodes administered for several days or weeks can have the most beneficial results and is very rarely associated with adverse health effects compared to common pharmacological interventions. However, the results, although very promising, are not yet consolidated. Above all, it is necessary to define exactly the level and dose of hypoxia necessary to obtain the best results. Also, the duration of the treatment (days, weeks, months) and especially the persistence of the results over time have yet to be established through well designed (randomized, placebo-controlled, and blinded) studies on large samples. Finally, it should be clearly defined which patients can best benefit from the treatment while minimizing any side effects and which tests, if any, should be performed before treatment.

Abbreviations

ARE	antioxidant responsive element
ATP	adenosine triphosphate
Bf	breathing frequency
CaO_2	arterial oxygen content
COPD	chronic obstructive pulmonary disease
$C\bar{v}O_2$	mixed venous oxygen content
DLCO	lung diffusion capacity for carbon monoxide
HC	hypoxia conditioning
HR	heart rate
IHC	intermittent hypoxia conditioning
Keap1	Kelch-like ECH-associated protein 1
Nrf2	nuclear factor-erythroid 2-related factor 2
O_2	oxygen
Q	cardiac output;
6MWT	6-min walking test
SpO_2	peripheral oxygen saturation
SV	stroke volume

VA/Qc   ventilation/perfusion ratio
VE   pulmonary ventilation
VO$_2$max   maximal oxygen uptake
VT   tidal volume

References

1. Mallet, R.T., et al., *Molecular mechanisms of high-altitude acclimatization.* Int J Mol Sci, 2023. **24**(2): p. 1698.
2. Cogo, A., *The lung at high altitude.* Multidiscip Respir Med, 2011. **6**(1): p. 14–15.
3. Swenson, E.R. and P. Bärtsch, *High-altitude pulmonary edema.* Compr Physiol, 2012. **2**(4): p. 2753–2773.
4. Tan, L., et al., *Effect of nocturnal oxygen therapy on nocturnal hypoxemia and sleep apnea among patients with chronic obstructive pulmonary disease traveling to 2048 meters: A randomized clinical trial.* JAMA Netw Open, 2020. **3**(6): p. e207940.
5. Coker, R.K., R. Shiner, and M.R. Partridge, *Is air travel safe for those with lung disease?* Eur Respir J, 2008. **32**(5): p. 1423–1424.
6. Ahmedzai, S., et al., *Managing passengers with stable respiratory disease planning air travel: British Thoracic Society recommendations.* Thorax, 2011. **66** (**Suppl 1**): p. i1–30.
7. Furian, M., et al., *Exercise performance of lowlanders with COPD at 2,590 m: Data from a randomized trial.* Respir, 2018. **95**(6): p. 422–432.
8. Furian, M., et al., *Efficacy of dexamethasone in preventing acute mountain sickness in COPD patients: Randomized trial.* Chest, 2018. **154**(4): p. 788–797.
9. Furian, M., et al., *Acute high altitude exposure, acclimatization and re-exposure on nocturnal breathing.* Front Physiol, 2022. **13**: p. 965021.
10. Ahmed, T. and B. Marchette, *Hypoxia enhances nonspecific bronchial reactivity.* Am Rev Respir Dis, 1985. **132**(4): p. 839–844.
11. Saito, H., et al., *Effect of mild hypoxia on airway responsiveness to methacholine in subjects with airway hyperresponsiveness.* Chest, 1999. **116**(6): p. 1653–1658.
12. Allegra, L., et al., *High altitude exposure reduces bronchial responsiveness to hypo-osmolar aerosol in lowland asthmatics.* Eur Respir J, 1995. **8**(11): p. 1842–1846.
13. Cogo, A., et al., *Bronchial asthma and airway hyperresponsiveness at high altitude.* Respiration, 1997. **64**(6): p. 444–449.
14. Stokes, S., et al., *Bronchial asthma on Mount Kilimanjaro is not a disadvantage,* in *Thorax.* 2008: England. p. 936–937.
15. Huismans, H.K., et al., *Asthma in patients climbing to high and extreme altitudes in the Tibetan Everest region.* J Asthma, 2010. **47**(6): p. 614–619.
16. Wu, T.Y., et al., *Who should not go high: chronic disease and work at altitude during construction of the Qinghai-Tibet railroad.* High Alt Med Biol, 2007. **8**(2): p. 88–107.
17. Seys, S.F., et al., *Effects of high altitude and cold air exposure on airway inflammation in patients with asthma.* Thorax, 2013. **68**(10): p. 906–913.
18. Doan, D. and A.M. Luks, *Wilderness and adventure travel with underlying asthma.* Wilderness Environ Med, 2014. **25**(2): p. 231–240.

19. Golan, Y., et al., *Asthma in adventure travelers: A prospective study evaluating the occurrence and risk factors for acute exacerbations.* Arch Intern Med, 2002. **162**(21): p. 2421–2426.
20. Schwarz, E.I., et al., *Blood pressure response to exposure to moderate altitude in patients with COPD.* Int J Chron Obstruct Pulmon Dis, 2019. **14**: p. 659–666.
21. Latshang, T.D., et al., *Sleep and breathing disturbances in patients with chronic obstructive pulmonary disease traveling to altitude: A randomized trial.* Sleep, 2019. **42**(1): 1–10.
22. Meszaros, M., et al., *Effect of nocturnal oxygen on blood pressure response to altitude exposure in COPD: Data from a randomized placebo-controlled cross-over trial.* Int J Chron Obstruct Pulmon Dis, 2021. **16**: p. 3503–3512.
23. Gutweniger, S., et al., *Effect of nocturnal oxygen therapy on exercise performance of COPD patients at 2048 m: Data from a randomized clinical trial.* Sci Rep, 2021. **11**(1): p. 20355.
24. Hackett, P.H. and R.C. Roach, *High-altitude illness.* N Engl J Med, 2001. **345**(2): p. 107–114.
25. Serebrovskaya, T.V., *Intermittent hypoxia research in the former Soviet Union and the Commonwealth of Independent States: History and review of the concept and selected applications.* High Alt Med Biol, 2002. **3**(2): p. 205–221.
26. Serebrovskaya, T.V. and L. Xi, *Intermittent hypoxia training as non-pharmacologic therapy for cardiovascular diseases: Practical analysis on methods and equipment.* Exp Biol Med (Maywood), 2016. **241**(15): p. 1708–1723.
27. Navarrete-Opazo, A. and G.S. Mitchell, *Therapeutic potential of intermittent hypoxia: A matter of dose.* Am J Physiol Regul Integr Comp Physiol, 2014. **307**(10): p. R1181–R1197.
28. Glazachev, O.S., et al., *Safety and efficacy of intermittent hypoxia conditioning as a new rehabilitation/ secondary prevention strategy for patients with cardiovascular diseases: A systematic review and meta-analysis.* Curr Cardiol Rev, 2021. DOI: 10.2174/1573403X17666210514005235
29. Viscor, G., et al., *Physiological and biological responses to short-term intermittent hypobaric hypoxia exposure: From sports and mountain medicine to new biomedical applications.* Front Physiol, 2018. **9**: p. 814.
30. Mallet, R.T., et al., *Cardioprotection by intermittent hypoxia conditioning: Evidence, mechanisms, and therapeutic potential.* Am J Physiol Heart Circ Physiol, 2018. **315**(2): p. H216–H232.
31. Lyamina, N.P., et al., *Normobaric hypoxia conditioning reduces blood pressure and normalizes nitric oxide synthesis in patients with arterial hypertension.* J Hypertens, 2011. **29**(11): p. 2265–2272.
32. Sprick, J.D., et al., *Ischaemic and hypoxic conditioning: potential for protection of vital organs.* Exp Physiol, 2019. **104**(3): p. 278–294.
33. Li, S., et al., *Preconditioning in neuroprotection: From hypoxia to ischemia.* Prog Neurobiol, 2017. **157**: p. 79–91.
34. Baillieul, S., et al., *Hypoxic conditioning and the central nervous system: A new therapeutic opportunity for brain and spinal cord injuries?* Experimental biology and medicine (Maywood, N.J.), 2017. **242**(11): p. 1198–1206.
35. Burtscher, J., et al., *Hypoxia and brain aging: Neurodegeneration or neuroprotection?* Ageing Res Rev, 2021. **68**: p. 101343.
36. Serebrovskaya, T.V. and L. Xi, *Intermittent hypoxia in childhood: The harmful consequences versus potential benefits of therapeutic uses.* Front Pediatr, 2015. **3**: p. 44.

37. Burtscher, M., et al., *Effects of interval hypoxia on exercise tolerance: Special focus on patients with CAD or COPD.* Sleep Breath, 2010. **14**(3): p. 209–220.
38. Vogtel, M. and A. Michels, *Role of intermittent hypoxia in the treatment of bronchial asthma and chronic obstructive pulmonary disease.* Curr Opin Allergy Clin Immunol, 2010. **10**(3): p. 206–213.
39. Redzhebova, O.K. and A. Chizhov, *[Results of utilization of intermittent normobaric hypoxia in patients with bronchial asthma and chronic obstructive bronchitis].* Fiziol Zh (1978), 1992. **38**(5): p. 39–42.
40. Serebrovskaia, T.V., et al., *[A method for intermittent hypoxic exposures in the combined treatment of bronchial asthma patients].* Lik Sprava, 1998(6): p. 104–108.
41. Serebrovskaya, T.V., R.J. Swanson, and E.E. Kolesnikova, *Intermittent hypoxia: mechanisms of action and some applications to bronchial asthma treatment.* J Physiol Pharmacol, 2003. **54** (**Suppl 1**): p. 35–41.
42. Broytman, O., et al., *Effects of chronic intermittent hypoxia on allergen-induced airway inflammation in rats.* Am J Respir Cell Mol Biol, 2015. **52**(2): p. 162–170.
43. Burtscher, M., et al., *Intermittent hypoxia increases exercise tolerance in patients at risk for or with mild COPD.* Respir Physiol Neurobiol, 2009. **165**(1): p. 97–103.
44. Haider, T., et al., *Interval hypoxic training improves autonomic cardiovascular and respiratory control in patients with mild chronic obstructive pulmonary disease.* J Hypertens, 2009. **27**(8): p. 1648–1654.
45. Burtscher, J., et al., *Adaptive responses to hypoxia and/or hyperoxia in humans.* Antioxid Redox Signal, 2022. **37**(13–15): p. 887–912.
46. Fu, Q. and B.D. Levine, *Exercise and the autonomic nervous system.* Handb Clin Neurol, 2013. **117**: p. 147–160.
47. Haider, T., et al., *Interval hypoxic training improves autonomic cardiovascular and respiratory control in patients with mild chronic obstructive pulmonary disease.* J Hypertens, 2009. **27**(8), p. 1648–1654.
48. Bernardi, L., et al., *Respiratory and cardiovascular adaptations to progressive hypoxia; effect of interval hypoxic training.* Eur Heart J, 2001. **22**(10): p. 879–886.
49. Kodama, S., et al., *Cardiorespiratory fitness as a quantitative predictor of all-cause mortality and cardiovascular events in healthy men and women: a meta-analysis.* JAMA, 2009. **301**(19): p. 2024–2035.
50. Burtscher, J. and M. Burtscher, *Run for your life: Tweaking the weekly physical activity volume for longevity.* Br J Sports Med, 2019. **54**(13), p. 759–760.
51. van Eeden, S.F. and D.D. Sin, *Oxidative stress in chronic obstructive pulmonary disease: a lung and systemic process,* Can Respir J. 2013. 20: p. 27–29.
52. Pialoux, V., et al., *Effects of exposure to intermittent hypoxia on oxidative stress and acute hypoxic ventilatory response in humans.* Am J Respir Crit Care Med, 2009. **180**(10): p. 1002–1009.
53. González-Candia, A., et al., *Cardioprotective antioxidant and anti-inflammatory mechanisms induced by intermittent hypobaric hypoxia.* Antioxidants (Basel), 2022. **11**(6).

SECTION 4

9

HYPOXIA AND OBESITY

Samuel Verges and Bengt Kayser

9.1 The burden of obesity

Obesity is characterized by excess body fat, marked by an increase in both the number and volume of adipocytes. Even though imperfect [1], body mass index (BMI; weight/height^2 in kg/m^2) provides a simple indirect evaluation of body composition, classifying individuals as overweight (BMI > 25 kg/m^2) or obese (BMI > 30 kg/m^2) [2]. The global prevalence of obesity nearly tripled between 1975 and 2016, with substantial rises in most countries, including low-income and middle-income nations. By 2016, worldwide more than 1.9 billion adults were overweight, 650 million were obese, and more than 2.8 million people die each year as a result of being overweight or obese [2]. Obesity, now recognized as a global pandemic by the World Health Organization, poses an important risk for chronic diseases such as heart disease, stroke, and several cancers. It also exacerbates the impact of other life-shortening conditions such as nonalcoholic fatty liver and diabetes mellitus [3, 4]. Beyond physical symptoms, obesity imposes psychological and social burdens including social stigma, low self-esteem, reduced mobility, and a poorer quality of life for many individuals.

The etiology of obesity is complex, primarily arising from a positive energy balance where energy intake exceeds energy expenditure. When energy balance is properly regulated, energy intake is adapted to energy expenditure to keep a constant body mass. For an average person, even a mere 1% error in energy balance can theoretically lead to ~1 kg change in fat mass within a year. Over a decade, a ~25 kcal excess daily energy intake (a little more than a sugar lump per day) would result in a 10-kg increase in fat mass.

DOI: 10.4324/9781003402879-14

While not all overweight or obese individuals are metabolically unhealthy, the majority are prone to develop a metabolically unhealthy phenotype over time. This phenotype is characterized by central obesity, hypertension, insulin resistance, atherogenic dyslipidemia, chronic inflammation, and an increased risk for all-cause mortality [5]. Managing obesity and its comorbidities is complex, and although pharmacological approaches show promises, lifestyle intervention programs focusing on regular physical activity, healthy nutrition, and weight reduction yield the best outcomes. However, adherence to lifestyle changes among individuals with obesity and overweight is generally low. Research into optimal multidimensional interventions, focusing on weight loss and improving associated comorbidities, remain crucial. With this goal, exposure to controlled doses of hypoxia, known as hypoxic conditioning, has been proposed as an original strategy for both managing and preventing obesity.

This chapter provides an overview of the two-sided interaction between hypoxia and obesity (Figure 9.1). On the one hand, hypoxia plays a role in

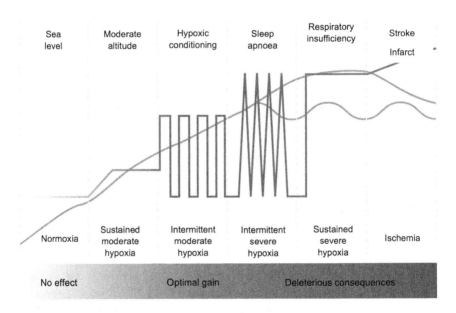

FIGURE 9.1   Schematic representation of the continuum from normoxia to severe hypoxia including exposure leading to hypoxic conditioning. Within this continuum, obesity can be associated with sustained local hypoxia (in adipose tissue) and intermittent severe hypoxia (due to sleep apnoea) with deleterious cardiovascular and metabolic consequences, but obesity can also show a reduced prevalence in populations at altitude and benefit from hypoxic conditioning strategies.

Adapted from [39].

the pathophysiology of obesity, especially in adipose tissue dysregulation, and the cardiovascular and metabolic consequences of sleep apnea. Obesity also appears to be a risk factor for mountain sickness during altitude exposure. On the other hand, prolonged altitude exposure data suggest that hypoxia may lead to a negative energy balance, resulting in a reduction of body mass. In recent decades, controlled doses of hypoxia have been used in clinical studies to improve the body composition and health status of individuals with obesity.

9.2 Hypoxia and the pathophysiology of obesity

Hypoxia is thought to contribute to the pathophysiological mechanisms underlying the deleterious cardiovascular and metabolic consequences of obesity. Regions of hypoxia in rapidly growing hypertrophic white adipose tissue may contribute to a state of chronic mild inflammation and metabolic dysregulation often seen in obesity, even though this contention remains debated [6]. Also, a prevalent problem in overweight and obese subjects is the occurrence of obstructive sleep apnea (OSA), characterized by nocturnal respiratory events leading to intermittent episodes of systemic hypoxia and hypercarbia with deleterious cardiovascular and metabolic consequences [7].

9.2.1 Hypoxia and white adipose tissue

White adipose tissue, more than just a highly efficient means for energy storage, is now recognized as an active endocrine organ releasing important regulatory adipokines such as leptin [6]. The excessive adipose tissue in obesity is associated with a state of permanent mild inflammation with increased circulating levels of inflammatory markers such as C-reactive protein, haptoglobin, interleukin-6, monocyte chemo-attractant protein-1, plasminogen activator inhibitor-1, and tumor necrosis factor-alpha. In this context, the hypertrophy of adipose tissues would lead to localized hypoxia inducing AMPK activation and local inflammation [6]. This hypothesis gains support from direct measurements of localized hypoxia in adipose tissue in obesity, the up-regulation of hypoxia-activated genes like the hypoxia-inducible factor-1 (HIF-1), vascular endothelial growth factor (VEGF), glucose transporter (GLUT1), heme-oxygenase and 3-phosphoinositide-dependent protein kinase-1, as well as increased levels of tissue lactate indicating the Pasteur effect [8].

HIF-1α plays a pivotal role in the response to hypoxia within white adipose tissue as in other tissues exposed to hypoxia. About 70 genes have been identified as being hypoxia-sensitive through HIF-1α and encompass those encoding several proteins involved in glucose and energy metabolism, cell proliferation, apoptosis, and angiogenesis [9]. In normoxic conditions, HIF-1α is continuously synthesized and degraded. However, under hypoxic conditions, such as those found in rapidly growing adipocytes, HIF-1α experiences stabilization and translocation. HIF-1α is expressed at higher levels in adipose tissue of obese rodents compared to lean, and its mRNA appears to be up-regulated in fat tissue and infiltrating macrophages of obese humans. This increase in HIF-1α expression may contribute to several hypoxic responses in white adipose tissue, including increased GLUT1 concentration, expression and secretion of inflammation-related adipokines, production of the angiogenic factor VEGF, and insulin resistance [6].

Adipokines produced in hypoxic adipocytes are involved in several important physiological and metabolic processes through autocrine, paracrine, and endocrine mechanisms. These adipokines influence insulin sensitivity, glucose homeostasis, angiogenesis, inflammation, immunity, food intake, and energy expenditure [10]. Leptin and adiponectin are the most prominent protein hormones secreted by adipocytes and are increased and reduced, respectively, in obese patients. The link between hypoxia, adipokines, inflammation, and energy balance is complex but probably plays a key role in obesity physiopathology [10–12].

9.2.2 Obesity, obstructive sleep apnea, and hypoxia

Obesity and OSA share a complex, bidirectional relationship marked by mutual causality. OSA is a disorder marked by reduced pharyngeal muscle tone during sleep, causing recurrent pharyngeal collapse and disrupting normal ventilation and sleep patterns [7]. These respiratory events trigger desaturation–reoxygenation sequences, resulting in intermittent hypoxemia. This, in turn, leads to oxidative stress, increased expression of adhesion molecules, activation of leukocytes, production of systemic inflammation, and vascular endothelium damage and dysfunction. Although hypoxic stress is considered the major mechanism responsible for OSA's cardiovascular, metabolic, and cerebral consequences, recent work also suggests a role for repeated exposure to high levels of CO_2 [13]. OSA is generally defined as five or more apneas–hypopneas per hour of sleep (i.e., the apnea–hypopnea index). With almost 1 billion affected people worldwide, OSA is highly prevalent, with rates ranging from 2% to 46% in the general population. Men, older age groups, and specific patient populations such as obese individuals exhibit higher OSA prevalence. Given the escalating incidence of obesity, the most important risk factor for OSA, it is anticipated that OSA prevalence will continue to rise.

9.3 Obesity and mountain sickness

Obesity seems to be a risk factor for acute mountain sickness (AMS). Data from the construction of the Qinghai–Tibet railroad suggests that obese persons are almost three times more susceptible to AMS compared to those with a normal BMI (97% vs. 37%) [14]. Hirata et al. [15] found that lean subjects (BMI < 22 kg/m^2) were less susceptible to AMS at 5,150 m than those who are standard or obese, with incidence rates of 22%, 54%, and 70%, respectively. Kayser [16] showed that male trekkers who suffered from AMS around 5,400 m had significantly higher BMI than those who were not sick. Ri-Li et al. [17] found that obesity predisposes to AMS in conditions of simulated hypoxia. The mechanisms predisposing obese individuals to AMS are unclear, but relative hypoventilation, especially during sleep, may play a role by accentuating hypoxemia [18].

Hypoxic exposure at altitude is known to increase pulmonary artery pressure, with this effect appearing accentuated in obese individuals showing higher pulmonary artery pressure than normal subjects at a given altitude [14]. Even at a moderate altitude (2,240 m), obese subjects showed a mean pulmonary artery pressure of ~30 mmHg, surpassing values in normal weight subjects (~15 mmHg) at the same altitude and exceeding the pulmonary artery pressure of normal weight Peruvians (~22 mmHg) living at higher altitude (3,730 m) [19]. At altitudes between 4,630 and 4,905 m, it has also been reported that subjects with a BMI > 28 kg/m^2 have higher mean pulmonary artery pressure (~31 mmHg) than those with a BMI of 25–27 kg/m^2 (~24 mmHg) and of 22–24 kg/m^2 (~22 mmHg) [14].

Altogether, these data suggest that individuals with obesity are more prone to develop health issues such as symptoms of AMS and pulmonary hypertension during exposure for several days to hypoxia at altitude.

9.4 Hypoxia and energy balance

Altitude, as a natural environment inducing hypoxic exposure, is often accompanied by weight loss. Studies have consistently reported loss of body mass during prolonged altitude sojourns at altitudes above 5,000–5,500 m [20]. The primary factor contributing to this weight loss appears to be a reduction in energy intake, possibly due to the anorexic effect of exposure to altitude. This effect may be amplified by increased energy expenditure resulting from increased physical activity during trekking. Conversely, a reduction in intestinal energy uptake, stemming from impaired intestinal function, probably plays a minor role if any [21].

9.4.1 Energy expenditure

In contrast to many other animals, humans acutely exposed to hypoxia show an increased resting metabolic rate (RMR) [22]. Mechanisms driving this elevation in hypoxia include an increased sympathetic activity [23], enhanced thyroid activity [24], and interleukin-6 level [25]. Over the first days of altitude exposure between 3,500 and 5,000 m, RMR was shown to increase by 10% to 28% [20].

In animals, acute hypoxia generally reduces physical activity, therefore inducing a reduction in energy expenditure. In humans, sojourns at altitude are often associated with increased physical activity levels (e.g., hiking) and therefore increased energy expenditure compared to a sedentary lifestyle. This increase in energy expenditure can contribute to an impaired energy balance and therefore reduced body (especially fat) mass at altitude. Sojourns at high altitude are also known to reduce fat-free mass [26], although there may be a potential threshold below which the effect of hypoxic exposure on muscle is limited [27].

9.4.2 Malabsorption

The question of whether altitude hypoxia induces malabsorption that may contribute to the negative energy balance at high altitude remains unclear. Some results suggested reduced energy digestibility in climbers at 6,300 m [28], but others did not (e.g., [29]). Intestinal flora changes during a high-altitude expedition might contribute to malabsorption, although determining the exact role of altitude, exertion, changes in nutrition, and exposure to different bacterial strains while traveling in foreign countries is difficult [30].

9.4.3 Energy intake

The main effect of hypoxia leading to a negative energy balance seems to be a reduction in energy intake from a lack of appetite. The regulation of appetite and food intake involves complex interactions between physiological and social factors [31]. The hypothalamus plays a key role by integrating neural, metabolic, and endocrine information about energy intake and expenditure. Leptin, mainly released by adipose tissue, and insulin, predominantly released by the pancreas, influence body mass regulation by stimulating the release of anorexigenic molecules in the hypothalamus. Changes in other (an)orexigenic factors under hypoxic/altitude conditions may affect the energy balance, such as NPY, ghrelin, galanin, and CCK, although their specific roles remain to be specified. Cytokines such as interleukin-6 and tumor necrosis factor-alpha are other potential key players of changes in energy balance due to hypoxia, exercise, and various pathological conditions including obesity.

At high altitudes, both energy and protein intake have been shown to be reduced by 20-40% [32]. Although differences in food availability (both quantitative and qualitative) can partly explain differences in energy intake between high altitude and sea level conditions, prolonged hypoxic exposure at high altitudes seems responsible for the reduced appetite and food intake and supports the contention of an anorexigenic effect of hypoxia [33].

Overall, the effects of hypoxia on energy balance observed at high altitudes, and especially the reduction in appetite, provide a physiological basis to consider hypoxic exposure as a means to induce a reduction in body mass, and therefore to manage obesity [34]. In addition to the effect of sojourn at high altitude on body composition, the lower prevalence of obesity in populations living at moderate altitude (even after accounting for important confounding factors such as temperature, diet, smoking, and physical activity) further supports the concept that exposure to hypoxia may be beneficial to prevent or decrease excessive body fat stores [35–37].

9.5 Hypoxic conditioning and obesity

Based on the effect of hypoxic exposure on energy balance and preclinical data indicating positive cardiometabolic effects of moderate hypoxia [38, 39], exposure to hypoxia has been proposed to treat metabolically unhealthy overweight or obese people (Figure 9.2). Such hypoxic conditioning (HC) could be an innovative therapeutic approach to complement best quality of care for overweight or obese persons with cardiometabolic disorders. HC is theoretically attractive for cardiovascular and metabolic improvements because the

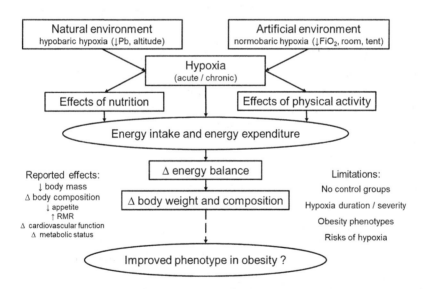

FIGURE 9.2   Schematic representation of the interactions linking obesity, hypoxia, physical activity, nutrition, and energy balance.

RMR, resting metabolic rate. From [79].

homeostatic perturbations induced by hypoxia are integrated via signaling pathways into alterations in gene expression and phenotype changes, remarkably similar to those induced by physical exercise [40]. Because of these similarities, athletes have for many years utilized natural or simulated altitude exposure as an additional training stimulus to enhance performance.

Only a few studies have assessed the effects of hypoxia in obese individuals during an actual sojourn at moderate altitude (1,700–2,650 m) [41–43]. Only one of these included a control group at low altitude [41], an important aspect of the study design to consider the potential placebo effect of such type of intervention (group sojourn, supervision, etc.). Only one of these studies [42] did not include a physical activity program at altitude, therefore enabling the evaluation of the specific effects of hypoxic exposure independent of any changes in physical activity. Although these studies reported some encouraging results like improved BMI [42, 44], cardiovascular status (i.e., reduced blood pressure [42, 43] and glucose and lipid metabolism [41, 43]) after moderate altitude exposure, further controlled studies should confirm any positive effects of altitude exposure, with or without physical activity, on the health status of obese individuals, taking into account comorbidities.

Despite the potential interest of actual altitude sojourns in the management of obesity, logistical limitations have prompted consideration of simulated altitude exposure as a potential treatment alternative. Replicating hypoxic conditions encountered at altitude can be achieved by reducing the oxygen concentration of inspired air, either through a mask connected to a gas mixing device (delivering a gas mixture with a reduced inspiratory oxygen fraction, FiO_2) or within a hypoxic room (or tent) with reduced oxygen partial pressure. HC sessions typically consist of repetitive, brief bouts of moderate (hypocapnic) hypoxia, interrupted by periods of normoxic recovery, achieved by altering inspiratory oxygen tension. Similar to methods used by athletes to increase their performance [45]; intermittent hypoxic exposure has been evaluated in pilot studies over the past years in the context of obesity, both passively (i.e., at rest, without exercise) during day time [46–49] or during sleep [50–52]. Workman and Basset [49] demonstrated that six sessions of 3-hour passive exposure to hypoxia (peripheral oxygen saturation, SpO_2 ~80%) increased energy expenditure and lipid oxidation in overweight males compared to sham normoxic sessions. Costalat et al. [47] showed in six overweight or obese individuals that ten 70-min long sessions of intermittent hypoxia (~15 deoxygenations to SpO_2 = 80%–reoxygenation cycles) over 2 weeks reduced blood lipid levels (LDLc) and lowered systolic blood pressure. In a randomized controlled study including an 8-week intervention with three 1-hour sessions per week of intermittent hypoxia (5 min–3 min) versus sustained hypoxia (SpO_2 75%) or normoxia, Chacaroun et al. [46] showed a significant reduction in diastolic blood pressure after the intervention but no change in body composition and metabolic status.

Instead of daytime hypoxic sessions, which may lead to a relatively low total dose of hypoxic exposure (typically three to five 1-hour sessions per week) and be difficult to integrate into daily activities, some authors have implemented in patients a strategy similar to the living high–training low strategy used in athletes, with nocturnal hypoxic exposure. Marlatt et al. [51] evaluated the effect of hypoxic exposure during night-time only (sleeping in a hypoxic tent at home with a FiO_2 of 0.15) in obese patients with type-II diabetes. In this uncontrolled study, 14 nights of hypoxic exposure significantly improved glucose tolerance. In a similar uncontrolled design with eight obese patients, nocturnal hypoxic exposure for 10 consecutive nights was shown to reduce body weight and improve fasting blood glucose and insulin sensitivity [50]. Only one randomized controlled study evaluated the effect of a 4-week living high (nocturnal FiO_2 0.147)–training low versus living low–training low programs in 35 adolescents (12–16 years) with obesity [52]. Despite similar aerobic exercise training and diet programs in both groups, adolescents spending the night in hypoxia showed larger reductions in body weight (–8.7 ± 2.2 kg versus –7.1 ± 2.2 kg) together with an increase of GLP-1, a satiety hormone possibly upregulated by interleukin-6. Implementing nocturnal hypoxic exposure in individuals with obesity and cardiometabolic disorders may increase the total hypoxic dose with little impact on habitual daily activities. However, it requires relatively sophisticated infrastructures, and nocturnal hypoxic exposure may induce significant sleep impairments (i.e., periodic breathing and reduced sleep quality [53]) that might be detrimental in the context of obesity.

Overall, these pilot studies suggest that intermittent hypoxic exposure (i.e., from 70 min to 12 h, every 24 h) at rest, even for relatively short periods (1–2 weeks) and without additional interventions (nutritional or physical activity) can induce positive metabolic changes. In a randomized crossover study, Van Maijel et al. [48] exposed 12 obese patients to three sessions of 2 hours of hypoxia (FiO_2 0.15) or normoxia for seven consecutive days, aiming to clarify the metabolic and molecular adaptations of HC in men with obesity. They provided the first tissue-specific (adipose tissue and skeletal muscle) measurements of reduced oxygen pressure during hypoxic exposure (FiO_2 0.15), confirming that inducing moderate hypoxemia at rest leads to significant tissue hypoxia. The authors also reported an increased reliance on glycolysis to ensure ATP production, associated with an upregulation of several inflammatory and metabolic pathways after the hypoxic program. Further studies are required to describe the metabolic pathways targeted by different types of passive hypoxic conditioning strategies to improve the health status of obese individuals.

Some studies that investigated the effect of acute exercise performed in hypoxia versus normoxia suggest that combining exercise training and hypoxic exposure might be an interesting option for the management of obesity. Bailey et al. [54] showed that when healthy males exercised in hypoxia (FiO_2 0.145), it more effectively reduced plasma ghrelin and appetite for the subsequent 2 h compared to normoxic exercise conditions. Mackenzie et al. [55] showed that when overweight or obese type II diabetic patients performed a 60-min exercise trial in hypoxia (FiO_2 0.146), it improved glucose tolerance and peripheral insulin sensitivity in the subsequent 4 h compared to a normoxic exercise trial. This suggests that repeated exercise (i.e., training) in hypoxia might provide additional benefits for obese individuals compared to normoxic exercise training.

Similar to strategies used by athletes in altitude training paradigms [45], recent randomized controlled studies have evaluated the combination of hypoxic exposure and exercise training in obese subjects. The interventions typically involved endurance whole-body exercise sessions (i.e., cycling or walking/running on a treadmill) lasting for 1 h, performed while breathing an hypoxic gas mixture with a FiO_2 close to 0.15 (i.e., simulating an altitude of 2,500 m), although some studies [56, 57] used lower FiO_2 close to 0.13 (i.e., equivalent to 3,500 m). Chacaroun et al. [56] proposed to clamp SpO_2 at ~80% during hypoxic sessions by individually and continuously adapting FiO_2 in order to minimize interindividual variability. Some active HC studies also combined endurance and strength exercises under hypoxic conditions [58–61]. Greater improvement in body weight or composition was observed following hypoxic exercise training in some [57, 61–64] but not all studies [56, 58–60, 65–67]. Most studies did not report greater improvement in metabolic status (e.g., lipid status, glucose tolerance, and insulin sensitivity) between hypoxic and normoxic exercise training [56, 58, 62, 64, 65, 68], although some observed greater improvements in lipid status [57, 59, 63] and glucose tolerance and insulin response [59]. Greater improvements in cardiovascular parameters (e.g., blood pressure) were reported by some [60, 61, 63] but not all [56, 57, 64, 66, 67] studies in hypoxia. Similarly, larger increase in maximal exercise performance were reported in some [56, 59, 60] but not all [58, 64, 66] studies, although in the latter the similar improvements between environments were obtained despite lower absolute workload during whole body exercise in hypoxia [64]. The feasibility and adherence to exercise training may be enhanced in obese individuals with musculoskeletal issues and experiencing pain that may be exacerbated with high absolute exercise power output [69].

High-intensity exercise, specifically interval or sprint training in hypoxia, has recently gained popularity in athletes since it may provide greater improvement in maximal exercise capacity compared to normoxia [70, 71]. It has also been hypothesized that hypoxic high-intensity interval training might positively impact energy balance by inhibiting appetite-stimulating hormones and reducing dietary intake compared to normoxic interventions [72]. Five randomized controlled trials evaluated the effect of hypoxic interval exercise training in obese individuals, with two studies using sprint training [73, 74], two using 1-min [75] or 2-min [76] interval training, and one comparing 3-min interval and sprint training programs [77]. The FiO_2 ranged from 0.17 to 0.12 and the program duration from 2 to 12 weeks (three to four sessions/week). Only one study reported greater improvement in body composition following hypoxic interval training for 12 weeks in obese females [73]. Maximal exercise capacity increased to a greater extent following hypoxic versus normoxic training in two studies only involving obese females [74, 77]. Camacho-Cardenosa et al. [77] found similar improvements in exercise capacity following interval and sprint hypoxic training, with the latter requiring only 29.6 min of exercise per session versus 41.5 min for the interval training. Further studies are required to elucidate the potential interest of interval and sprint training programs in hypoxia, considering factors such as exercise protocol, hypoxia severity, and the subjects' characteristics (e.g., sex differences).

Overall, the divergent outcomes in the effects of active HC on obesity may arise from differences in the amount (session duration and number of sessions per week), modality, and intensity (e.g., low-intensity endurance, high-intensity interval or strength training) of exercise training and hypoxic exposure. In addition, the incorporation of nutritional interventions alongside exercise and hypoxic interventions is essential to achieve clinically relevant improvements in body weight in obese individuals. In a systematic review and meta-analysis that included 13 randomized controlled studies on overweight or obese individuals, Ramos-Campo et al. [78] concluded that hypoxic conditioning may lead to greater reductions in triglycerides and muscle growth than normoxic intervention, with similar changes in body weight. Future studies should need to elucidate the optimal role of HC in obesity prevention and management (Figure 9.2).

Abbreviations

AMS	acute mountain sickness
BMI	body mass index
FiO_2	inspiratory oxygen fraction
GLUT1	glucose transporter
HC	hypoxic conditioning
HIF-1	hypoxia-inducible factor-1
OSA	obstructive sleep apnea
RMR	resting metabolic rate
SpO_2	peripheral oxygen saturation
VEGF	vascular endothelial growth factor.

References

1. Prentice, A.M. and S.A. Jebb, *Beyond body mass index.* Obes Rev, 2001. **2**(3): p. 141–147.
2. World Health Organization, *Obesity and overweight - fact sheet 311.* 2016. http://www.who.int/mediacentre/factsheets/fs311/en/index.html
3. Flegal, K.M., et al., *Association of all-cause mortality with overweight and obesity using standard body mass index categories: A systematic review and meta-analysis.* JAMA, 2013. **309**(1): p. 71–82.
4. Guh, D.P., et al., *The incidence of co-morbidities related to obesity and overweight: A systematic review and meta-analysis.* BMC Public Health, 2009. **9**: p. 88.
5. Abdelaal, M., C.W. le Roux, and N.G. Docherty, *Morbidity and mortality associated with obesity.* Ann Transl Med, 2017. **5**(7): p. 161.
6. Trayhurn, P., B. Wang, and I.S. Wood, *Hypoxia in adipose tissue: A basis for the dysregulation of tissue function in obesity?* Br J Nutr, 2008. **100**(2): p. 227–235.
7. Levy, P., et al., *Obstructive sleep apnoea syndrome.* Nat Rev Dis Primers, 2015. **1**: p. 15015.
8. Ye, J., *Emerging role of adipose tissue hypoxia in obesity and insulin resistance.* Int J Obes (Lond), 2009. **33**(1): p. 54–66.
9. Semenza, G.L., *HIF-1 and mechanisms of hypoxia sensing.* Curr Opin Cell Biol, 2001. **13**(2): p. 167–171.
10. Trayhurn, P., *Hypoxia and adipose tissue function and dysfunction in obesity.* Physiol Rev, 2013. **93**(1): p. 1–21.
11. Steiner, A.A. and A.A. Romanovsky, *Leptin: At the crossroads of energy balance and systemic inflammation.* Prog Lipid Res, 2007. **46**(2): p. 89–107.
12. Thaler, J.P., et al., *Hypothalamic inflammation and energy homeostasis: Resolving the paradox.* Front Neuroendocrinol, 2010. **31**(1): p. 79–84.
13. Levy, P., et al., *Intermittent hypoxia and sleep-disordered breathing: Current concepts and perspectives.* Eur Respir J, 2008. **32**(4): p. 1082–1095.
14. Wu, T.Y., et al., *Who should not go high: Chronic disease and work at altitude during construction of the Qinghai–Tibet railroad.* High Alt Med Biol, 2007. **8**(2): p. 88–107.
15. Hirata, K., S. Masuyama, and A. Saito, *Obesity as risk factor for acute mountain sickness.* Lancet, 1989. **2**(8670): p. 1040–1041.
16. Kayser, B., *Acute mountain sickness in western tourists around the Thorong Pass (5400m) in Nepal.* J Wilderness Med, 1991. **2**: p. 110–117.
17. Ri-Li, G., et al., *Obesity: Associations with acute mountain sickness.* Ann Intern Med, 2003. **139**(4): p. 253–257.
18. Hackett, P.H. and R.C. Roach, *High-altitude illness.* N Engl J Med, 2001. **345**(2): p. 107–114.
19. Lupi-Herrera, E., et al., *Behavior of the pulmonary circulation in the grossly obese patient. Pathogenesis of pulmonary arterial hypertension at an altitude of 2,240 meters.* Chest, 1980. **78**(4): p. 553–558.
20. Kayser, B., *Nutrition and energetics of exercise at altitude. Theory and possible practical implications.* Sports Med, 1994. **17**(5): p. 309–323.
21. Westerterp, K.R. and B. Kayser, *Body mass regulation at altitude.* Eur J Gastroenterol Hepatol, 2006. **18**(1): p. 1–3.
22. Butterfield, G.E., et al., *Increased energy intake minimizes weight loss in men at high altitude.* J Appl Physiol, 1992. **72**(5): p. 1741–1748.

23. Moore, L.G., et al., *Propranolol blocks metabolic rate increase but not ventilatory acclimatization to 4300 m*. Respir Physiol, 1987. 70(2): p. 195–204.
24. Hamad, N. and S.P.L. Travis, *Weight loss at high altitude: Pathophysiology and practical implications*. Eur J Gastroenter Hepat, 2006. 18(1): p. 5–10.
25. Wallenius, V., et al., *Interleukin-6-deficient mice develop mature-onset obesity*. Nat Med, 2002. 8(1): p. 75–79.
26. Berryman, C.E., et al., *Severe negative energy balance during 21 d at high altitude decreases fat-free mass regardless of dietary protein intake: A randomized controlled trial*. FASEB J, 2018. 32(2): p. 894–905.
27. D'Hulst, G. and L. Deldicque, *Human skeletal muscle wasting in hypoxia: A matter of hypoxic dose?* J Appl Physiol (1985), 2017. 122(2): p. 406–408.
28. Boyer, S.J. and F.D. Blume, *Weight-loss and changes in body-composition at high altitude*. J Appl Physiol, 1984. 57(5): p. 1580–1585.
29. Westerterp, K.R., et al., *Operation Everest III: Energy and water balance*. Pflugers Arch, 2000. 439(4): p. 483–488.
30. Kleessen, B., et al., *Microbial and immunological responses relative to high-altitude exposure in mountaineers*. Med Sci Sports Exer, 2005. 37(8): p. 1313–1318.
31. Wynne, K., et al., *Appetite control*. J Endocrinol, 2005. 184(2): p. 291–318.
32. Rose, M.S., et al., *Operation Everest. II: Nutrition and body composition*. J Appl Physiol, 1988. 65(6): p. 2545–2551.
33. Westerterp-Plantenga, M.S., et al., *Appetite at "high altitude" [Operation Everest III (Comex-'97)]: A simulated ascent of Mount Everest*. J Appl Physiol, 1999. 87(1): p. 391–399.
34. Dunnwald, T., et al., *Body composition and body weight changes at different altitude levels: A systematic review and meta-analysis*. Front Physiol, 2019. 10: p. 430.
35. Lopez-Pascual, A., et al., *Living at a geographically higher elevation is associated with lower risk of metabolic syndrome: Prospective analysis of the SUN cohort*. Front Physiol, 2016. 7: p. 658.
36. Voss, J.D., et al., *Association of elevation, urbanization and ambient temperature with obesity prevalence in the United States*. Int J Obes (Lond), 2013. 37: p. 1407–1412.
37. Woolcott, O.O., et al., *Inverse association between altitude and obesity: A prevalence study among andean and low-altitude adult individuals of Peru*. Obesity (Silver Spring), 2016. 24(4): p. 929–937.
38. Kayser, B. and S. Verges, *Hypoxia, energy balance and obesity: From pathophysiological mechanisms to new treatment strategies*. Obes Rev, 2013. 14: p. 579–592.
39. Verges, S., et al., *Hypoxic conditioning as a new therapeutic modality*. Front Pediatr, 2015. 3: p. 58.
40. Fluck, M., *Functional, structural and molecular plasticity of mammalian skeletal muscle in response to exercise stimuli*. J Exp Biol, 2006. 209(Pt 12): p. 2239–2248.
41. Gutwenger, I., et al., *Pilot study on the effects of a 2-week hiking vacation at moderate versus low altitude on plasma parameters of carbohydrate and lipid metabolism in patients with metabolic syndrome*. BMC Res Notes, 2015. 8: p. 103.
42. Lippl, F.J., et al., *Hypobaric hypoxia causes body weight reduction in obese subjects*. Obesity (Silver Spring), 2010. 18(4): p. 675–681.

43. Schobersberger, W., et al., *Austrian Moderate Altitude Study 2000 (AMAS 2000). The effects of moderate altitude (1,700 m) on cardiovascular and metabolic variables in patients with metabolic syndrome.* Eur J Appl Physiol, 2003. **88**(6): p. 506–514.

44. Gunga, H.C., et al., *Austrian Moderate Altitude Study (AMAS 2000): Fluid shifts, erythropoiesis, and angiogenesis in patients with metabolic syndrome at moderate altitude (congruent with 1700 m).* Eur J Appl Physiol, 2003. **88**(6): p. 497–505.

45. Millet, G.P., et al., *Combining hypoxic methods for peak performance.* Sports Med, 2010. **40**(1): p. 1–25.

46. Chacaroun, S., et al., *Cardiovascular and metabolic responses to passive hypoxic conditioning in overweight and mildly obese individuals.* Am J Physiol Regul Integr Comp Physiol, 2020. **319**(2): p. R211–R222.

47. Costalat, G., et al., *Intermittent hypoxia revisited: a promising non-pharmaceutical strategy to reduce cardio-metabolic risk factors?* Sleep Breath, 2018. **22**(1): p. 267–271.

48. van Meijel, R.L.J., et al., *Mild intermittent hypoxia exposure induces metabolic and molecular adaptations in men with obesity.* Mol Metab, 2021. **53**: p. 101287.

49. Workman, C. and F.A. Basset, *Post-metabolic response to passive normobaric hypoxic exposure in sedentary overweight males: A pilot study.* Nutr Metab (Lond), 2012. **9**(1): p. 103.

50. Lecoultre, V., et al., *Ten nights of moderate hypoxia improves insulin sensitivity in obese humans.* Diabetes Care, 2013. **36**(12): p. e197–e178.

51. Marlatt, K.L., et al., *Two weeks of moderate hypoxia improves glucose tolerance in individuals with type 2 diabetes.* Int J Obes (Lond), 2020. **44**(3): p. 744–747.

52. Yang, Q., et al., *"Living high-training low" improved weight loss and glucagon-like peptide-1 level in a 4-week weight loss program in adolescents with obesity: A pilot study.* Medicine (Baltimore), 2018. **97**(8): p. e9943.

53. Bloch, K.E., et al., *Sleep at high altitude: Guesses and facts.* J Appl Physiol (1985), 2015. **119**(12): p. 1466–1480.

54. Bailey, D.P., et al., *Appetite and gut hormone responses to moderate-intensity continuous exercise versus high-intensity interval exercise, in normoxic and hypoxic conditions.* Appetite, 2015. **89**: p. 237–245.

55. Mackenzie, R., et al., *Acute hypoxia and exercise improve insulin sensitivity (S(I) (2*)) in individuals with type 2 diabetes.* Diabetes Metab Res Rev, 2011. **27**(1): p. 94–101.

56. Chacaroun, S., et al., *Hypoxic exercise training to improve exercise capacity in obese individuals.* Med Sci Sports Exerc, 2020. **52**(8): p. 1641–1649.

57. Lee, J.H. and C.K. Kim, *Effects of 12 weeks aerobic training in hypoxia on body composition and fat metabolism in obese adults.* Int J Sports Sci Med, 2017. **1**(1): p. 10–16.

58. Britto, F.A., et al., *Effects of a 30-week combined training program in normoxia and in hypoxia on exercise performance and health-related parameters in obese adolescents: a pilot study.* J Sports Med Phys Fitness, 2020. **60**(4): p. 601–609.

59. De Groote, Estelle, et al., *Hypoxic training improves normoxic glucose tolerance in adolescents with obesity.* Med Sci Sports Exerc, 2018. **50**(11): p. 2200–2208.

60. Gonzalez-Muniesa, P., et al., *Impact of intermittent hypoxia and exercise on blood pressure and metabolic features from obese subjects suffering sleep apnea-hypopnea syndrome.* J Physiol Biochem, 2015. **71**(3): p. 589–599.

61. Kong, Z., Y. Zang, and Y. Hu, *Normobaric hypoxia training causes more weight loss than normoxia training after a 4-week residential camp for obese young adults.* Sleep Breath, 2014. 18(3): p. 591–597.

62. Netzer, N.C., R. Chytra, and T. Kupper, *Low intense physical exercise in normobaric hypoxia leads to more weight loss in obese people than low intense physical exercise in normobaric sham hypoxia.* Sleep Breath, 2008. 12(2): p. 129–134.

63. Park, H.Y. and K. Lim, *The effects of aerobic exercise at hypoxic condition during 6 weeks on body composition, blood pressure, arterial stiffness, and blood lipid level in obese women.* Int J Sports Sci Med, 2017. 1(1): p. 1–5.

64. Wiesner, S., et al., *Influences of normobaric hypoxia training on physical fitness and metabolic risk markers in overweight to obese subjects.* Obesity (Silver Spring), 2009. 18(1): p. 116–120.

65. Fernandez Menendez, A., et al., *Effects of short-term normobaric hypoxic walking training on energetics and mechanics of gait in adults with obesity.* Obesity (Silver Spring), 2018. 26(5): p. 819–827.

66. Gatterer, H., et al., *Normobaric intermittent hypoxia over 8 months does not reduce body weight and metabolic risk factors: A randomized, single blind, placebo-controlled study in normobaric hypoxia and normobaric sham hypoxia.* Obes Facts, 2015. 8(3): p. 200–209.

67. Klug, L., et al., *Normobaric hypoxic conditioning in men with metabolic syndrome.* Physiol Rep, 2018. 6(24): p. e13949.

68. Rausch, L.K., et al., *Adiponectin, leptin and visfatin in hypoxia and its effect for weight loss in obesity.* Front Endocrinol (Lausanne), 2018. 9: p. 615.

69. Hobbins, L., et al., *Normobaric hypoxic conditioning to maximize weight loss and ameliorate cardio-metabolic health in obese populations: a systematic review.* Am J Physiol Regul Integr Comp Physiol, 2017. 313(3): p. R251–R264.

70. Faiss, R., O. Girard, and G.P. Millet, *Advancing hypoxic training in team sports: from intermittent hypoxic training to repeated sprint training in hypoxia.* Br J Sports Med, 2013. 47(1): p. i45–i50.

71. Westmacott, A., et al., *High-intensity interval training (HIIT) in hypoxia improves maximal aerobic capacity more than HIIT in normoxia: A systematic review, meta-analysis, and meta-regression.* Int J Environ Res Public Health, 2022. 19(21): 14261.

72. Chen, C.Y., et al., *A sports nutrition perspective on the impacts of hypoxic high-intensity interval training (HIIT) on appetite regulatory mechanisms: A narrative review of the current evidence.* Int J Environ Res Public Health, 2022. 19(3): 1736.

73. Camacho-Cardenosa, A., et al., *Effects of high-intensity interval training under normobaric hypoxia on cardiometabolic risk markers in overweight/obese women.* High Alt Med Biol, 2018. 19(4): p. 356–366.

74. Kong, Z., et al., *High-intensity interval training in normobaric hypoxia improves cardiorespiratory fitness in overweight Chinese young women.* Front Physiol, 2017. 8: p. 175.

75. Ghaith, A., et al., *Hypoxic high-intensity interval training in individuals with overweight and obesity.* Am J Physiol Regul Integr Comp Physiol, 2022. 323(5): p. R700–R709.

76. Hobbins, L., et al., *Acute psycho-physiological responses to perceptually regulated hypoxic and normoxic interval walks in overweight-to-obese adults.* J Sci Med Sport, 2021. 24(5): p. 481–487.

77. Camacho-Cardenosa, A., et al., *Repeated sprint in hypoxia as a time-metabolic efficient strategy to improve physical fitness of obese women.* Eur J Appl Physiol, 2020. **120**(5): p. 1051–1061.
78. Ramos-Campo, D.J., et al., *Additive stress of normobaric hypoxic conditioning to improve body mass loss and cardiometabolic markers in individuals with overweight or obesity: A systematic review and meta-analysis.* Physiol Behav, 2019. **207**: p. 28–40.
79. Kayser, B. and S. Verges, *Hypoxia, energy balance, and obesity: An update.* Obes Rev, 2021. **22**(2): p. e13192.

10

METABOLIC DISORDERS: METABOLIC SYNDROME AND TYPE 2 DIABETES

Tobias Dünnwald and Martin Burtscher

10.1 Epidemiology and clinical relevance of metabolic disorders (metabolic syndrome and type 2 diabetes)

10.1.1 Prevalence and diagnosis of metabolic syndrome and type 2 diabetes

According to recent data reported from the World Health Organization (WHO), more than 1 billion people worldwide are obese (body mass index [BMI] $\geq$30 kg/m^2, data from 2016), affecting 650 million adults, while 340 million adolescents and 39 million children are obese or overweight, and this number is still increasing [1]. As obesity is a component of metabolic syndrome (MetS) and a risk factor for type 2 diabetes (T2D) these disorders are increasing too. Diagnosis of MetS commonly includes abdominal obesity, increased fasting plasma glucose and fasting serum insulin, elevated arterial blood pressure, and dyslipidemia (e.g., elevated triglycerides and decreased high-density lipoprotein cholesterol, HDL-C). Diagnosis of T2D can be made based on a fasting plasma glucose concentration $\geq$ 7.0 mmol/l (126 mg/dL). Based on global data from 28 million individuals, the MetS prevalence varied from 12.5% to 31.4% depending on the diagnostic criteria [2]. In the 10th edition of the International Diabetes Federation (IDF) *Diabetes Atlas*, the global prevalence of diabetes was shown to have increased from 285 million in 2010 to 537 million cases in 2021 among adults aged between 20 and 79 years and was projected to further increase in this population to 643 million in 2030 to 784 million cases in 2045 (IDF 2021; https://www.diabetesatlas.org).

DOI: 10.4324/9781003402879-15

10.1.2 MetS and related health consequences

Obesity represents a major risk factor for MetS and is interlinked with all other components of MetS, namely, elevated blood glucose levels, dyslipidemia (high triglycerides and low HDL cholesterol), and systemic hypertension. Unhealthy lifestyle behaviors, in particular physical inactivity and unhealthy diet, impact all components of MetS. Conversely, sufficient amounts of physical activity and a healthy diet render the development of MetS unlikely and are thus considered protective factors [3]. Moreover, as favorable lifestyle behavior is associated with socioeconomic factors, MetS is much more prevalent in people with poor socioeconomic status [4]. Besides these lifestyle factors, poor sleep quality and duration, for example due to obstructive sleep apnea (OSA) [5] and chronic inflammation, which is characterized by high levels of inflammatory markers like C-reactive protein (CRP), interleukin-6 (IL-6), and tumor necrosis factor (TNF), were shown to play important roles in the development of MetS [6].

Clinical consequences of MetS primarily include a higher risk for cardio- and cerebrovascular diseases (e.g., coronary atherosclerosis, myocardial infarction, heart failure, ischemic and hemorrhagic stroke), T2D, and dementia [7–10]. It has been estimated that the population-attributable fraction for the MetS is about 12–17% for cardiovascular disease and 30–52% for diabetes [8].

10.1.3 T2D and related health consequences

T2D is a public health concern seriously impacting on human life and health expenditures. T2D affects functional capacities and quality of life, resulting in considerable morbidity and premature mortality [11]. Unhealthy diets and physical inactivity, often associated with obesity and elevated fasting plasma glucose, are characteristic features of current epidemiological trends of diabetes, which are aggravated by the aging of the human population [12]. While infections, hypo- and hyperglycemic states, and sometimes life-threatening emergencies represent acute complications, chronic complications affect almost all organs, in particular causing diabetic neuropathy, nephropathy, retinopathy, and vasculopathy, not rarely resulting in diabetic foot syndrome, vision loss, heart attacks, and stroke. For example, a 1-year observation found that the prevalence of acute and chronic complications was 13.3% and 73.1%, respectively [13].

10.1.4 Nonpharmacological measures and potentially related mechanisms for the prevention and treatment of MetS and T2D

Adopting a healthy lifestyle (healthy diet and regular physical activity) is crucial in the prevention and treatment of both MetS and T2D, for example by supporting weight control, physical fitness, and glucose homeostasis and reducing low-grade inflammation. Obesity may lead to the development of a chronic low-grade inflammation due to an imbalance of the expression of pro- and anti-inflammatory adipokines, whose secretion is adversely affected by adipose tissue dysfunction [14]. Chronic inflammation, a hallmark of MetS and T2D, has repeatedly been demonstrated to be partially counteracted by exercise prevention programs including aerobic and strength exercises [3, 15]. Exercise training may reduce systemic inflammation in these conditions by an elevated uptake of free fatty acids (FFA) into the skeletal muscle, resulting in lower plasma FFA levels and Toll-like receptor activation [16]. In addition, regular exercise (and dietary restriction) may improve mitochondrial dysfunction in MetS and T2D and promote anti-inflammatory effects [17].

Recently, hypoxia conditioning (HC) has been suggested as a promising complementary measure in the prevention and therapy of MetS and T2D, for instance by improving disturbed autonomic regulatory processes and systemic inflammation [18–20].

10.2 Hypoxia conditioning in metabolic disorders

Health-related adaptation to controlled hypoxia in subjects with metabolic diseases were examined in studies applying HC either under resting conditions (continuously or intermittently) or in combination with structured exercise. Figure 10.1 indicates possible favorable effects from passive HC that patients with metabolic disorders may benefit from (adapted from [21]).

10.2.1 Passive HC in prediabetes and T2D

In patients with T2D, already a single one-hour session of breathing intermittent hypoxia (IH; fractional inspired oxygen concentration (FiO$_2$): 13%, 5×6 min hypoxia interspersed by 6 min of normoxia) promoted glucose lowering accompanied by improved cardiorespiratory reflexes [20]. Likewise, diminished circulating blood concentrations and improved insulin sensitivity were reported following 1 h of continuous hypoxia (FiO$_2$: 14.6%) in T2D subjects [22]. Exposure of prediabetes patients to hypoxia for several weeks (FiO$_2$: 12%, 4×5 min hypoxia alternating with 5 min normoxia, 3×/week) enhanced oral glucose tolerance (2 h post oral glucose tolerance test [OGTT]) [23], with fasting glucose concentrations and glucose tolerance still being improved after one month [23]. In addition, tolerance to hypoxia was reported to be beneficially affected (i.e., less reduction in arterial blood oxygen saturation [SaO$_2$], lower heart rate [HR] and systolic blood pressure [SBP] for a given hypoxic stimulus) while hypoxia inducible factor 1α (HIF-1α) mRNA expression in blood leucocytes progressively increased

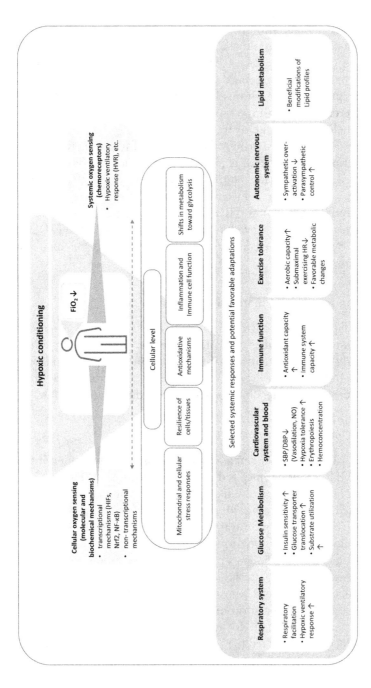

FIGURE 10.1 Physiological responses to passive hypoxia conditioning and resulting potential beneficial effects relevant for metabolic syndrome and type 2 diabetes.

DBP: diastolic blood pressure; FiO$_2$, fraction of inspired oxygen, HIF, hypoxia-inducible factor; HR, heart rate; NF-κB, nuclear factor-κB; NO, nitric oxide Nrf2, nuclear factor erythroid 2-related factor 2; SBP, systolic blood pressure.

(Figure based on Burtscher et al. [21]).

6.5-fold [23]. Further analysis in these patients demonstrated lower post OGTT blood insulin levels, indicating improved insulin sensitivity [24]. Replacing the 5-min normoxic phases by 3-min inhalation of 36% oxygen, the same authors found both IH protocols to similarly improve glucose homeostasis, tolerance to hypoxia, and the blood lipid profile [25]. Improved 2-h glucose tolerance in T2D patients was also reported following 14 nights of continuous hypoxia (FiO$_2$: 15%, 7–12 h/night) [26].

10.2.2 Passive HC in overweight, obesity, and MetS

Effects of passive HC in overweight/obese subjects or individuals suffering from MetS are somewhat conflicting. In overweight subjects, acute exposure for 1 h to continuous hypoxia (FiO$_2$: 15.5% or 12.5%) was ineffective in altering glucose homeostasis, insulin sensitivity, as well as inflammatory and oxidative stress markers [27]. It has been suggested that the absence of an effect may be due, at least in part, to the patients' initial normal glycemic control [27]. Likewise, postprandial glucose concentrations and insulin response remained unchanged following passive hypoxia exposure for 3×30 min during a 7.5-h period [28]. Exposing male overweight subjects to 3 h of continuous hypoxia (individually adjusted peripheral oxygen saturation, SpO$_2$, of 80%), either once or repeatedly per day over 7 days, increased energy expenditure and led to a shift in fuel utilization from glucose to fat oxidation [29].

Implementation of considerably longer total hypoxia exposure times, (3×2 h of intermittent hypoxia (FiO$_2$: 15%) separated by 1 h of normoxia per day for 7 days) led to a shift toward carbohydrate oxidation (fasting and postprandial) together with increased lactate concentrations without affecting insulin sensitivity in overweight/obese subjects [30]. Although acute IH exposure for 70 min (FiO$_2$: 10%) significantly reduced blood glucose levels in overweight and obese subjects, the initially beneficial effects disappeared following 10 consecutive sessions of IH (5×/week, 2 weeks) [31]. Yet, after 2 weeks, low-density lipoprotein-cholesterol (LDL-C) and subsequently the LDL-C to HDL-C ratio decreased, accompanied by a reduction in SBP [31]. The hypotensive effect was attributed to alterations on the endothelium (e.g., increased bioavailability of nitric oxide [NO]) instead of to an increased sensitivity of the baroreceptors, as cardiac autonomic indices and heart rate did not change [31]. Moreover, in overweight and mildly obese subjects, 8 weeks of either intermittent or continuous hypoxia (3×1 h/week, SpO$_2$: 75%, IH: 7 cycles of 5 min of hypoxia alternating 3 min of normoxia) decreased diastolic blood pressure (DBP), while no effects on glucose metabolism, lipid profiles, anthropometry, or vasculature were observed [32].

10.2.3 Effects of HC in combination with physical exercise in prediabetes and T2D

Theoretically, and as recently reviewed in more detail [33, 34], exercise-induced muscle deoxygenation may be intensified by concomitant exposure to moderate hypoxia, inducing a total increase in hypoxemia, with potential beneficial effects on glucose homeostasis. Therefore, in T2D patients, one single 60-min cycling bout performed during hypoxia (FiO_2: 14.6%, at ~50–55% VO_2max) improved insulin sensitivity more than exercising at equal absolute workload in normoxia [22]. In a subsequent though uncontrolled study conducted under similar conditions, 60- and 40-min but not 20-min hypoxic exercise bouts reduced fasting glucose levels, with most pronounced effects following the 60-min session [35]. Furthermore, blood glucose lowering was reported being more efficient following 60 min of continuous exercise (FiO_2: 14.7%, 90% at lactate threshold [LT]) compared to 60 min of interval hypoxic exercise (120% at LT; 5 min hypoxia/5 min passive recovery); however, acute effects were not different to the normoxic control group (i.e., interval exercise only) [36]. Conversely, cycling for 1 h in hypoxia (FiO_2: 14.0%, HR corresponding to 55% of normoxic VO_2max) had no impact on fasting glucose concentrations but compromised glucose tolerance in prediabetic subjects [37]. Aside from glucose metabolism alterations, Brinkmann et al. showed that central molecules involved in angiogenesis such as pro-angiogenic vascular endothelial growth factor (VEGF) were upregulated following 40 min of hypoxic but not normoxic exercise in T2D subjects, yet exercise-induced effects were not significantly different between the conditions [38].

Only a few studies investigated the effects of repeated exercise bouts in subjects with dysregulated glucose tolerance or T2D, also demonstrating no clear differences between normoxic and hypoxic exercise [39, 40].

10.2.4 Effects of HC in combination with exercise in overweight, obesity, and MetS

Glucose homeostasis: Combined endurance and strength training in hypoxia (FiO_2: 15%, 50-60 min 3×/week, 6 weeks), but not in normoxia, increased glucose tolerance and decreased postprandial plasma insulin levels in obese adolescents, although changes were not significantly different between conditions [41]. While the relative exercise intensity was the same, insulin sensitivity (e.g., homeostasis model assessment-insulin resistance, Homa-IR) improved under both conditions [41]. In addition, in obese men with MetS, a 6-week endurance intervention (FiO_2: 15%, 3×60 min/week at 50–60% of HRmax) significantly enhanced myocellular insulin sensitivity determined by a hyperinsulinemic euglycemic clamp [42]. Similarly, in overweight subjects, an 8-week hypoxic training improved insulin sensitivity [43] whereas a 4-week hypoxic training in elderly overweight to obese subjects reduced fasting insulin and improved the HOMA index [44]. Notably, in the latter three studies, improvements in glucose metabolism were not significantly different to the training in normoxia.

In contrast, hypoxic training in obese individuals with an individual adjusted SpO_2 to 80% (75% of HRmax, 3×45 min/week, 8 weeks) did not change fasting glucose and insulin concentrations [45]. Likewise, in MetS patients, a 6-week running intervention in hypoxia (FiO_2: 15%; 3×/week, 50-60% of HRmax) was ineffective in altering glucose concentrations, HbA1c, or glucose tolerance [46]. Combining hypoxic endurance and strength training in obese individuals suffering from sleep apnea, glucose homeostasis (FiO_2: 16%, 2×60 min/week, 8 weeks) [47] and insulin sensitivity (FiO_2: 15%, 1 h/week, 30 weeks) remained unchanged [48].

Body weight, body composition and lipid profiles: Several studies demonstrated more pronounced reductions in body weight or improvements in body composition (e.g., higher fat loss) following hypoxic training [44, 49–51]. Contrastingly, other investigations showed similar improvements after training in normoxia and hypoxia [41, 46–48] or reported no effects on these outcomes at all [43, 45, 52, 53]. Here, exercise intensity was suggested to be a critical factor for the divergent findings. A recent meta-analysis of randomized-controlled trials (mainly 3–4 weeks) performed in obese and overweight subjects demonstrated similar beneficial effects on body weight, fat mass, anthropometric parameters (e.g., waist to hip ratio), lipid profile (i.e., lower LDLc) as well as on SBP and DBP following training under hypoxic or normoxic conditions [54]. Notably, additive effects of hypoxia were reported for the decrease in triglycerides as well as the increase in muscle mass [54].

Cardiorespiratory fitness: Cardiorespiratory fitness (CRF; e.g., estimated by the assessment of VO_2max) represents an independent risk factor for cardiovascular diseases [55] and is also linked to the development of the MetS [56]. Results from studies implementing low-to-moderate intensity exercise in obese subjects showed that more pronounced improvements in CRF occurred after hypoxic compared to normoxic training [45], while others demonstrated similar effects under the two conditions [41, 44, 48]. Conversely, CRF was reported to remain unchanged following hypoxic and normoxic training in obese subjects [52], in those with sleep apnea syndrome [47], and in individuals with MetS [46]. Interestingly, despite lower absolute training workload (–20%) in hypoxia, implementation of high-intensity interval exercise in training programs revealed either additive effects of hypoxia in obese (FiO_2: 17%, 12 weeks) [57] and overweight women (FiO_2: 15%, 5 weeks) [58], or at least similar improvements compared to normoxia in overweight and obese subjects (FiO_2: ~12%, 8 weeks) [59].

In summary, available research indicates that, especially in individuals with higher levels of metabolic impairment (i.e., T2D), acute and prolonged passive HC can importantly benefit glycemic control, although more well-designed studies are essential to confirm these preliminary findings. There is currently no clear evidence for increased effectiveness of exercise training in hypoxia compared to training in normoxia in metabolic diseases. However, even though several studies implemented lower absolute exercise intensities during training in hypoxia, comparable positive effects on disease specific health outcomes (i.e., glucose metabolism, body weight/composition, lipid profile, CRF) were reported. Nevertheless, it has to be considered that several external and internal factors may modify these outcomes, including exercise- and hypoxic dose (i.e., intensity, duration and frequency), behavior (i.e., food intake and physical activity), extent of metabolic impairment, as well as individual variation in the response to hypoxia (incorporating glucoregulatory hormone responses).

10.3 Conclusions

Metabolic disorders like MetS and T2D represent major public health challenges worldwide. Modifications of lifestyle behaviors (healthy diet and sufficient regular physical activity [1, 60]) are primary measures to prevent or treat these disorders. Besides pharmacological strategies, novel research findings indicate that the application of hypoxia conditioning could beneficially complement lifestyle changes. As CRF is commonly reduced in people with MetS and/or T2D, passive HC or the combination with exercise could be used to partially substitute and/or increase the motivation and tolerance for physical activity.

Abbreviations

BMI	body mass index
CRF	cardiorespiratory fitness
CRP	C-reactive protein
DBP	diastolic blood pressure
FFA	free fatty acid
FiO_2	fraction of inspired oxygen
HC	hypoxia conditioning
IDF	International Diabetes Federation
HDL	high-density lipoprotein
HIF-1α	hypoxia inducible factor 1α
HOMA-IR	homeostasis model assessment-insulin resistance
HR	heart rate
IL-6	interleukin-6
LDL	low-density lipoprotein
Mets	metabolic syndrome
LT	lactate threshold

NO   nitric oxide
OGTT   oral glucose tolerance test
OSA   obstructive sleep apnea
O_2 oxygen
SaO_2 arterial blood oxygen saturation
SBP   systolic blood pressure
SpO_2 peripheral oxygen saturation
T2D   type 2 diabetes
TNF   tumor necrosis factor
VEGF   vascular endothelial growth factor
VO_2max maximal oxygen uptake
WHO   World Health Organization.

References

1. WHO. *World Health Organization— Facts sheet on obesity and overweight.* 2021, January 30, 2024. https://www.who.int/news-room/fact-sheets/detail/obesity-and-overweight
2. Noubiap, J.J., et al., *Geographic distribution of metabolic syndrome and its components in the general adult population: A meta-analysis of global data from 28 million individuals.* Diabetes Res Clin Pract, 2022. **188**: p. 109924.
3. Nilsson, P.M., J. Tuomilehto, and L. Rydén, *The metabolic syndrome: What is it and how should it be managed?* Eur J Prev Cardiol, 2019. **26**(2): p. 33–46.
4. Blanquet, M., et al., *Socio-economics status and metabolic syndrome: A meta-analysis.* Diabetes Metab Syndr, 2019. **13**(3): p. 1805–1812.
5. Qian, Y., et al., *Obstructive sleep apnea predicts risk of metabolic syndrome independently of obesity: A meta-analysis.* Arch Med Sci, 2016. **12**(5): p. 1077–1087.
6. Reddy, P., et al., *Metabolic syndrome is an inflammatory disorder: A conspiracy between adipose tissue and phagocytes.* Clin Chim Acta, 2019. **496**: p. 35–44.
7. Tune, J.D., et al., *Cardiovascular consequences of metabolic syndrome.* Transl Res, 2017. **183**: p. 57–70.
8. Ford, E.S., *Risks for all-cause mortality, cardiovascular disease, and diabetes associated with the metabolic syndrome: A summary of the evidence.* Diabetes Care, 2005. **28**(7): p. 1769–1778.
9. Li, X., et al., *Metabolic syndrome and stroke: A meta-analysis of prospective cohort studies.* J Clin Neurosci, 2017. **40**: p. 34–38.
10. Pal, K., et al., *Mild cognitive impairment and progression to dementia in people with diabetes, prediabetes and metabolic syndrome: A systematic review and meta-analysis.* Soc Psychiatry Psychiatr Epidemiol, 2018. **53**(11): p. 1149–1160.
11. Ramtahal, R., et al., *Prevalence of self-reported sleep duration and sleep habits in type 2 diabetes patients in South Trinidad.* J Epidemiol Glob Health, 2015. **5**(1): p. S35–43.
12. Khan, M.A.B., et al., *Epidemiology of type 2 diabetes: Global burden of disease and forecasted trends.* J Epidemiol Glob Health, 2020. **10**(1): p. 107–111.

13. Chamine, I., et al., *Acute and chronic diabetes-related complications among patients with diabetes receiving care in community health centers*. Diabetes Care. 2022: p. e141–e143.
14. Gregor, M.F. and G.S. Hotamisligil, *Inflammatory mechanisms in obesity*. Annu Rev Immunol, 2011. **29**: p. 415–445.
15. Balducci, S., et al., *Anti-inflammatory effect of exercise training in subjects with type 2 diabetes and the metabolic syndrome is dependent on exercise modalities and independent of weight loss*. Nutr Metab Cardiovasc Dis, 2010. **20**(8): p. 608–617.
16. Rada, I., et al., *Toll like receptor expression induced by exercise in obesity and metabolic syndrome: A systematic review*. Exerc Immunol Rev, 2018. **24**: p. 60–71.
17. Forte, M., et al., *Molecular mechanisms underlying the beneficial effects of exercise and dietary interventions in the prevention of cardiometabolic diseases*. J Cardiovasc Med (Hagerstown), 2023. **24**(Suppl 1): p. e3–e14.
18. Verges, S., et al., *Hypoxic conditioning as a new therapeutic modality*. Front Pediatr, 2015. **3**: p. 58.
19. Timon, R., et al., *Effect of intermittent hypoxic conditioning on inflammatory biomarkers in older adults*. Exp Gerontol, 2021. **152**: p. 111478.
20. Duennwald, T., et al., *Effects of a single bout of interval hypoxia on cardiorespiratory control and blood glucose in patients with type 2 diabetes*. Diabetes Care, 2013. **36**(8): p. 2183–2189.
21. Burtscher, J., et al., *Mechanisms underlying the health benefits of intermittent hypoxia conditioning*. J Physiol, 2023. https://doi.org/10.1113/JP285230
22. Mackenzie, R., et al., *Acute hypoxia and exercise improve insulin sensitivity (S(I) (2*)) in individuals with type 2 diabetes*. Diabetes Metab Res Rev, 2011. **27**(1): p. 94–101.
23. Serebrovska, T.V., et al., *Intermittent hypoxia training in prediabetes patients: Beneficial effects on glucose homeostasis, hypoxia tolerance and gene expression*. Exp Biol Med (Maywood), 2017. **242**(15): p. 1542–1552.
24. Serebrovska, T.V., et al., *Effects of intermittent hypoxia training on leukocyte pyruvate dehydrogenase kinase 1 (PDK-1) mRNA expression and blood insulin level in prediabetes patients*. Eur J Appl Physiol, 2019. **119**(3): p. 813–823.
25. Serebrovska, T.V., et al., *Intermittent hypoxia/hyperoxia versus intermittent hypoxia/normoxia: Comparative study in prediabetes*. High Alt Med Biol, 2019. **20**(4): p. 383–391.
26. Marlatt, K.L., et al., *Two weeks of moderate hypoxia improves glucose tolerance in individuals with type 2 diabetes*. Int J Obes (Lond), 2020. **44**(3): p. 744–747.
27. Corbett, J., et al., *Effect of different levels of acute hypoxia on subsequent oral glucose tolerance in males with overweight: A balanced cross-over pilot feasibility study*. Physiol Rep, 2023. **11**(9): p. e15623.
28. Morishima, T., et al., *Impact of exercise and moderate hypoxia on glycemic regulation and substrate oxidation pattern*. PLoS One, 2014. **9**(10): p. e108629.
29. Workman, C. and F.A. Basset, *Post-metabolic response to passive normobaric hypoxic exposure in sedentary overweight males: a pilot study*. Nutr Metab (Lond), 2012. **9**(1): p. 103.
30. van Meijel, R.L.J., et al., *Mild intermittent hypoxia exposure induces metabolic and molecular adaptations in men with obesity*. Mol Metab, 2021. **53**: p. 101287.

31. Costalat, G., et al., *Intermittent hypoxia revisited: A promising non-pharmaceutical strategy to reduce cardio-metabolic risk factors?* Sleep Breath, 2018. **22**(1): p. 267–271.

32. Chacaroun, S., et al., *Cardiovascular and metabolic responses to passive hypoxic conditioning in overweight and mildly obese individuals.* Am J Physiol Regul Integr Comp Physiol, 2020. **319**(2): p. R211–R222.

33. van Hulten, V., R.L.J. van Meijel, and G.H. Goossens, *The impact of hypoxia exposure on glucose homeostasis in metabolically compromised humans: A systematic review.* Rev Endocr Metab Disord, 2021. **22**(2): p. 471–483.

34. Soo, J., et al., *The role of exercise and hypoxia on glucose transport and regulation.* Eur J Appl Physiol, 2023. **123**(6): p. 1147–1165.

35. Mackenzie, R., et al., *The effect of hypoxia and work intensity on insulin resistance in type 2 diabetes.* J Clin Endocrinol Metab, 2012. **97**(1): p. 155–162.

36. Mackenzie, R., et al., *Intermittent exercise with and without hypoxia improves insulin sensitivity in individuals with type 2 diabetes.* J Clin Endocrinol Metab, 2012. **97**(4): p. E546–E555.

37. De Groote, E., et al., *Effect of hypoxic exercise on glucose tolerance in healthy and prediabetic adults.* Am J Physiol Endocrinol Metab, 2021. **320**(1): p. E43–E54.

38. Brinkmann, C., et al., *Hypoxia and hyperoxia affect serum angiogenic regulators in T2DM men during cycling.* Int J Sports Med, 2017. **38**(2): p. 92–98.

39. van Meijel, R.L.J., E.E. Blaak, and G.H. Goossens, *Effects of hypoxic exercise on 24-hour glucose profile and substrate metabolism in overweight and obese men with impaired glucose metabolism.* Am J Physiol Endocrinol Metab, 2023. **324**(2): p. E135–E143.

40. Schreuder, T.H., et al., *Impact of hypoxic versus normoxic training on physical fitness and vasculature in diabetes.* High Alt Med Biol, 2014. **15**(3): p. 349–355.

41. De Groote, E., et al., *Hypoxic training improves normoxic glucose tolerance in adolescents with obesity.* Med Sci Sports Exerc, 2018. **50**(11): p. 2200–2208.

42. Mai, K., et al., *Hypoxia and exercise interactions on skeletal muscle insulin sensitivity in obese subjects with metabolic syndrome: Results of a randomized controlled trial.* Int J Obes (Lond), 2020. **44**(5): p. 1119–1128.

43. Chobanyan-Jürgens, K., et al., *Influences of hypoxia exercise on whole-body insulin sensitivity and oxidative metabolism in older individuals.* J Clin Endocrinol Metab, 2019. **104**(11): p. 5238–5248.

44. Wiesner, S., et al., *Influences of normobaric hypoxia training on physical fitness and metabolic risk markers in overweight to obese subjects.* Obesity (Silver Spring), 2010. **18**(1): p. 116–120.

45. Chacaroun, S., et al., *Hypoxic exercise training to improve exercise capacity in obese individuals.* Med Sci Sports Exerc, 2020. **52**(8): p. 1641–1649.

46. Klug, L., et al., *Normobaric hypoxic conditioning in men with metabolic syndrome.* Physiol Rep, 2018. **6**(24): p. e13949.

47. González-Muniesa, P., et al., *Impact of intermittent hypoxia and exercise on blood pressure and metabolic features from obese subjects suffering sleep apnea-hypopnea syndrome.* J Physiol Biochem, 2015. **71**(3): p. 589–599.

48. Britto, F.A., et al., *Effects of a 30-week combined training program in normoxia and in hypoxia on exercise performance and health-related parameters in obese adolescents: A pilot study.* J Sports Med Phys Fitness, 2020. **60**(4): p. 601–609.

49. Camacho-Cardenosa, A., et al., *High-intensity interval training in normobaric hypoxia leads to greater body fat loss in overweight/obese women than high-intensity interval training in normoxia.* Front Physiol, 2018. **9**: p. 60.

50. Kong, Z., Y. Zang, and Y. Hu, *Normobaric hypoxia training causes more weight loss than normoxia training after a 4-week residential camp for obese young adults.* Sleep Breath, 2014. **18**(3): p. 591–597.

51. Park, H.Y., et al., *Twelve weeks of exercise modality in hypoxia enhances health-related function in obese older Korean men: A randomized controlled trial.* Geriatr Gerontol Int, 2019. **19**(4): p. 311–316.

52. Gatterer, H., et al., *Normobaric intermittent hypoxia over 8 months does not reduce body weight and metabolic risk factors: A randomized, single blind, placebo-controlled study in normobaric hypoxia and normobaric sham hypoxia.* Obes Facts, 2015. **8**(3): p. 200–209.

53. Hobbins, L., et al., *Short-term perceptually regulated interval-walk training in hypoxia and normoxia in overweight-to-obese adults.* J Sports Sci Med, 2021. **20**(1): p. 45–51.

54. Ramos-Campo, D.J., et al., *Additive stress of normobaric hypoxic conditioning to improve body mass loss and cardiometabolic markers in individuals with overweight or obesity: A systematic review and meta-analysis.* Physiol Behav, 2019. **207**: p. 28–40.

55. Myers, J., et al., *Physical activity and cardiorespiratory fitness as major markers of cardiovascular risk: Their independent and interwoven importance to health status.* Prog Cardiovasc Dis, 2015. **57**(4): p. 306–314.

56. Duncan, G.E., *Exercise, fitness, and cardiovascular disease risk in type 2 diabetes and the metabolic syndrome.* Curr Diab Rep, 2006. **6**(1): p. 29–35.

57. Camacho-Cardenosa, A., et al., *Repeated sprint in hypoxia as a time-metabolic efficient strategy to improve physical fitness of obese women.* Eur J Appl Physiol, 2020. **120**(5): p. 1051–1061.

58. Kong, Z., et al., *High-intensity interval training in normobaric hypoxia improves cardiorespiratory fitness in overweight Chinese young women.* Front Physiol, 2017. **8**: p. 175.

59. Ghaith, A., et al., *Hypoxic high-intensity interval training in individuals with overweight and obesity.* Am J Physiol Regul Integr Comp Physiol, 2022. **323**(5): p. R700–R709.

60. WHO, *World Health Organization—fact sheets on physical activity* 2022, January 30, 2024. https://www.who.int/news-room/fact-sheets/detail/physical-activity

SECTION 5

11

INTERMITTENT HYPOXIA CONDITIONING FOR THERAPY OF SYSTEMIC HYPERTENSION

H. Fred Downey, Nadezhda P. Lyamina, Svetlana V. Lyamina and Eugenia Manukhina

11.1 Introduction

To most clinicians and many physiologists, the terms "hypertension" and "intermittent hypoxia" bring to mind obstructive sleep apnea. In fact, the severe intermittent hypoxia caused during frequent obstructive sleep apnea over a long period does produce hypertension due to sympathetic activation and impairment of the baroreflex and chemoreflex [1, 2]. However, for more than 40 years, studies have shown that more mild, therapeutic intermittent hypoxia conditioning (IHC) is antihypertensive.

In spite of advances in pharmacological therapy, hypertension remains a serious disease and a risk factor for other cardiovascular diseases [3]. Drug interactions and side effects are an increasing problem that confounds pharmacological treatment of arterial hypertension (AH) [4, 5]. Thus, complementary therapies, such as IHC, must be considered. Since reoxygenation is an integral component of IHC, new studies have combined IHC with intermittent hyperoxia (IHHC). This chapter aims to acquaint the reader with the history of therapeutic IHC or IHHC in hypertensive patients and with studies in animals that have provided insight into mechanisms of IHC's antihypertensive action.

11.2 IHC therapy for hypertension

Following Meerson et al.'s initial report in 1971 of an antihypertensive effect of high altitude in rats [6], Katiukhin et al. [7] in 1979 reported decreased blood pressure (BP) of patients with stage 1 AH after exposure to hypobaric hypoxia in a hypobaric chamber. In 1989, Chizhov et al. [8] and Evgen'eva et al. [9] reported antihypertensive benefits of normobaric IHC in

DOI: 10.4324/9781003402879-17

pregnant women. Potievskaia and Chizhov [10] reported pronounced antihypertensive and emotional benefits in 71% of patients treated with normobaric IHC in 1992. In 1993, Aleshin et al. [11] reported a decline in BP of 22 treated patients. In the same year, Vorob'ev et al. [12] reported that normobaric IHC had a pronounced antihypertensive effect in 87% of the patients that persisted for 6 months in 84% of the patients. Later (1994) this group reported similar findings in >120 patients [13].

In the first use of 24-hour monitoring of BP in IHC research, Simonenko et al. [14] reported in 2003 that positive changes in the 24-hour BP profile were significantly more evident in patients treated with normobaric IHC and antihypertensive drugs than in patients treated with drugs alone. Mukharliamov et al. [15] also found that IHC improved the efficacy of prescribed antihypertensive medications (2006). In 2011, Tin'kov et al. [16] reported that hypobaric IHC reduced systolic and diastolic BP by 14% and 8%, respectively, in postmenopausal women with AH. Lyamina et al. [17] observed decreased BP following normobaric IHC treatment of patients with stage 1 AH also in 2011. More recently (2020), Muangritdech et al [18] found that normobaric IHC significantly reduced systolic BP, and that the effect persisted for 6 weeks. To summarize, reports have consistently shown that hypobaric and normobaric IHC reduce BP in hypertensive patients. This was confirmed by a recent meta-analysis [1].

Since dynamic exercise has been shown to be antihypertensive [20], studies have investigated the possibility of a synergistic antihypertensive effect of IHC and exercise. However, when Muangritdech et al. [18] added normobaric IHC during exercise to hypertensive patients, they found no added effect compared to IHC alone. In contrast, Lizamore et al. [21] reported that IHC combined with exercise lowered systolic BP in untrained, normotensive subjects. Also, Behrendt et al. [22] found that IHC prior to aerobic exercise reduced cardiovascular risk factors, including BP, in geriatric patients.

Although not administered specifically as therapy for AH, IHC has been shown to reduce BP in studies of aging and in patients with comorbidities. For example, Burtscher et al. [23] found that 3 weeks of normobaric IHC decreased exercise systolic BP in elderly men with and without coronary artery disease. Shatilo et al. [23] reported that normobaric IHC improved exercise performance and reduced BP of healthy senior men whether or not the men routinely exercised or avoided exercise. Korkushko et al. [25] treated aged cardiac patients with normobaric IHC. Systolic BP was reduced by 6% and cardiac variables improved. Kong et al. [26] reported that IHC combined with exercise lowered systolic and mean BP in normotensive, obese subjects more than exercise alone. IHC also resulted in more weight loss. Costalat et al. [27] reported reduced systolic, but not diastolic, BP in overweight and obese subjects. Other cardiovascular risk factors were reduced. Chacaroun et al. [28] treated sedentary, obese patients with IHC and found a significant decrease in diastolic BP and in heart rate variability, but no significant changes in body weight index, vascular function, blood glucose, insulin, or lipid profile. In a recent study, Panza et al. [29] found that 3 weeks of normobaric IHC reduced systolic and diastolic BP by about 8% each in patients whose AH was associated with their obstructive sleep apnea. In summary, IHC appears safe for elderly patients and for patients with comorbidities, and it reduces BP. For many such patients, especially load-compromised ones, IHC may be a viable alternative to exercise for reducing BP and other cardiovascular risk factors.

In an early study of IHHC, Glazachev et al. [30] treated metabolic syndrome patients and observed a tendency for systolic BP to decrease along with a significant decrease in diastolic BP. Body weight decreased along with decreased total cholesterol and low-density lipoproteins. Dudnik et al. [31] found that BP was not altered in older, comorbid cardiac outpatients treated with IHHC, although cardiorespiratory fitness improved. On the other hand, Bestavashvili et al. [32] reported that after IHHC, systolic and diastolic BP of patients with metabolic syndrome significantly decreased. Behrendt et al. [22] treated geriatric patients with IHHC and observed reduced systolic BP. However, the effects of IHHC and exercise were not additive. Since IHHC has not been used to treat hypertension specifically, such studies seem warranted.

In summary, IHC and IHHC should be considered an effective and safe alternative therapy for AH, especially for patients who cannot or will not exercise. However, many questions must be addressed before use of IHC or IHHC can become a routine antihypertensive therapy. For example, what is the optimal treatment strategy? What is an ideal maintenance program?

11.3 Antihypertensive mechanisms of IHC

Among mechanisms of IHC's antihypertensive effect (Figure 11.1), nitric oxide (NO) appears to be the most studied.

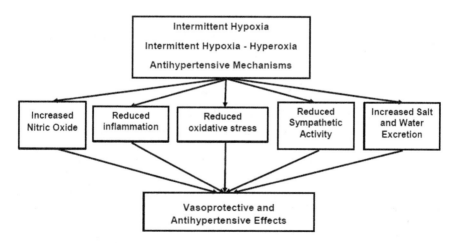

FIGURE 11.1   Vasoprotective and antihypertensive effects of IHC and IHHC.

The central role of NO in the antihypertensive effect of IHC is illustrated in Figure 11.2.

Hypoxia is a major factor that influences NO production. Hypoxia increases hypoxia-inducible factor 1 [33], which activates expression of NO synthases, inducible NO synthase [34], neuronal NO synthase [35], and endothelial NO synthase. [35]. IHC also increases Ca^{2+} entry into cells through L-type Ca^{2+} channels [37] and thereby activates endothelial NO synthase (eNOS) in

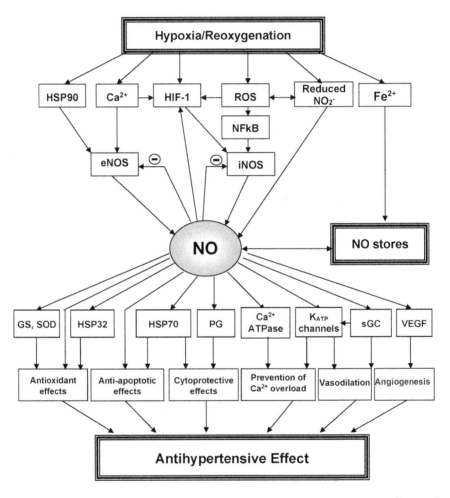

FIGURE 11.2   Nitric oxide (NO)-dependent mechanisms in protective effects of adaptation to hypoxia. See text for details.

NO_2^- = nitrite; NOS = NO synthase; iNOS = inducible NOS; cNOS = constitutive NOS; SOD = superoxide dismutase; GS = glutathione; HSP = heat shock protein; HIF-1 = hypoxia-inducible factor 1; ROS = reactive oxygen species; PG = prostaglandins; VEGF = vascular endothelium growth factor.

vascular endothelium [38]. During hypoxia, nitrite is reduced to bioactive NO and becomes an alternative, NOS-independent, source of NO [39]. Moreover, hypoxia induces heat shock protein (HSP) 90 [40], which binds to eNOS to increase NO production [41]. The transcription factor nuclear factor-κB is activated by reactive oxygen species generated during IHC [42], and it contributes to inducible nitric oxide synthase gene expression [43].

With increased NO production, there is a potential danger of nitrosative stress, as excessive NO reacts with superoxide to form toxic peroxynitrite [44]. This danger is alleviated by NO storage [45]. NO is stored in relatively stable complexes and transported to tissues, where it is released to cause vasodilation [45, 46].

NO enhances antioxidant defenses [47], including synthesis of the antioxidants glutathione [48] and superoxide dismutase [49] and by scavenging toxic free radicals [50]. NO increases the expression and activity of HSP32, which enhances protection against oxidative injury [51]. NO also increases expression of HSP70 [52], which has anti-apoptotic [53] action and blocks proinflammatory processes [54]. In addition, NO stimulates synthesis of cytoprotective prostaglandins PGE_2 and PGI_2 through activation of cyclooxygenases [55, 56].

NO increases synthesis of cyclic guanosine monophosphate GMP (cGMP) [57], and cGMP-dependent kinases phosphorylate several regulatory proteins and modulate ion channels [58, 59], including K_{ATP} channels [60]. The resulting potassium efflux decreases Ca^{2+} influx, resulting in vasodilation [60]. Also, Gao et al. [61] found that IHC facilitated baroreceptor function by opening K_{ATP} channels in the carotid sinus. NO also mediates activation of soluble guanylyl cyclase, which is critical in the cGMP signaling pathway that results in vascular relaxation [62].

NO enhances vascular endothelial growth factor (VEGF) expression, and synthesis of this factor is required for execution of the IHC-mediated angiogenic effect in endothelial cells [63]. An antihypertensive effect of hypoxia-stimulated angiogenesis in brain has been demonstrated [64]. Angiogenesis may reduce total peripheral resistance and BP.

In addition to NO-mediated mechanisms, other antihypertensive mechanisms are activated by IHC (Figure 11.1). Hypertension is often associated with activation of chronic inflammation [65]. Along with its antihypertensive effect, IHC produces a pronounced anti-inflammatory effect [66]. In a recent study, Chen et al. [67] concluded that IHC decreased BP in hypertensive rats by "inhibiting renin-angiotensin (Ang) system activity, downregulating the Ang-converting enzyme (ACE) – Ang II – Ang II receptor type 1 axis, and upregulating the ACE2 – (Ang1–7) – Mas receptor axis." The result of these processes was less vascular remodeling and fibrosis, as well as reduced inflammation.

Oxidative stress is an essential component of AH pathogenesis [68]. While excessive reactive oxygen species production is cytotoxic, lower concentrations produced after each hypoxic exposure and reoxygenation activate defense mechanisms, including nuclear factor erythroid 2-related factor 2, a transcriptional factor for the expression of antioxidant and anti-inflammatory enzymes [69, 70]. Furthermore, IHC increases activities and expression of antioxidant enzymes, including superoxide dismutase, catalase, and glutathione peroxidase [71, 72]. These antioxidant defenses are effective, since Susta et al. [73] found that neither IHC nor IHHC decreased oxidative stress or impaired antioxidant defenses.

IHC suppresses both basal and stress-induced sympathetic activation [29, 74] with a resultant decrease in BP [29, 75, 76]. Also, IHC reduced the content and turnover of norepinephrine in the hypothalamus, brainstem, frontal cortex, and striatum [76]. Panza et al. (29) also reported increased parasympathetic activity after IHC in patients with OSA.

The ability of the kidneys to balance the excretion and supply of water and electrolytes is critical for BP control [77]. Early studies showed that the antihypertensive effect of IHC was associated with increased water and salt excretion in hypertensive rats [6, 77, 78]. In fact, in 1981 Meerson et al. suggested that increased water and salt excretion is the main antihypertensive mechanism of IHC [79]. However, this antihypertensive effect of IHC seems to have received no further attention.

11.4 Limitations of IHC and IHHC as antihypertensive therapies

Studies of the antihypertensive effects of IHC and IHHC have been single-site with relative small numbers of patients and with little or no follow-up. Clearly, multicenter, large-scale, randomized, controlled trials are needed to investigate the efficacy of IHC and IHHC on blood pressure in individuals with hypertension. In addition, studies are needed to define the optimal antihypertensive dose and treatment regimen and to compare specifically the antihypertensive effect of IHC and with that of IHHC. Finally, no information is available to aid in patient selection or exclusion for antihypertensive therapy with IHC or IHHC.

11.5 Conclusions

Reports have consistently shown that hypobaric and normobaric IHC and IHHC reduce BP in hypertensive patients and patients with comorbidities. The antihypertensive mechanisms of IHC and IHHC include increased production of NO, anti-inflammatory action, increased activity and expression of antioxidant enzymes, suppressed basal and stress-induced sympathetic activation, and increased water and salt excretion. Uncertainties remain about the optimal dose, treatment regimen, and duration of the antihypertensive effect of IHC and IHHC.

Acknowledgment

This publication was a part of the State Assignment of the Institute of General Pathology and Pathophysiology # FGFU-2022-0011, "Identification of significant bio-indicators for various disorders of body function" and the State Assignment of the Moscow Centre for Research and Practice in Medical Rehabilitation, Restorative and Sports Medicine # 123041300012-28.04.2023, "Optimization of individual programs for complex rehabilitation of patients with various somatic pathologies."

Abbreviations

ACE	angiotensin-converting enzyme
AH	arterial hypertension
Ang	angiotensin
BP	blood pressure
cGMP	cyclic guanosine monophosphate
eNOS	endothelial NO synthase
GMP	guanosine monophosphate
HSP	heat shock protein
IHC	intermittent hypoxia conditioning
IHHC	intermittent hypoxia-hyperoxia conditioning
NO	nitric oxide.

References

1. Serebrovskaya TV, Manukhina EB, Smith ML, Downey HF, Mallet RT. *Intermittent hypoxia: cause of or therapy for systemic hypertension?* Exp Biol Med (Maywood). 2008. **233**: 627–650.
2. Seravalle G, Grassi G. *Sleep apnea and hypertension*. High Blood Press Cardiovasc Prev. 2022. **29**: 23–31.
3. NCD Risk Factor Collaboration (NCD-RisC). *Worldwide trends in hypertension prevalence and progress in treatment and control from 1990 to 2019: A pooled analysis of 1201 population-representative studies with 104 million participants.* Lancet. 2021. **398**: 957–980.
4. Shalaeva EV, Messerli FH. *What is resistant arterial hypertension?* Blood Press. 2023. **32**: 2185457.
5. Polaczyk M, et al. *Multiple drug intolerance in patients with arterial hypertension: prevalence and determining factors.* Pol Arch Intern Med. 2023 **133**: 16399.
6. Meerson FZ, et al. *[Preventive effect of preliminary adaptation to high [altitude] hypoxia on the development of DOC-salt hypertension in rats].* Kardiologiia. 1971. **11**: 14–22. Russian.

7. Katiukhin VN, Shliakhto EV, Shuĭskaia GA. *[Effect of discontinuous high-altitude barotherapy on the hemodynamics in arterial hypertension]*. Kardiologiia. 1979. **19**: 107–108. Russian.

8. Aia C, Evgen'eva IA, Karash IuM. *[Kinetics of oxygen metabolism in pregnant women with high risk of developing late toxemia during intermittent normo-baric hypoxia]*. Akush Ginekol (Mosk). 1989. **5**: 17–20. Russian.

9. Evgen'eva IA, Karash IuM, Aia C. *[Preventive use of intermittent normobaric hypoxic hypoxia in pregnant women at high risk of developing late toxicosis]*. Akush Ginekol (Mosk). 1989. **6**: 50–53. Russian.

10. Potievskaia VI, Aia C. *[Effect of intermittent normobaric hypoxia on dynamics of disease state in patients with hypertension]*. Fiziol Zh 1992. **38**: 53–57. Russian.

11. Aleshin IA, et al. *[The nondrug treatment of hypertension patients by their adaptation to periodic hypoxia in a barochamber]*. Ter Arkh. 1993. **65**: 23–29. Russian.

12. Vorob'ev LP, Chizhov AIA, Potievskaia VI. *[The evaluation of the efficacy of adaptation to intermittent normobaric hypoxia as a method for treating hyper-tension]*. Vopr Kurortol Fizioter Lech Fiz Kult. 1993 **5**: 9–12. Russian.

13. Vorob'ev LP, Chizhov AIA, Potievskaia VI. *[The possibilities of using intermit-tent normobaric hypoxia for treating hypertension patients]*. Ter Arkh. 1994. **66**: 12–15. Russian.

14. Simonenko VB, et al. *[Effects of adaptation to intermittent normobaric hypoxia on the results of 24-hour monitoring of arterial pressure in hypertensive patients]*. Klin Med (Mosk). 2003 **81**: 22–25. Russian.

15. Mukharliamov Fiu, et al. *[Interval hypoxic training in arterial hypertension]*. Vopr Kurortol Fizioter Lech Fiz Kult. 2006 **2**: 5–6. Russian.

16. Tin'kov AN, Konstantinova OD, Kshniaseva SK. *[Efficacy of hypobaric hypoxia in the treatment of arterial hypertension in postmenopausal women]*. Ter Arkh. 2011. **83**: 16–19. Russian.

17. Lyamina NP, et al. *Normobaric hypoxia conditioning reduces blood pressure and normalizes nitric oxide synthesis in patients with arterial hypertension*. J Hypertens. 2011. **11**: 2265–2272.

18. Muangritdech N, et al. *Hypoxic training improves blood pressure, nitric oxide and hypoxia-inducible factor-1 alpha in hypertensive patients*. Eur J Appl Physiol. 2020 **120**: 1815–1826.

19. Glazachev OS, et al. *Safety and efficacy of intermittent hypoxia conditioning as a new rehabilitation / secondary prevention strategy for patients with cardiovas-cular diseases: A systematic review and meta-analysis*. Curr Cardiol Rev. 2021. **17**: e051121193317.

20. Edwards JJ, et al. *Exercise training and resting blood pressure: A large-scale pairwise and network meta-analysis of randomized controlled trials*. Br J Sports Med. 2023. **57**: 1335–1336.

21. Lizamore CA, Stoner L, Kathiravel Y. *Does intermittent hypoxic exposure enhance the cardioprotective effect of exercise in an inactive population?* Front Physiol. 2022. **13**: 1005113.

22. Behrendt T, et al. *Influence of acute and chronic intermittent hypoxic-hyperoxic exposure prior to aerobic exercise on cardiovascular risk factors in geriatric patients-a randomized controlled trial*. Front Physiol. 2022. **13**: 1043536.

23. Burtscher M, et al. *Intermittent hypoxia increases exercise tolerance in elderly men with and without coronary artery disease.* Int J Cardiol. 2004. **96**: 247–254.

24. Shatilo VB, et al. *Effects of intermittent hypoxia training on exercise performance, hemodynamics, and ventilation in healthy senior men.* High Alt Med Biol. 2008. **9**: 43–52.

25. Korkushko OV, Shatilo VB, Ishchuk VA. *[Effectiveness of intermittent normabaric hypoxic trainings in elderly patients with coronary artery disease].* Adv Gerontol. 2010. **23**: 476–482. Russian.

26. Kong Z, Zang Y, Hu Y. *Normobaric hypoxia training causes more weight loss than normoxia training after a 4-week residential camp for obese young adults.* Sleep Breath. 2014. **18**: 591–597.

27. Costalat G, et al. *Intermittent hypoxia revisited: A promising non-pharmaceutical strategy to reduce cardio-metabolic risk factors?* Sleep Breath. 2018. **22**: 267–271.

28. Chacaroun S, et al. *Cardiovascular and metabolic responses to passive hypoxic conditioning in overweight and mildly obese individuals.* Am J Physiol Regul Integr Comp Physiol. 2020. **319**: R211–R222.

29. Panza GS, et al. *Daily exposure to mild intermittent hypoxia reduces blood pressure in male patients with obstructive sleep apnea and hypertension.* Am J Respir Crit Care Med. 2022. **205**: 949–958.

30. Glazachev OS, et al. *[Interval hypoxic-hyperoxic training in the treatment of the metabolic syndrome].* Eksp Klin Gastroenterol. 2010. 7: 51–56. Russian.

31. Dudnik E, Zagaynaya E, Glazachev OS, Susta D. *Intermittent hypoxia-hyperoxia conditioning improves cardiorespiratory fitness in older comorbid cardiac outpatients without hematological changes: A randomized controlled trial.* High Alt Med Biol. 2018 **19**: 339–343.

32. Bestavashvili A, Glazachev O, Bestavashvili A, Suvorov A, Zhang Y, Zhang X, Rozhkov A, Kuznetsova N, Pavlov C, Glushenkov D, Kopylov P. *Intermittent hypoxic-hyperoxic exposures effects in patients with metabolic syndrome: Correction of cardiovascular and metabolic profile.* Biomedicines. 2022 **10**: 566.

33. Afsar B, Afsar RE. *Hypoxia-inducible factors and essential hypertension: Narrative review of experimental and clinical data.* Pharmacol Rep. 2023. **75**: 861–875.

34. Robinson MA, et al. *Oxygen-dependent regulation of nitric oxide production by inducible nitric oxide synthase.* Free Radic Biol Med. 2011. **51**: 1952–1965.

35. Li G, et al. *Up-regulation of neuronal nitric oxide synthase expression by cobalt chloride through a HIF-1α mechanism in neuroblastoma cells.* Neuromolecular Med. 2015. 17: 443–453.

36. Coulet F, et al. *Identification of hypoxia-response element in the human endothelial nitric-oxide synthase gene promoter.* J Biol Chem. 2003. 278: 46230–46240.

37. Macdonald WA, Hool LC. *The effect of acute hypoxia on excitability in the heart and the L-type calcium channel as a therapeutic target.* Curr Drug Discov Technol. 2008. 5:302–311.

38. Lin S, et al. *Sustained endothelial nitric-oxide synthase activation requires capacitative Ca^{2+} entry.* J Biol Chem. 2000. **275**: 17979–17985.

39. Lundberg JO, Weitzberg E. *NO-synthase independent NO generation in mammals.* Biochem Biophys Res Commun. 2010. **396**: 39–45.

40. Almgren CM, Olson LE. *Moderate hypoxia increases heat shock protein 90 expression in excised rat aorta.* J Vasc Res. 1999. **36**: 363–371.

41. Garcia-Cardena G, Fan R, Shah V, Sorrentino R, Cirino G, Papapetropoulos A, Sessa WC. *Dynamic activation of endothelial nitric oxide synthase by HSP90.* Nature 1998. **392**: 821–824.
42. Cummins EP, Taylor CT. *Hypoxia-responsive transcription factors.* Pflugers Arch. 2005. **450**: 363–371.
43. Pautz A, et al. *Regulation of the expression of inducible nitric oxide synthase.* Nitric Oxide. 2010. **23**: 75–93.
44. Beckman JS, Koppenol WH. *Nitric oxide, superoxide, and peroxynitrite: The good, the bad, and ugly.* Am J Physiol. 1996. **271**: C1424–C1437.
45. Manukhina EB, et al. *Production and storage of nitric oxide in adaptation to hypoxia.* Nitric Oxide. 1999. **3**: 393–401.
46. Richardson DR, Lok HC. *The nitric oxide-iron interplay in mammalian cells: Transport and storage of dinitrosyl iron complexes.* Biochim Biophys Acta. 2008. **1780**: 638–651.
47. Sazontova TG, Arkhipenko YuV. *Membranoprotective effects of adaptation in the heart and skeletal muscles.* In Hargens A, Takeda N, Signal PK, Eds. *Adaptation Biology and Medicine. Volume 4: Current Concepts.* New Delhi: Narosa, pp. 112–123, 2005.
48. Dhakshinamoorthy S, Porter AG. *Nitric oxide-induced transcriptional up-regulation of protective genes by Nrf2 via the antioxidant response element counteracts apoptosis of neuroblastoma cells.* J Biol Chem. 2004. **279**: 20096–20107.
49. Fukai T, et al. *Regulation of the vascular extracellular superoxide dismutase by nitric oxide and exercise training.* J Clin Invest. 2000. **105**: 1631–1639.
50. Xu KY, et al. *Nitric oxide protects cardiac sarcolemmal membrane enzyme function and ion active transport against ischemia-induced inactivation.* J Biol Chem. 2003. **278**: 41798–41803.
51. Takahashi K et al. *Expression of heme oxygenase isozyme mRNAs in the human brain and induction of heme oxygenase-1 by nitric oxide donors.* J Neurochem. 1996. **67**: 482–489.
52. Xu Q, Hu Y, Kleindienst R, Wick G. *Nitric oxide induces heat-shock protein 70 expression in vascular smooth muscle cells via activation of heat shock factor 1.* J Clin Invest. 1997. **100**: 1089–1097.
53. Mosser DD, et al. *Role of the human heat shock protein hsp70 in protection against stress-induced apoptosis.* Mol Cell Biol. 1997, **17**: 5317–5327.
54. Manucha W. *HSP70 family in the renal inflammatory response.* Inflamm Allergy Drug Targets. 2014. **13**: 235–240.
55. Mollace V, et al. *Modulation of prostaglandin biosynthesis by nitric oxide and nitric oxide donors.* Pharmacol Rev. 2005. **57**: 217–252.
56. Kim SF. *The nitric oxide-mediated regulation of prostaglandin signaling in medicine.* Vitam Horm. 2014. **96**: 211–245.
57. Ignarro LJ. *Biosynthesis and metabolism of endothelium-derived nitric oxide.* Annu Rev Toxicol. 1990. **30**: 535–560.
58. Bredt DS, Snyder SH. *Nitric oxide, a physiological messenger molecule.* Annu Rev Biochem. 1954. **63**: 175–195.
59. Waldron GJ, Cole WC. *Activation of vascular smooth muscle K+ channels by endothelium-derived relaxing factors.* Clin Exp Pharmacol Physiol. 1999. **26**: 180–184.

60. Cohen MV, Yang XM, Downey JM. *Nitric oxide is a preconditioning mimetic and cardioprotectant and is the basis of many available infarct-sparing strategies.* Cardiovasc Res. 2006. **70**: 231–239.
61. Gao L, et al. *Facilitation of chronic intermittent hypobaric hypoxia on carotid sinus baroreflex in anesthetized rats.* Chin J Physiol. 2012. **55**: 62–70.
62. Mónica FZ, Bian K, Murad F. *The endothelium-dependent nitric oxide-cgmp pathway.* Adv Pharmacol. 2016. **77**: 1–27.
63. Cooke JP. *NO and angiogenesis.* Atheroscler Suppl. 2003. **4**: 53–60.
64. Manukhina EB, et al. *Intermittent hypoxia training protects cerebrovascular function in Alzheimer's disease.* Exp Biol Med 2016. **241**: 1351–1363.
65. Krzemińska J, Wronka M, Młynarska E, Franczyk B, and Rysz J. *Arterial hypertension-oxidative stress and inflammation.* Antioxidants (Basel). 2022. **11**: 172.
66. González-Candia A, et al. *Cardioprotective antioxidant and anti-inflammatory mechanisms induced by intermittent hypobaric hypoxia.* Antioxidants (Basel). 2022. **11**:1043.
67. Chen H, et al. *Chronic intermittent hypobaric hypoxia decreases high blood pressure by stabilizing the vascular renin-angiotensin system in spontaneously hypertensive rats.* Front Physiol. 2021. **12**: 639454.
68. Rotariu D, et al. *Oxidative stress: Complex pathological issues concerning the hallmark of cardiovascular and metabolic disorders.* Biomed Pharmacother. 2022. **152**: 113238.
69. Gonchar O, Mankovska I. *Moderate hypoxia/hyperoxia attenuates acute hypoxia-induced oxidative damage and improves antioxidant defense in lung mitochondria.* Acta Physiol Hung. 2012. **99**: 436–446.
70. Mallet RT, et al. *Cardioprotection by intermittent hypoxia conditioning: Evidence, mechanisms, and therapeutic potential.* Am J Physiol Heart Circ Physiol. 2018. **315**: H216–H232.
71. Herrera EA, et al. *Ω3 supplementation and intermittent hypobaric hypoxia induce cardioprotection enhancing antioxidant mechanisms in adult rats.* Mar Drugs. 2015. **13**: 838–860.
72. Aguilar M, et al. *Mechanisms of cardiovascular protection associated with intermittent hypobaric hypoxia exposure in a rat model: Role of oxidative stress.* Int J Mol Sci. 2018. **19**: 366.
73. Susta D, et al. *Redox homeostasis in humans exposed to intermittent hypoxia-normoxia and to intermittent hypoxia-hyperoxia.* High Alt Med Biol. 2020. **21**: 45–51.
74. Melin A, Fauchier L, Dubuis E, Obert P, Bonnet P. *Heart rate variability in rats acclimatized to high altitude.* High Alt Med Biol. 2003. **3**: 375–387.
75. Guan Y., et al. *Chronic intermittent hypobaric hypoxia antagonizes renal vascular hypertension by enhancement of vasorelaxation via activating BKCa.* Life Sci. 2016. **157**: 74–81.
76. Henley WN, Bellush LL, Tucker A. *Sympathetic and metabolic correlates of hypoxic moderation of spontaneous hypertension in the rat.* Proc Soc Exp Biol Med. 1989. **192**: 114–120.
77. Kitada K, Nishiyama A. *Revisiting blood pressure and body fluid status.* Clin Sci (Lond). 2023. **137**: 755–767.

78. Potievskaia VI. *[Mechanisms of therapeutic and preventive effects of adaptation to hypoxia in arterial hypertension]*. Fiziol Zh. 1993. **2–3**: 94–107. Russian.
79. Meerson FZ, Barbarash NA, Gia D, Prokina NS. *Rol' natriǔureza v profilakticheskom éffekte adaptatsii k gipoksii pri nasledstvennoǐ gipertonii [Role of natriuresis in the prophylactic effect of adaptation to hypoxia in hereditary hypertension]*. Kardiologiia. 1981. 7: 25–32. Russian.

12

INTERMITTENT HYPOXIA EFFECTIVE SYSTEMIC MODALITY FOR CARDIAC REHABILITATION

Robert T. Mallet, Konrad Mayer and Lei Xi

12.1 Benefits and limitations of conventional cardiac rehabilitation programs

Cardiac rehabilitation fosters recovery from myocardial infarction (MI), cardiac surgery, or other acute events and lowers cardiovascular morbidity and mortality [1, 2]. Rehabilitation programs combine lifestyle education, counseling, and supervised physical activity to optimize recovery of cardiac function and ward off additional cardiac events. Cardiac rehabilitation's short-term benefits include increased functional capacity and decreased pathophysiological and psychological manifestations of chronic heart disease [3]. Over the long term, cardiac rehabilitation may slow the progression of coronary artery disease (CAD), lowering the risk of myocardial reinfarction and sudden cardiac death [4].

Despite its efficacy, participation in cardiac rehabilitation is persistently low. Only 14–35% of heart attack survivors in the United States receive cardiac rehabilitation [5], and women are only half as likely as men to complete rehabilitation [6]. Mental and physical disabilities, heart failure, pulmonary disease, or unwillingness to exercise are potential roadblocks to cardiac rehabilitation. For such patients, an alternative regimen is essential to promote cardiovascular health. Mounting evidence supports cyclic breathing of moderately hypoxic gas, alternated with room air (intermittent hypoxia: IH) or moderately hyperoxic gas (intermittent hypoxia–hyperoxia: IHH) as a solitary modality for cardiac rehabilitation or a co-treatment to augment the benefits of physical exercise.

DOI: 10.4324/9781003402879-18

12.2 Hypoxia–normoxia (IHC) and hypoxia–hyperoxia (IHHC) programs improve fitness and endurance

The benefits of IHC include improved exercise tolerance, prolonged time to exhaustion [7], and increased cardiac parasympathetic activity, which slows heart rate and limits tachyarrhythmias [8, 9]. In healthy human subjects, 60-min IHC sessions increased heart rate variability, indicating enhanced parasympathetic control of cardiac rhythm, while 60-min sustained hypoxia lowered heart rate variability [10].

Saeed et al. studied older adults (ages 42–70) with chronic, stable heart failure with reduced left ventricular ejection fraction (LVEF), who completed ten 3–4 h sessions of hypoxia equivalent to 2,700 m altitude. Four weeks later, exercise tolerance, skeletal muscle strength, and quality of life score were increased versus the respective baselines. Hypoxia training also effected persistent increases in LVEF and peak O_2 consumption (VO_{2peak}), a measure of cardiopulmonary fitness [11]. In elderly patients with CAD, a 15-session IHHC regimen (5–7 cycles/session alternating 4–6 min at 10–12% FIO_2 and 3 min at 30–35% FIO_2) improved quality of life and exercise tolerance, lowered the incidence and severity of angina pectoris, and raised VO_{2peak} by 3.5 ml $O_2 \cdot min^{-1} \cdot kg^{-1}$ [12], an increase auguring favorable outcomes [13].

In ischemic heart disease patients with angina pectoris, a 3-week, 15-session IHHC program increased VO_{2peak}/kg and patient-perceived quality of life. Notably, VO_{2peak}/kg remained elevated one month after IHHC [14]. In a meta-analysis of eight clinical studies, IHHC consistently increased exercise tolerance and VO_{2peak} [15]. Thus, IHC and IHHC programs proved efficacious and safe in healthy adults [10, 16] and patients with cardiovascular disease [11, 12, 14, 15].

Dudnik et al. [17] compared cardiorespiratory fitness in CAD patients 1–2 weeks after an 8-week physical exercise program or 4 weeks after a 5-week, 15-session IHHC regimen alternating 4–6 min hypoxia (11–12% FIO_2) and 3 min hyperoxia (33% FIO_2) for 5–7 cycles/session. IHHC increased VO_{2peak} by 43%, but the exercise program produced a nonsignificant upward trend. IHHC improved cardiorespiratory fitness at least as effectively as physical exercise in CAD patients without altering blood O_2-carrying capacity [17]. These findings support the application of IHHC to rehabilitate patients who cannot exercise.

12.3 Combining intermittent hypoxia with exercise

Because IHC and IHHC are administered noninvasively, for example via facemask or altitude chamber [18], they are readily applied during exercise. The possibility that concurrent IHC or IHHC may accentuate the benefits of physical exercise was tested in healthy subjects undertaking cycling training [19, 20] and in elderly physiotherapy patients [21, 22]. Wang et al. studied combined hypoxia and cycling exercise in healthy, sedentary men [19, 20] exercising at 50% of maximum workload for 30 min/day, 5 days/week for 4 weeks while breathing 21% or 15% O_2. Before training, exercising while breathing 12% O_2 lowered cardiac output as well as exercising muscle blood flow and O_2 delivery, but hypoxia-enhanced physiotherapy prevented these effects [20].

The benefits of complementary IHHC on physical fitness and cognitive function were assessed in elderly adults undergoing multimodal physiotherapy [21]. Combined IHHC and physiotherapy increased cognitive function and effected a greater improvement in functional exercise capacity [21], although, in a subsequent study, IHHC did not augment perceived health and mobility versus physiotherapy alone [22].

Glazachev et al. [23] studied patients with clinically stable CAD who completed a 15-session IHHC program alternating 3 min 10–12% FIO_2 and 3 min 30–35% FIO_2 for 5–7 cycles/session. The IHHC regimen effected cardiorespiratory and hemodynamic improvements which were more substantial one month later. Exercise cessation due to angina pectoris was delayed appreciably after IHHC, and even further at one-month follow-up, while self-assessed angina burden decreased. The IHHC program lowered arterial pressure and resting heart rate and increased LVEF and VO_{2peak}.

Nowak-Lis et al. studied patients recovering from MI and coronary angioplasty [24] who completed 24 sessions of 40 min interval cycling while breathing room air or mildly hypoxic (16.8% FIO_2) gas. Relative to room air exercise, the hypoxia exercise regimen increased exercise duration, VO_{2peak}, maximum heart rate, and systolic arterial pressure (SAP) during exercise testing, without altering resting arterial pressures or heart rate. Ultrasonography revealed a modest increase in LVEF when hypoxia was added to the exercise regimen.

12.4 Intermittent hypoxia augments muscle perfusion, cardiac remodeling, and capillarization

Hypoxia elicits adaptations that increase O_2 delivery to skeletal muscle and myocardium. At the cellular level, hypoxia mobilizes hypoxia-inducible factor-1 (HIF-1), a powerful transcription factor controlling an extensive gene program that increases tolerance to decreased O_2 availability (Figure 12.1) [25]. HIF-1 activates the synthesis of erythropoietin, vascular endothelial growth factor (VEGF) membrane glucose transporters, and glycolytic enzymes. Preclinical and clinical evidence implicates these adaptations in IHC- and IHHC-induced cardioprotection.

Xu et al. evaluated the impact of hypoxia on myocardial remodeling and revascularization in a rat MI model [26]. When initiated after 7 days of coronary artery ligation, 4 weeks of hypobaric (5,000 m) hypoxia (6 h/day)

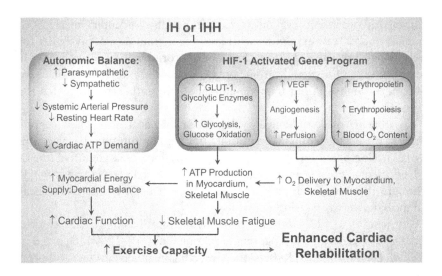

FIGURE 12.1   Mechanisms whereby intermittent hypoxia–normoxia (IH) and intermittent hypoxia–hyperoxia (IHH) exposures increase exercise capacity and effectiveness of cardiac rehabilitation. IHC/IHHC shifts autonomic balance in favor of parasympathetic activity, which, by decreasing heart rate and systemic arterial pressure, lowers myocardial energy demand. IHC/IHHC also activates HIF-1-driven expression of genes encoding glucose transporter 1 (GLUT-1) and the entire glycolytic enzyme sequence, increasing the capacity for ATP-generating glucose catabolism in myocardium and skeletal muscle. HIF-1 also activates genes encoding vascular endothelial growth factor (VEGF), which promotes angiogenesis, and erythropoietin. Erythropoietin and VEGF increase O_2 delivery to myocardium and skeletal muscle to support oxidative phosphorylation. Improved ATP supply:demand balance improves cardiac mechanical function and skeletal muscle contractile function, thereby increasing the patient's capacity for physical rehabilitation.

suppressed fibrosis and cardiomyocyte apoptosis in the ischemic myocardium, decreased infarct volume by 25–30%, attenuated left ventricular dilation, and partially preserved LVEF. Hypoxia doubled VEGF content and increased capillary density by 60% in the peri-infarct zone but increased neither VEGF nor capillary density in non-infarcted hearts. The contributions of angiogenesis to improved cardiac performance and cardioprotection were not determined. In rabbits, a similar hypobaric (4,000 m) hypoxia program (1 h/day, 5 days/week for 4 weeks) also begun at 7 days after initiation of coronary artery occlusion reduced infarct volume by 28% and attenuated increases in left ventricular end-systolic and end-diastolic diameters and decrease in LVEF [27]. Coronary occlusion alone increased serum VEGF by 51%, while hypoxia increased circulating VEGF by 112%. In rats and rabbits, hypobaric hypoxia initiated after a week of coronary occlusion augmented VEGF activity and myocardial capillarization, partially preserved LVEF, and attenuated infarct volume and cardiac remodeling.

Sedentary men underwent cycling training while breathing 15% or 21% O_2 for 30 min/day, 5 days/week for 5 weeks. Compared with normoxic training, hypoxia-enhanced training produced greater increases in aerobic capacity, cardiac output, and O_2 delivery to the exercising muscle [19]. Hypoxic training augmented circulating endothelial and cardiomyocyte progenitor cells and their proliferative capacities and increased circulating pro-angiogenic factors stromal cell-derived factor-1 and matrix metalloproteinase-9. After normoxic training, acute exercise while breathing 12% O_2 lowered cardiac output and perfusion of the active muscle, but hypoxia-enhanced training maintained cardiac output and muscle perfusion during acute hypoxic exercise [20].

Del Pilar Valle et al. [28] evaluated the long-term impact of hypobaric hypoxia training (14 weekly sessions of 4,200 m simulated altitude) on myocardial perfusion in six older men (≥53 years), all lifelong lowlanders with severe, stable CAD. Six months later, myocardial blood flow assessed by ^{99}Tc Sestamibi imaging was increased, and hypoperfusion stress score lowered, versus pre-training. None of the men showed evidence of impaired myocardial perfusion. Thus, hypobaric hypoxia effected persistent improvements in myocardial perfusion.

Elderly adults often are anemic, increasing their risk of falling and limiting their exercise capacity and cardiorespiratory fitness [29]. IHC programs may offer a nonexercise alternative to increase hemoglobin [30, 31] and tissue O_2 delivery [32] via erythropoiesis. Indeed, brief exposures to 10–14% FIO_2 alternated with 21% FIO_2 increased blood oxygenated hemoglobin and red cell and plasma volumes, paralleling increased VO_{2max} in sedentary patients with CAD [33] or chronic obstructive pulmonary disease [34]. IHC and IHHC effect moderate, gradual increases in hematocrit and blood hemoglobin [31], thereby avoiding blood hyperviscosity.

12.5 Intermittent hypoxia and cardiac risk factors: hyperglycemia, hyperlipidemia

Diabetes mellitus and its associated hyperglycemia and inflammation are major cardiovascular disease risk factors. Type 2 diabetics generally exercise less than their nondiabetic counterparts, so the possibility that IHC/IHHC may provide an alternative means of improving glycemic control merits attention [30]. In prediabetic older adults (ages 48–70), a nine-session (4 cycles of 5 min 12% O_2 and 5 min room air) IHC program lowered fasting serum glucose and improved glucose tolerance, especially a month later, and blunted tachycardic and pressor responses to acute hypoxia [16]. In a subsequent study [35], prediabetic older adults completed 15 IHC or IHHC sessions (4 cycles of 5 min 12% O_2 and either 5 min room air or 3 min 33% O_2). IHC and IHHC attenuated O_2 desaturation during acute 12% O_2 exposure and lowered serum glucose during fasting and at 2 h of oral glucose tolerance test.

Although the mechanisms mediating the improved glucose management effected by IHC/IHHC are not yet clear, activation of HIF-1 and its hypoxia-adaptive gene program is likely to be pivotal (Figure 12.1). HIF-1 activates genes encoding glucose transporter GLUT1 [36, 37] and the complete glycolytic enzyme sequence [38, 39]. Increased glucose uptake provides a substrate for glycogen synthesis and the glycolytic machinery. Indeed, IHC increased skeletal muscle glycogen content in diabetic rats [40]. Increased glycogen could enhance exercise capacity by augmenting the fuel supply for anaerobic glycolysis in exercising muscle (Figure 12.1).

A 4-week program of twice-daily 3-h swim sessions while breathing 14% O_2 increased myocardial glycogen content by 67% in male rats, while swim exercise alone increased glycogen by 45% [36]. Hypoxia, swimming, or the combination increased myocardial content of glucose transporter GLUT4 by 40–70%, but only hypoxia increased myocardial GLUT1 content. Thus, moderate hypoxia combined with swimming exercise increased myocardial capacity to import and store glucose more effectively than swimming alone.

Intermittent hypoxia also may help manage another cardiovascular risk factor, hyperlipidemia. Tin'kov and Aksenov [41] applied 22 daily 3 h bouts of moderate hypobaric hypoxia to men with hyperlipidemia and CAD who had survived an MI or had experienced cardiac ischemic episodes. IHC lowered serum total and low-density lipoprotein (LDL) cholesterol, increased high-density lipoprotein (HDL) cholesterol, and lowered the coefficient of atherogenicity [(total cholesterol – HDL cholesterol)/HDL cholesterol]; these effects lasted 6 months before subsiding.

Costalat et al. evaluated serum lipids and carbohydrates in overweight and obese adults (ages 56 ± 10 years) completing 10 IHC sessions of cyclic hypoxia (FIO_2 10%)–reoxygenation producing 80% mean arterial O_2 saturation for 70 min. Although the first IHC session lowered serum glucose and increased serum lactate, both returned to their baselines by the 10th session. In contrast, reductions in serum LDL concentration and LDL/HDL ratio were sustained over the entire IHC program, while SAP declined by ~10 mmHg [42].

In prediabetic older adults, both IHC and IHHC lowered serum total and LDL cholesterol, and these benefits persisted at least one month after IHC or IHHC [35]. In CAD patients [23], an IHHC program that alleviated exercise-induced angina and improved cardiopulmonary and hemodynamic function lowered serum glucose, total cholesterol, and LDL concentrations one month post-IHHC versus the respective baselines. A 15-session IHHC program ameliorated lipid profile and inflammation biomarkers in adults with metabolic syndrome [43]. A meta-analysis of 38 clinical hypoxia studies revealed that IHC and IHHC improved quality of life, cognitive function, and physical performance; increased red cell mass; decreased SAP; and lowered serum glucose, LDL, total cholesterol, and inflammatory factors [44].

Although the preponderance of clinical evidence indicates metabolic benefits of IHC/IHHC training, the evidence is not unequivocal. In overweight or obese adults, neither 24 sessions of 60 min sustained hypoxia (FIO$_2$ 11±1%) nor IHC (7 cycles of 5 min 10±1% O$_2$ and 3 min room air) affected body mass index or serum concentrations of glucose, lipoproteins, nitric oxide (NO) metabolites, or oxidative stress biomarker malondialdehyde [45]. Why hypoxia failed to improve glycemic control, normalize serum lipids and lipoproteins, and boost NO production is unclear. Studies comparing the effects of IHC/IHHC in lean versus overweight or obese subjects are urgently needed.

12.6 Intermittent hypoxia for cardiac rehabilitation: limitations and safety considerations

Despite their myriad benefits in patients with heart disease, IHC and IHHC may be stressful to the O$_2$-dependent myocardium. Consequently, IHC is not risk-free, particularly during the early post-MI period [46]. Safety concerns include systemic hypotension due to hypoxia-induced vasodilation, heightened risk of hemoconcentration and thrombosis, and cardiac rhythm disturbances. Li et al. studied the impact of moderate hypoxia combined with running exercise on circulating antioxidants and oxidative stress biomarkers in young adult marathoners during alternating high- and moderate-intensity running while breathing either 21% or 14.4% FIO$_2$ [47]. Serum antioxidant capacity fell more sharply and cardiac troponin I increased only after hypoxic exercise, indicating that moderate hypoxia intensified cardiac stress during dynamic exercise. These findings in healthy, endurance-conditioned athletes underscore the importance of carefully designing cardiac rehabilitation programs combining exercise and hypoxia to limit myocardial demand in patients recovering from adverse cardiac events.

On the other hand, the moderate hypoxia of IHC and IHHC programs is likely safer than more protracted or severe hypoxia episodes. In elderly patients with CAD completing 15 IHHC sessions, adverse effects including dyspnea, dizziness, palpitations, and headache were moderate and uncommon, affecting only 4 of the 27 patients, and were relieved by slightly increasing FIO$_2$ without interrupting the sessions [23]. Angina occurred in only 6 of 408 sessions [23]. Importantly, the IHHC regimen was well-tolerated and produced no adverse outcomes [12]. Mild hypoxia (16.8% FIO$_2$) also proved to be safe and well-tolerated in post-MI patients with stable CAD undergoing cycling exercise for cardiac rehabilitation [24].

12.7 Future directions

Despite mounting evidence that IHC and IHHC enhance cardiac rehabilitation, important questions remain regarding their practical application. The possibility that combining physical exercise with IHC/IHHC might effect more rapid or robust cardiac recovery, thereby attaining rehabilitation objectives in fewer sessions, merits attention, as does the concept that IHC/IHHC programs might bridge the patient from major cardiac events to physical rehabilitation. Timely initiation of cardiac rehabilitation is associated with increased program adherence [48] and improved cardiovascular recovery [49]. However, MI survivors, especially those with significant comorbidities or physical frailty [50], may be unable to exercise at first. IHC/IHHC, which can be administered with the patient comfortably seated, is less demanding than conventional cardiac rehabilitation, helping patients progress until they can undertake physical exercise.

Abbreviations

CAD	coronary artery disease
FIO_2	fraction of inspired O_2
HDL	high-density lipoprotein
GLUT	glucose transporter
HIF	hypoxia-inducible factor
IHC	intermittent hypoxia conditioning
IHHC	intermittent hypoxia-hyperoxia conditioning
LDL	low-density lipoprotein
LVEF	left ventricular ejection fraction
MI	myocardial infarction
SAP	systolic arterial pressure
VEGF	vascular endothelial growth factor
VO_{2peak}	peak whole-body O_2 consumption.

References

1. Hammill, B.G., et al., *Relationship between cardiac rehabilitation and long-term risks of death and myocardial infarction among elderly Medicare beneficiaries.* Circulation, 2010. **121**: p. 63–70.
2. Martin, B.J., et al., *Cardiac rehabilitation attendance and outcomes in coronary artery disease patients.* Circulation, 2012. **126**: p. 677–687.
3. Taylor, R.S., H.M. Dalal, and S.T.J. McDonagh, *The role of cardiac rehabilitation in improving cardiovascular outcomes.* Nat Rev Cardiol, 2022. **19**: p. 180–194.
4. Dalal, H.M., P. Doherty, and R.S. Taylor, *Cardiac rehabilitation.* BMJ, 2015. **351**: p. h5000.
5. Balady, G.J., et al., *Referral, enrollment, and delivery of cardiac rehabilitation/ secondary prevention programs at clinical centers and beyond: A presidential advisory from the American Heart Association.* Circulation, 2011. **124**: p. 2951–2960.

6. Resurreccion, D.M., et al., *Reasons for dropout from cardiac rehabilitation programs in women: A qualitative study.* PLoS One, 2018. **13**: p. e0200636.

7. Lizamore, C.A. and M.J. Hamlin, *The use of simulated altitude techniques for beneficial cardiovascular health outcomes in nonathletic, sedentary, and clinical populations: A literature review.* High Alt Med Biol, 2017. **18**: p. 305–321.

8. Dyavanapalli, J., *Novel approaches to restore parasympathetic activity to the heart in cardiorespiratory diseases.* Am J Physiol Heart Circ Physiol, 2020. **319**: p. H1153–H1161.

9. Schomer, A.C., et al., *Vagus nerve stimulation reduces cardiac electrical instability assessed by quantitative T-wave alternans analysis in patients with drug-resistant focal epilepsy.* Epilepsia, 2014. **55**: p. 1996–2002.

10. Chacaroun, S., et al., *Physiological responses to two hypoxic conditioning strategies in healthy subjects.* Front Physiol, 2016. **7**: p. 675.

11. Saeed, O., et al., *Improved exercise performance and skeletal muscle strength after simulated altitude exposure: A novel approach for patients with chronic heart failure.* J Card Fail, 2012. **18**: p. 387–391.

12. Glazachev, O.S., et al., *[Adaptation to dosed hypoxia-hyperoxia as a factor in improving the quality of life of elderly patients with cardiac pathology.].* Adv Gerontol, 2019. **32**: p. 145–151.

13. Myers, J., et al., *Exercise capacity and mortality among men referred for exercise testing.* N Engl J Med, 2002. **346**: p. 793–801.

14. Syrkin, A.L., et al., *[Adaptation to intermittent hypoxia-hyperoxia in the rehabilitation of patients with ischemic heart disease: Exercise tolerance and quality of life].* Kardiologiia, 2017. **57**: p. 10–16.

15. Behrendt, T., et al., *Effects of intermittent hypoxia-hyperoxia on performance- and health-related outcomes in humans: A systematic review.* Sports Med Open, 2022. **8**: p. 70.

16. Serebrovska, T.V., et al., *Intermittent hypoxia training in prediabetes patients: Beneficial effects on glucose homeostasis, hypoxia tolerance and gene expression.* Exp Biol Med (Maywood), 2017. **242**: p. 1542–1552.

17. Dudnik, E., et al., *Intermittent hypoxia-hyperoxia conditioning improves cardiorespiratory fitness in older comorbid cardiac outpatients without hematological changes: A randomized controlled trial.* High Alt Med Biol, 2018. **19**: p. 339–343.

18. Serebrovskaya, T.V. and L. Xi, *Intermittent hypoxia training as non-pharmacologic therapy for cardiovascular diseases: Practical analysis on methods and equipment.* Exp Biol Med (Maywood), 2016. **241**: p. 1708–1723.

19. Wang, J.S., et al., *Hypoxic exercise training improves cardiac/muscular hemodynamics and is associated with modulated circulating progenitor cells in sedentary men.* Int J Cardiol, 2014. **170**: p. 315–323.

20. Wang, J.S., et al., *Effects of normoxic and hypoxic exercise regimens on cardiac, muscular, and cerebral hemodynamics suppressed by severe hypoxia in humans.* J Appl Physiol (1985), 2010. **109**: p. 219–229.

21. Bayer, U., et al., *[Adaptation to intermittent hypoxia-hyperoxia improves cognitive performance and exercise tolerance in elderly].* Adv Gerontol, 2017. **30**: p. 255–261.

22. Bayer, U., et al., *Effects of intermittent hypoxia-hyperoxia on mobility and perceived health in geriatric patients performing a multimodal training intervention: a randomized controlled trial.* BMC Geriatr, 2019. **19**: p. 167.

23. Glazachev, O., et al., *Adaptations following an intermittent hypoxia-hyperoxia training in coronary artery disease patients: A controlled study*. Clin Cardiol, 2017. **40**: p. 370–376.

24. Nowak-Lis, A., et al., *The use of artificial hypoxia in endurance training in patients after myocardial infarction*. Int J Environ Res Public Health, 2021. **18**: p. 1633.

25. Semenza, G.L., *Expression of hypoxia-inducible factor 1: Mechanisms and consequences*. Biochem Pharmacol, 2000. **59**: p. 47–53.

26. Xu, W.Q., et al., *Therapeutic effect of intermittent hypobaric hypoxia on myocardial infarction in rats*. Basic Res Cardiol, 2011. **106**: p. 329–342.

27. Wan, C.X., et al., *Hypoxia training attenuates left ventricular remodeling in rabbit with myocardial infarction*. J Geriatr Cardiol, 2014. **11**: p. 237–244.

28. del Pilar Valle, M., et al., *Improvement of myocardial perfusion in coronary patients after intermittent hypobaric hypoxia*. J Nucl Cardiol, 2006. **13**: p. 69–74.

29. Burtscher, M., *Exercise limitations by the oxygen delivery and utilization systems in aging and disease: Coordinated adaptation and deadaptation of the lung–heart muscle axis—a mini-review*. Gerontology, 2013. **59**: p. 289–296.

30. Leone, R.J. and S. Lalande, *Intermittent hypoxia as a means to improve aerobic capacity in type 2 diabetes*. Med Hypotheses, 2017. **100**: p. 59–63.

31. Tobin, B., G. Costalat, and G.M.C. Renshaw, *Intermittent not continuous hypoxia provoked haematological adaptations in healthy seniors: Hypoxic pattern may hold the key*. Eur J Appl Physiol, 2020. **120**: p. 707–718.

32. Verges, S., et al., *Hypoxic conditioning as a new therapeutic modality*. Front Pediatr, 2015. **3**: p. 58.

33. Burtscher, M., et al., *Intermittent hypoxia increases exercise tolerance in elderly men with and without coronary artery disease*. Int J Cardiol, 2004. **96**: p. 247–254.

34. Burtscher, M., et al., *Intermittent hypoxia increases exercise tolerance in patients at risk for or with mild COPD*. Respir Physiol Neurobiol, 2009. **165**: p. 97–103.

35. Serebrovska, T.V., et al., *Intermittent hypoxia/hyperoxia versus intermittent hypoxia/normoxia: Comparative study in prediabetes*. High Alt Med Biol, 2019. **20**: p. 383–391.

36. Chou, S.W., et al., *Effect of systemic hypoxia on GLUT4 protein expression in exercised rat heart*. Jpn J Physiol, 2004. **54**: p. 357–363.

37. Varela-Guruceaga, M., et al., *Effect of hypoxia on caveolae-related protein expression and insulin signaling in adipocytes*. Mol Cell Endocrinol, 2018. **473**: p. 257–267.

38. Kierans, S.J. and C.T. Taylor, *Regulation of glycolysis by the hypoxia-inducible factor (HIF): Implications for cellular physiology*. J Physiol, 2021. **599**: p. 23–37.

39. Mechlovich, D., et al., *The novel multi-target iron chelator, M30 modulates HIF-1alpha-related glycolytic genes and insulin signaling pathway in the frontal cortex of APP/PS1 Alzheimer's disease mice*. Curr Alzheimer Res, 2014. **11**: p. 119–127.

40. Chen, X., et al., *Intermittent hypoxia maintains glycemia in streptozotocin-induced diabetic rats*. Cell Stress Chaperones, 2016. **21**: p. 515–522.

41. Tin'kov, A.N. and V.A. Aksenov, *Effects of intermittent hypobaric hypoxia on blood lipid concentrations in male coronary heart disease patients*. High Alt Med Biol, 2002. **3**: p. 277–282.

42. Costalat, G., et al., *Intermittent hypoxia revisited: A promising non-pharmaceutical strategy to reduce cardio-metabolic risk factors?* Sleep Breath, 2018. **22**: p. 267–271.

43. Bestavashvili, A.A., et al., *The effects of intermittent hypoxic-hyperoxic exposures on lipid profile and inflammation in patients with metabolic syndrome.* Front Cardiovasc Med, 2021. **8**: p. 700826.

44. Tessema, B., et al., *Effects of intermittent hypoxia in training regimes and in obstructive sleep apnea on aging biomarkers and age-related diseases: A systematic review.* Front Aging Neurosci, 2022. **14**: p. 878278.

45. Chacaroun, S., et al., *Cardiovascular and metabolic responses to passive hypoxic conditioning in overweight and mildly obese individuals.* Am J Physiol Regul Integr Comp Physiol, 2020. **319**: p. R211–R222.

46. Sanchis-Gomar, F., J. Vina, and G. Lippi, *Intermittent hypobaric hypoxia applicability in myocardial infarction prevention and recovery.* J Cell Mol Med, 2012. **16**: p. 1150–1154.

47. Li, F., et al., *The impact of intermittent exercise in a hypoxic environment on redox status and cardiac troponin release in the serum of well-trained marathon runners.* Eur J Appl Physiol, 2016. **116**: p. 2045–2051.

48. Russell, K.L., et al., *Cardiac rehabilitation wait times: Effect on enrollment.* J Cardiopulm Rehabil Prev, 2011. **31**: p. 373–377.

49. Fell, J., V. Dale, and P. Doherty, *Does the timing of cardiac rehabilitation impact fitness outcomes? An observational analysis.* Open Heart, 2016. **3**: p. e000369.

50. Baldasseroni, S., et al., *Predictors of physical frailty improvement in older patients enrolled in a multidisciplinary cardiac rehabilitation program.* Heart Vessels, 2023. **38**: p. 1056–1064.

SECTION 6

13

LOAD-COMPROMISED INDIVIDUALS

Mohammed Ihsan and Olivier Girard

13.1 Introduction

Load-compromised individuals (LCI) represent a diverse clinical population facing challenges in weight-bearing activities due to factors including injuries, medical conditions, or disabilities. This group encompasses individuals with musculoskeletal injuries, arthritis, osteoporosis, neurological disorders, chronic pain, obesity, and other health issues. Conventional exercise programs often prove impractical and may potentially worsen their conditions, risking prolonged physical inactivity and adverse consequences. Therefore, it becomes imperative to explore non-exercise or exercise-complementary therapeutic strategies to enhance functional capacity and overall well-being.

Hypoxic conditioning (HC) emerges as a promising intervention to increase cardiovascular or musculoskeletal intensity without a corresponding elevation in the mechanical load on the locomotor system. HC involves exposure to systemic and/or localized hypoxia, reducing oxygen supply to tissues due to decreased arterial blood O_2 saturation. This exposure can occur at rest (passive) or combined with exercise (active) [1]. While athletes have long utilized training in deprived-O_2 conditions, emerging work demonstrates its potential in clinical and rehabilitation settings. For instance, in obese [2] and geriatric [3] populations, aerobic activity performed in hypoxic conditions (FiO_2 = 14.5–15.3%, simulating ~3,000 m of altitude) can elicit physiological responses comparable to normoxic exercise, despite a 7–25% reduction in external load. Furthermore, localized hypoxia modalities, such as blood flow restriction (BFR), combined with low-load aerobic or resistance exercise (RE), lead to significant muscle hypertrophy and strength gains across various age groups and clinical conditions [4–6]. These findings position HC as

DOI: 10.4324/9781003402879-20

a clinically relevant rehabilitation tool to mitigate mechanical load (i.e., reduced cycling power output or walking/jogging velocity) while preserving the essential physiological stimulus needed for meaningful adaptations. This perspective suggests a potential paradigm shift toward achieving equivalent or greater physiological benefits with reduced mechanical effort, challenging the traditional notion of requiring greater mechanical exertion for enhanced physiological adaptations. This shift holds promise for improved exercise tolerance, increased enjoyment, and improved training compliance compared with conventional programs without HC.

Integrating HC into the exercise regimens of LCIs offers multiple pathways for rehabilitation, health maintenance, and performance enhancement. HC techniques, whether localized or systemic, can be employed passively or in conjunction with RE or aerobic activities (Figure 13.1). Understanding the intricate interplay between HC modalities, their impact on internal and external loads, the stage of rehabilitation, and physiological responses in LCIs enables researchers and healthcare professionals to formulate precise, evidence-based interventions to optimize outcomes. It is imperative for exercise physiologists and sport scientists to explore ways to reduce potentially harmful forces on weight-bearing joints during locomotion tasks. This makes the design of strategies to minimize exercise-induced pain or discomfort an important therapeutic target for LCIs. This chapter aims to provide a proof-of-concept overview of incorporating HC into exercise programs tailored for LCIs.

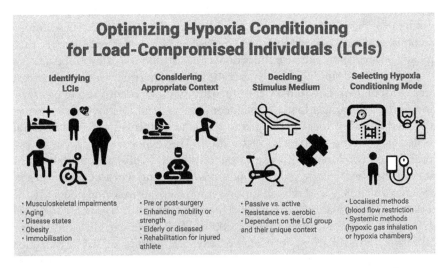

FIGURE 13.1 Overview of the therapeutic application of hypoxia conditioning (HC) considering type of LCI, context (e.g., rehabilitation stage), selection of stimulus medium, and HC mode.

13.2 Passive hypoxia conditioning: Minimal effort, meaningful gains?

Developments in passive HC research reveal a compelling phenomenon where positive clinical outcomes can be realized without engaging in contractile activity. This enables the formulation and delivery of clinical or rehabilitation programs tailored for LCIs, especially those facing movement limitations during post-surgery recovery, patients with neurological conditions, or those with advanced musculoskeletal ailments (e.g., severe arthritis or osteoporosis). Passive HC emerges as a potential solution for these patient groups, helping alleviate some of the deleterious health impacts associated with inactivity. However, the choice between localized or systemic HC delivery requires careful consideration, taking into account the specific rehabilitation stage and characteristics of the patient population.

While the use of systemic whole-body HC has not been firmly established across all patient groups, it has proven effective in several populations. Within passive systemic HC methods, simulated altitude exposure can be administered via normobaric hypoxia chambers or by breathing hypoxic air using valved face masks, typically with hypoxia severity levels of 12–15% FiO_2 [7, 8]. Continuous 1 h exposures using these HC methods have demonstrated improvements in both maximal and submaximal exercise performance in healthy sedentary men following a 4-week (5 sessions per week) treatment period [8]. However, severe HC (i.e., 12% FiO_2) seemed to elevate mean arterial pressure response to exercise and diminish vascular function, possibly due to increased oxidative stress impairing vascular hemodynamics and function [8]. This highlights potential drawbacks of prolonged continuous delivery, especially with severe hypoxia level. Conversely, intermittent delivery (i.e., 5–9 cycles of 3–5 min hypoxic-normoxia breathing intervals), albeit comparable in treatment duration (3 weeks), frequency (5 sessions per week), and hypoxia severity (12–15% FiO_2), has been shown to improve indices of maximal and submaximal exercise capacity. Additionally, it contributes to improvements in blood profile, resting blood pressures, and respiratory function in patients with mild chronic obstructive pulmonary disease [7].

Instead of applying arbitrary % FiO_2 levels, some studies adopt an individualized approach, administering hypoxia intensity based on percentage of O_2 saturation (SpO_2). Short-term treatments (i.e., 7 days) lasting 3 h each while maintaining SpO_2 at 80% have demonstrated increased metabolic rate and a shift in substrate utilization toward lipid-based energy stores [9]. This has implications for promoting weight loss over extended applications in sedentary overweight individuals [9]. Further, Chacaroun et al. [10] compared continuous (~60 min) and intermittent (i.e., 7 cycles of 5-min hypoxia and 3-min normoxia) delivery of hypoxia clamped at SpO_2 levels (i.e., 75%) among class 1 obese individuals, reporting similar improvements in cardiovascular and respiratory indices. This occurred despite the total hypoxic exposure duration during intermittent delivery being ~40% shorter than during continuous delivery [10].

Localized HC, particularly BFR, has shown significant potential as a passive modality for improving musculoskeletal function, especially in various post-surgery recovery scenarios. For instance, continuous BFR (200–240 mmHg) over 10–14 days substantially minimized lower leg muscle atrophy and strength loss in patients recovering from anterior cruciate ligament reconstruction or individuals undergoing 14 days of cast immobilization [11, 12]. Individualized occlusion pressures (e.g., 80% of the patient's SBP) has been recommended to determine appropriate occlusion pressures [13]. This approach, administered over ~11 days, has been shown to minimize muscle atrophy in elderly coma patients admitted to the intensive care unit [14]. However, while higher occlusion pressures are commonly recommended during passive applications [13], even occlusion pressures as low as 50 mmHg were effective in averting the decline in muscle strength and mass. Kubota et al. [15] showed that 5 sets of 5-min BFR cycles interspersed with 3-min recovery, performed twice a day (morning and afternoon), prevented the decline in knee extensor–flexor muscle torque during 2 weeks of cast immobilization in healthy males.

Passive HC provides a potent avenue for individuals facing physical limitations or medical conditions restricting their exercise capacity. For frail and deconditioned patients, as well as those unable to engage in traditional exercise, passive HC can serve as an initial step in their rehabilitation journey. This goal is to improve overall health and fitness, laying the foundation for eventual participation and fully benefits from exercise-based rehabilitation programs. The ability to achieve health and performance gains with minimal or no contractile activity marks a paradigm shift, particularly in cases of post-surgery recovery or severe musculoskeletal ailments. While both localized and systemic passive HC appear effective, the choice of delivery is a crucial consideration, hinging on available resources, the patient's specific needs, and the stage of rehabilitation.

13.3 Optimising the relationship between relative and absolute workloads through hypoxia conditioning for load-compromised individuals

Hypoxia conditioning is a useful tool to augment the relative intensity effect when faced with a fixed absolute workload or, conversely, lower the magnitude of absolute workload when confronted with a fixed relative intensity. This attribute holds significant promise for LCIs transitioning from complete immobilization or unloading, as they are cautiously reintroduced to progressive loading of their locomotor system. This scenario finds relevance in various contexts, including athletes recovering from injuries, where the injured limb can undergo progressive loading even when the individual may not be ready for heavy training. Integrating hypoxia into their rehabilitation program allows them to train at a higher relative intensity compared with normoxic conditions, even when the absolute workload remains conservative. This approach aims to minimize the risk of reinjury and facilitate the recovery process.

13.3.1 Systemic hypoxia conditioning in endurance and resistance exercise

It is well accepted that aerobic performance and capacity decrease with increasing systemic hypoxia due to the reduced partial pressure of O_2 in inspired air [16, 17]. This decline may vary among individuals, with a ~6.3% reduction in maximal oxygen uptake (VO_{2max}) per 1,000 m among endurance-trained individuals, and likely lower in untrained individuals [17, 18]. Consequently, the submaximal VO_2 required for a given absolute workload now represents a greater fraction of the reduced VO_{2max}, resulting in heightened physiological and perceptual responses (16). Likewise, exercising at a given physiological intensity (e.g., 75% $\dot{V}O_{2max}$) will result in reduced external power [19]. This concept has been well demonstrated among geriatric patients with multiple comorbidities, where continuous aerobic exercise in hypoxia substantially decreased absolute workload (i.e., a 25% decrease in mean power), despite similar relative intensities (e.g., %VO_{2max}) and comparable physiological responses [3].

Systemic HC can also be utilized during RE to enhance internal load, although research on this training modality among LCIs is lacking. As a proof of concept, when relative intensities were kept similar (i.e., %1RM), HC (3,100–3,400 m or SpO_2 ~88%) resulted in greater increases in maximal absolute and relative muscle squat strength [20] or leg press muscular endurance [21], indicating an enhanced training stimulus. Moreover, five weeks (three sessions per week) of low load (i.e., 20% 1RM) RE has been shown to improve muscle strength and endurance to a greater extent when performed in hypoxia (SpO_2 ~80%) compared with normoxia [22, 23]. These findings highlight the potential of such modalities in conjunction with low-load training, which is highly relevant for LCIs transitioning into load-bearing exercises.

13.3.2 Localized hypoxia conditioning in endurance and resistance exercise

Localised HC methods can effectively enhance physiological strain while sustaining low levels of mechanical output. For instance, a predetermined tolerable mechanical load (e.g., walking speed or cycling power) can be set and the extent of physiological strain manipulated by applying varying levels of BFR. Applying BFR at 60% AOP at walking speeds of 6 to 7.2 km·h1^{-1} increases cardiorespiratory responses compared with unrestricted equivalents [24]. To optimize internal intensity, it is also possible to apply heart rate (HR) clamps and mitigate external workload through manipulating %AOPs. For instance, with HR clamped at the first ventilatory threshold, BFR applied above 45% AOP has been shown to substantially reduce external power, alongside increased muscle deoxygenation and blood pooling, with more pronounced changes evident at 75% AOP [25]. However, caution must be taken to ensure that HC is well-tolerated by LCIs, who may already experience discomfort due to injury and excessive ground reaction forces. Perceptual measures of perceived exertion and discomfort can be considerably heightened during walking with BFR [24], even when using occlusion pressures as low as 30% AOP [25]. One way to circumvent this may be to prescribe or control exercise intensity based on perceptual indices [1]. Ensuring that HC is perceptually well-tolerated is an important consideration for LCIs to ensure exercise compliance.

Localized HC in the form of BFR has proven effective in enhancing intramuscular stress during RE. External loads are typically maintained at 20% to 40% 1RM [13], while intramuscular metabolic responses may be enhanced by manipulating occlusive pressure. In support, studies report increased muscle activity, muscle deoxygenation, fatigability, pronounced inorganic phosphate accumulation, and greater intramuscular pH reductions following the inclusion of BFR (i.e., 100 to 120 mmHg) during knee extensors or plantar flexors, despite the exercise tasks being performed at the same relative intensities (i.e., 20% 1RM) [26, 27]. However, it is important to acknowledge that while localized HC can augment the intramuscular stress response to low loads, the enhanced response is not equivalent to performing RE at higher intensities. Studies have reported higher muscle activation and greater lactate accumulation between RE performed at 70% 1RM compared with 15 to 20% 1RM with BFR [28, 29].

Determining the appropriate level of occlusion pressure concerning external load is an important consideration, as increased metabolic alterations have been postulated as a potential mechanism of muscle hypertrophy following BFR RE [30, 31]. The acute decline in maximal voluntary contraction torque immediately following exercise is believed to represent the extent of metabolic fatigue and the stimulus for adaptation following BFR RE [32]. Studies have reported that 80–90% of AOP resulted in greater strength loss compared with AOPs of 40–50% for RE loads of 15–20% 1RM, but this relationship was not evident when RE intensity was 30% 1RM [32]. With loads ≥ 30% 1RM, the applied load itself is purportedly sufficient to significantly limit blood flow, mitigating the effects of occlusion pressure [32].

13.4 Adaptations to exercise and hypoxia conditioning among load compromised individuals

Muscle atrophy is a common concern for many LCIs due to their limited ability to adequately load their musculoskeletal system. Both systemic and localized HC modalities have proven effective in reducing mechanical loading while preserving physiological strain. The implications of these approaches for averting muscle atrophy in various clinical populations will be explored.

13.4.1 Blood flow restriction (BFR) in resistance and aerobic exercise: A multifaceted approach

Localized HC methods, particularly the use of BFR, offer a versatile solution for addressing muscle atrophy concerns in LCIs. In older individuals (> 50 years), the incorporation of BFR with low-load RE substantially increased muscle mass compared with identically matched low-load RE alone (~12% versus 2.5%) [6]. It is noteworthy that the strength gains conferred by including BFR were lower compared with high-load RE (~24% versus 14%), although increases in muscle mass following both modes of training were similar (~6.2% versus 4.2%) [6]. These studies typically involved frequencies of two to three sessions per week, lasting at least 4 weeks and extending up to 12 weeks [33–39]. Most of them utilized training intensities of 20–30% 1RM [33, 34, 36–39], with some exploring upper limits of 30–50% 1RM [35]. It is recommended that occlusion pressures be set based on individual arterial occlusion pressure (AOP), with pressures ranging between 40% and 80% of AOP having evidence to support their efficacy [35]. However, higher occlusion pressure (80% AOP) may be necessary to induce meaningful physiological changes when performing RE at low intensities (20% 1RM) [40]. Although at higher workloads of 30–40% 1RM, there seems to be no effect of cuff pressures, as similar muscle hypertrophy levels were evident between AOPs of 40% compared with 80–90% at workloads of 30–40% 1RM [40, 41].

Studies have also reported comparable increases in muscle mass (~2.3%) and strength (~13%) following the inclusion of BFR during aerobic exercises such as walking, compared with equivalent walking alone [6]. For instance, among older individuals (>60 y), BFR has been shown to improve various leg strength measures (6–22%) and muscle mass or volume (3–10%) when applied during treadmill walking (20 min at 67 m/min or 45% HR reserve) performed for 4–5 days per week over a span of 6–10 weeks [42–44].

In other LCI cohorts with musculoskeletal impairments, training parameters such as duration (4–6 weeks), frequency (three sessions per week), and exercise intensity (30% 1RM) were reportedly similar [45–48] to the approaches applied to the aforementioned elderly cohorts. However, distinctions were noted in studies focusing on post-surgery rehabilitation following anterior cruciate ligament reconstruction [49–52] or other post-operative treatment [53]. In these studies, training frequency seemed higher, with five to seven sessions per week with one to three sessions daily in most [49, 50, 53] but not all cases [51, 52]. Likewise, within these cohorts, while the inclusion of BFR during low-load RE can produce greater adaptations in muscular strength compared with low-load RE alone, the strength gains following BFR appear to be smaller in magnitude than those achieved with high-load RE [4].

These findings reaffirm that the mechanical stimulus is the most potent factor for strength gains. However, in LCIs where low-load training is the feasible option, supplementing with BFR during aerobic or RE can result in greater gains in muscle mass and strength, leading to progressive return to heavy-load exercise.

13.4.2 Hypoxia conditioning and cardiovascular fitness

While localized HC such as BFR effectively improves muscle mass and strength during aerobic exercise and RE, its effectiveness in enhancing cardiovascular fitness is not firmly established. Recent work indicates heightened cardiovascular responses when incorporating BFR during cycling exercises, implying potential improvements in cardiovascular function. In contrast, in older individuals, Abe et al. [42] reported no changes in VO_2max following 6 weeks of treadmill walking (20 min sessions, 5 days per week) with BFR. However, when extending the training duration to 10 weeks with similar participant cohorts and exercise models, both BFR and non-BFR training groups showed ~9–10% increases in VO_2max [43].

Engaging in exercise under normobaric hypoxia is a well-established systemic HC model to improve cardiovascular fitness. This model provides an effective and quantifiable means to modify the relative–absolute workload relationship. However, research on the use of systemic HC has primarily focused on obese individuals, where it is purported to improve cardiometabolic heath and promote weight loss [54]. Regarding cardiovascular fitness, an eight-week aerobic training regimen (three sessions per week) in hypoxia (80% SpO_2 or FiO_2 13%) demonstrated an 8–9% improvement in VO_{2max} and corresponding mechanical power in overweight and obese individuals [55]. Moreover, in class 1 obese individuals, a three-week program (3 sessions per week, each lasting 60 min) at a preferred walking speed elicited lower speeds (7–9%) in hypoxia (~3,000 m) compared with normoxia. Nevertheless, comparable post-training improvements were observed in walking speed, perceived exertion, metabolic risk factors, and walking mechanics [2]. Conversely, aerobic exercise performed over 6 weeks (three sessions per week at 50–60% maximal HR) in either normobaric normoxia or hypoxia (15% FiO_2, ~2,500 m) resulted in minimal changes in VO_2max, peak workload, or lactate threshold among individuals with metabolic syndrome [56].

13.5 Concluding remarks

Hypoxia conditioning emerges as a promising tool to facilitate the transition from injury, immobilization, or post-operative care to increased engagement in conventional physical activity and loading (Figure 13.1). It allows LCIs to exercise at higher relative intensities while maintaining a conservative absolute workload, minimizing the risk of reinjury and enabling a gradual return to high-load exercise routines. Localized methods such as BFR demonstrate remarkable efficacy in promoting improvements in muscle mass and muscle strength, proving effective against muscle atrophy in LCIs. However, the use of BFR during aerobic exercise on cardiovascular fitness requires further investigation. Systemic HC, especially in normobaric hypoxia, has shown benefits in enhancing cardiovascular fitness in athletic populations, yet its applicability and potential benefits among LCIs remain a promising but minimally explored area.

In conclusion, the integration of HC holds promise for optimizing the rehabilitation and recovery of LCIs. It provides innovative solutions for health and performance enhancement while minimizing the limitations posed by load restrictions. Continued research focusing on central cardiovascular adaptations following localized and systemic HC in LCIs is expected to contribute significantly to well-being and physical capabilities.

Abbreviations

AOP	arterial occlusion pressure
BFR	blood flow restriction
FiO_2	fraction of inspired oxygen
HC	hypoxic conditioning
HR	heart rate
LCI	load compromised individuals
RE	resistance exercise
RM	repetition maximum
SpO_2	oxygen saturation
VO_{2max}	maximal oxygen uptake.

References

1. Girard O, Matic Girard I, Peeling P. Hypoxic conditioning: A novel therapeutic solution for load-compromised individuals to achieve similar exercise benefits by doing less mechanical work! Br J Sports Med. 2021;55(17):944–5.
2. Fernández Menéndez A, Saudan G, Sperisen L, Hans D, Saubade M, Millet GP, et al. Effects of short-term normobaric hypoxic walking training on energetics and mechanics of gait in adults with obesity. Obesity. 2018;26(5):819–27.
3. Pramsohler S, Burtscher M, Faulhaber M, Gatterer H, Rausch L, Eliasson A, et al. Endurance training in normobaric hypoxia imposes less physical stress for geriatric rehabilitation. Front Physiol. 2017;8:514.

4. Hughes L, Paton B, Rosenblatt B, Gissane C, Patterson SD. Blood flow restriction training in clinical musculoskeletal rehabilitation: A systematic review and meta-analysis. Br J Sports Med. 2017;51(13):1003–11.
5. Slysz J, Stultz J, Burr JF. The efficacy of blood flow restricted exercise: A systematic review & meta-analysis. J Sci Med Sport. 2016;19(8):669–75.
6. Centner C, Wiegel P, Gollhofer A, König D. Effects of blood flow restriction training on muscular strength and hypertrophy in older individuals: A systematic review and meta-analysis. Sport Med. 2019;49(1):95–108.
7. Burtscher M, Haider T, Domej W, Linser T, Gatterer H, Faulhaber M, et al. Intermittent hypoxia increases exercise tolerance in patients at risk for or with mild COPD. Respir Physiol Neurobiol. 2009;165(1):97–103.
8. Wang JS, Chen LY, Fu LL, Chen ML, Wong MK. Effects of moderate and severe intermittent hypoxia on vascular endothelial function and haemodynamic control in sedentary men. Eur J Appl Physiol. 2007;100(2):127–35.
9. Workman C, Basset FA. Post-metabolic response to passive normobaric hypoxic exposure in sedendary overweight males: A pilot study. Nutr Metab. 2012; 9(1):103.
10. Chacaroun S, Borowik A, Doutreleau S, Belaidi E, Wuyam B, Tamisier R, et al. Cardiovascular and metabolic responses to passive hypoxic conditioning in overweight and mildly obese individuals. Am J Physiol Regul Integr Comp Physiol. 2020;319(2):R211–R222.
11. Takarada Y, Takazawa H, Ishii N. Applications of vascular occlusion diminish disuse atrophy. Med Sci Sports Exerc. 2000;32(12):2035–2039.
12. Kubota A, Sakuraba K, Sawaki K, Sumide T, Tamura Y. Prevention of disuse muscular weakness by restriction of blood flow. Med Sci Sports Exerc. 2008; 40(3):529–534.
13. Patterson SD, Hughes L, Warmington S, Burr J, Scott BR, Owens J, et al. Blood flow restriction exercise position stand: Considerations of methodology, application, and safety. Front Physiol. 2019;10:533.
14. Barbalho M, Rocha AC, Seus TL, Raiol R, Del Vecchio FB, Coswig VS. Addition of blood flow restriction to passive mobilization reduces the rate of muscle wasting in elderly patients in the intensive care unit: A within-patient randomized trial. Clin Rehabil. 2019;33(2):233–240.
15. Kubota A, Sakuraba K, Koh S, Ogura Y, Tamura Y. Blood flow restriction by low compressive force prevents disuse muscular weakness. J Sci Med Sport. 2011; 14(2):95–99.
16. Fulco CS, Rock PB, Cymerman A. Maximal and submaximal exercise performance at altitude. Aviat Sp Environ Med. 1998;69(8):793–801.
17. Wehrlin JP, Hallén J. Linear decrease in VO_{2max} and performance with increasing altitude in endurance athletes. Eur J Appl Physiol. 2006;96(4):404–412.
18. Woorons X, Richalet JP. Modelling the relationships between arterial oxygen saturation, exercise intensity and the level of aerobic performance in acute hypoxia. Eur J Appl Physiol. 2021;121(7):1993–2003.
19. Li Y, Li J, Atakan MM, Wang Z, Hu Y, Nazif M, et al. Methods to match high-intensity interval exercise intensity in hypoxia and normoxia: A pilot study. J Exerc Sci Fit. 2022 Jan;20(1):70–6.
20. Mathew MW, Billaut F, Walker EJ, Petersen AC, Sweeting AJ, Aughey RJ. Heavy resistance training in hypoxia enhances 1RM squat performance. Front Physiol. 2016;7:502.
21. Kon M, Ohiwa N, Honda A, Matsubayashi T, Ikeda T, Akimoto T, et al. Effects of systemic hypoxia on human muscular adaptations to resistance exercise training. Physiol Rep. 2014;2(6):1–13.

22. Manimmanakorn A, Manimmanakorn N, Taylor R, Draper N, Billaut F, Shearman JP, et al. Effects of resistance training combined with vascular occlusion or hypoxia on neuromuscular function in athletes. Eur J Appl Physiol. 2013; 113(7):1767–74.

23. Manimmanakorn A, Hamlin MJ, Ross JJ, Taylor R, Manimmanakorn N. Effects of low-load resistance training combined with blood flow restriction or hypoxia on muscle function and performance in netball athletes. J Sci Med Sport. 2013; 16(4):337–42.

24. Walden TP, Girard O, Scott BR, Jonson AM, Peiffer JJ. Low- to moderate-intensity blood flow restricted walking is not an acute equivalent for unrestricted jogging in young active adults. Eur J Sport Sci. 2023;23(8):1560–1569.

25. Li SN, Ihsan M, Shaykevich A, Girard O. Exercise responses to heart rate clamped cycling with graded blood flow restriction. J Sci Med Sport. 2023;26(8): 434–439.

26. Kolind A, Mikkel I, Jeppe G, Henrik B, Jakob L. Effects of low load exercise with and without blood-flow restriction on microvascular oxygenation, muscle excitability and perceived pain. Eur J Sport Sci. 2023;23(4):542–551.

27. Suga T, Okita K, Morita N, Yokota T, Horiuchi M, Takada S, et al. Intramuscular metabolism during low-intensity resistance exercise with blood flow restriction. J Appl Physiol. 2009; 109(4):1119–1124.

28. Freitas EDS, Miller RM, Heishman AD, Ferreira-Júnior JB, Araújo JP, Bemben MG, et al. Acute physiological responses to resistance exercise with continuous versus intermittent blood flow restriction: A randomized controlled trial. Front Physiol. 2020;11;132.

29. Jessee MB, Buckner SL, Mattocks KT, Dankel SJ, Mouser JG, Bell ZW, et al. Blood flow restriction augments the skeletal muscle response during very low-load resistance exercise to volitional failure. Physiol Int. 2019;106(2):180–93.

30. Pearson SJ, Hussain SR. A review on the mechanisms of blood-flow restriction resistance training-induced muscle hypertrophy. Sport Med. 2015;45(2): 187–200.

31. Loenneke JP, Fahs CA, Wilson JM, Bemben MG. Blood flow restriction: The metabolite/volume threshold theory. Med Hypotheses. 2011;77(5):748–52.

32. De Queiros VS, De França IM, Trybulski R. Myoelectric activity and fatigue in low-load resistance exercise with different pressure of blood flow restriction: A systematic review and meta-analysis. Front Physiol. 2021;12:786752.

33. Karabulut M, Abe T, Sato Y, Bemben MG. The effects of low-intensity resistance training with vascular restriction on leg muscle strength in older men. Eur J Appl Physiol. 2010;108(1):147–55.

34. Shimizu R, Hotta K, Yamamoto S, Matsumoto T, Kamiya K, Kato M, et al. Low-intensity resistance training with blood flow restriction improves vascular endothelial function and peripheral blood circulation in healthy elderly people. Eur J Appl Physiol. 2016;116(4):749–57.

35. Cook SB, LaRoche DP, Villa MR, Barile H, Manini TM. Blood flow restricted resistance training in older adults at risk of mobility limitations. Exp Gerontol. 2017;99:138–45.

36. Libardi CA, Chacon-Mikahil MPT, Cavaglieri CR, Tricoli V, Roschel H, Vechin FC, et al. Effect of concurrent training with blood flow restriction in the elderly. Int J Sports Med. 2015;36(5):395–9.

37. Thiebaud RS, Loenneke JP, Fahs CA, Rossow LM, Kim D, Abe T, et al. The effects of elastic band resistance training combined with blood flow restriction on strength, total bone-free lean body mass and muscle thickness in postmenopausal women. Clin Physiol Funct Imaging. 2013;33(5):344–52.

38. Vechin FC, Libardi CA, Conceição MS, Damas FR, Lixandrão ME, Berton RPB, et al. Comparisons between low-intensity resistance training with blood flow restriction and high-intensity resistance training on quadriceps muscle mass and strength in elderly. J Strength Cond Res. 2015;29(4):1071–6.
39. Patterson SD, Ferguson RA. Enhancing strength and postocclusive calf blood flow in older people with training with blood-flow restriction. J Aging Phys Act. 2011;19(3):201–13.
40. Lixandrão ME, Ugrinowitsch C, Laurentino G, Libardi CA, Aihara AY, Cardoso FN, et al. Effects of exercise intensity and occlusion pressure after 12 weeks of resistance training with blood-flow restriction. Eur J Appl Physiol. 2015;115(12): 2471–80.
41. Counts BR, Dankel SJ, Barnett BE, Kim D, Mouser JG, Allen KM, et al. Influence of relative blood flow restriction pressure on muscle activation and muscle adaptation. Muscle Nerve. 2016;53(3):438–45.
42. Abe T, Sakamaki M, Fujita S, Ozaki H, Sugaya M, Sato Y, et al. Effects of low-intensity walk training with restricted leg blood flow on muscle strength and aerobic capacity in older adults. J Geriatr Phys Ther. 2010;33(1):34–40.
43. Ozaki H, Sakamaki M, Yasuda T, Fujita S, Ogasawara R, Sugaya M, et al. Increases in thigh muscle volume and strength by walk training with leg blood flow reduction in older participants. Journals Gerontol A Biol Sci Med Sci. 2011;66(3):257–63.
44. Ozaki H, Miyachi M, Nakajima T, Abe T. Effects of 10 weeks walk training with leg blood flow reduction on carotid arterial compliance and muscle size in the elderly adults. Angiology. 2011;62(1):81–6.
45. Bryk FF, Dos Reis AC, Fingerhut D, Araujo T, Schutzer M, de Cury RPL, et al. Exercises with partial vascular occlusion in patients with knee osteoarthritis: A randomized clinical trial. Knee Surg Sports Traumatol Arthrosc. 2016;24(5): 1580–6.
46. Segal NA, Williams GN, Davis MC, Wallace RB, Mikesky AE. Efficacy of blood flow-restricted, low-load resistance training in women with risk factors for symptomatic knee osteoarthritis. PM R. 2015;7(4):376–84.
47. Segal N, Davis MD, Mikesky AE. Efficacy of blood flow-restricted low-load resistance training for quadriceps strengthening in men at risk of symptomatic knee osteoarthritis. Geriatr Orthop Surg Rehabil. 2015;6(3):160–7.
48. Mattar MA, Gualano B, Perandini LA, Shinjo SK, Lima FR, Sá-Pinto AL, et al. Safety and possible effects of low-intensity resistance training associated with partial blood flow restriction in polymyositis and dermatomyositis. Arthritis Res Ther. 2014;16(5):473.
49. Ohta H, Kurosawa H, Ikeda H, Iwase Y, Satou N, Nakamura S. Low-load resistance muscular training with moderate restriction of blood flow after anterior cruciate ligament reconstruction. Acta Orthop Scand. 2003;74(1):62–8.
50. Iversen E, Røstad V, Larmo A. Intermittent blood flow restriction does not reduce atrophy following anterior cruciate ligament reconstruction. J Sport Health Sci. 2016;5(1):115–8.
51. Lambert B, Hedt CA, Jack RA, Moreno M, Delgado D, Harris JD, et al. Blood flow restriction therapy preserves whole limb bone and muscle following ACL reconstruction. Orthop J Sport Med. 2019;7(3_suppl2):2325967119S0019.
52. Jack RA, Lambert BS, Hedt CA, Delgado D, Goble H, McCulloch PC. Blood flow restriction therapy preserves lower extremity bone and muscle mass after ACL reconstruction. Sports Health. 2023;15(3):361–71.
53. Fan Y, Bai D, Cheng C, Tian G. The effectiveness and safety of blood flow restriction training for the post-operation treatment of distal radius fracture. Ann Med. 2023;55(2):2240329.

54. Girard O, Malatesta D, Millet GP. Walking in hypoxia: An efficient treatment to lessen mechanical constraints and improve health in obese individuals? Front Physiol. 2017;8:73.
55. Chacaroun S, Borowik A, Vega-Escamilla Y, Gonzalez I, Doutreleau S, Wuyam B, Belaidi E, et al. hypoxic exercise training to improve exercise capacity in obese individuals. Med Sci Sports Exerc. 2020;52(8):1641–9.
56. Klug L, Mähler A, Rakova N, Mai K, Schulz-Menger J, Rahn G, et al. Normobaric hypoxic conditioning in men with metabolic syndrome. Physiol Rep. 2018;6(24): 1–14.

SECTION 7

14

APPLICATIONS FROM BEFORE BIRTH TO HIGH AGE

Johannes Burtscher, Lutz Schega, Tom Behrendt and Tadej Debevec

14.1 Hypoxia in early life—risks and opportunities

Oxygen concentrations play important roles in mammalian embryo development, with the hypoxia response orchestrating hypoxia inducible factors (HIFs) guiding gene expression and morphogenesis. Many developing tissues, including the heart, gut, and skeleton, are physiologically hypoxic throughout development, also due to insufficient support of oxygen by the developing vasculature to the growing—and therefore highly energy-demanding—organs.

Conversely, cardiovascular or placental deficits as well as environmental or ambient hypoxia may trigger pathological developments.

14.1.1 Risks of early life hypoxia

Pre- and perinatal pathological hypoxia can exert far-reaching consequences in many physiological systems that may last a lifetime. For example, it can be particularly detrimental for the brain, may impair brain plasticity, and may increase the susceptibility to several neurological dysfunctions and diseases, including neurodegenerative diseases such as dementia (Chapter 5). Moreover, the potential detrimental and far-reaching effects of hypoxia related to premature birth, and associated treatment strategies, are noteworthy. Clear evidence indicates that prematurity independently modulates the development and maturation of virtually all physiological systems, with a particular impact on respiratory, cardiopulmonary, and cardiovascular function [1]. Given that cardiorespiratory factors play a pivotal role in the modulation of hypoxia adaptation, prematurity might influence subsequent physiological

DOI: 10.4324/9781003402879-22

and functional responses to environmental hypoxia stress later in life. This idea is supported by research suggesting differential hypoxia-related ventilatory, micro-vascular, and oxidative stress responses in prematurely born individuals [2]. Therefore, it is essential to explore the applicability and efficiency of hypoxia interventions in this population.

14.1.2 Potentials of modulating ambient oxygen in early life

In contrast to the risks associated with early-life hypoxia, recent research has revealed unexpected potential in reducing ambient oxygen levels to modulate susceptibility to brain diseases. Leigh syndrome, a mitochondrial disease-causing pediatric neurodegeneration, can result from a mutation in the *NDUFs4* gene, encoding a protein of complex I in the mitochondrial respirational chain. Mice with targeted mutations in *NDUFs4*, replicating some of the features of Leigh disease, have shown benefits from chronic exposure to ambient hypoxia with an inspired oxygen fraction (F_iO_2) of 11% (starting from 30 days after birth). This exposure prevented many symptoms, increased survival [3], and even reversed neuropathology [4]. On the other hand, chronic hyperoxia (55% oxygen) exacerbated the disease [3], while milder hypoxia (17% oxygen) or an intermittent protocol (one block of 11% oxygen for 10 hours per day, the rest at 21%) did not induce the same benefits [4]. The same authors later demonstrated that deficits in mitochondrial respiration led to brain hyperoxia, a condition that could be reversed by ambient hypoxia, even without activating HIFs [5].

14.2 Hypoxia and aging—hypoxia conditioning as an anti-aging strategy?

Aging is associated with a progressive decline in functional abilities. Depending on the applied dose, hypoxia can either contribute to the deterioration of some functions, or conversely, hypoxia conditioning may counteract certain consequences of aging and potentially aging itself.

HIFs and reactive oxygen species are central mediators of hypoxia adaptations, orchestrating the remodeling of cellular environments and metabolism via regulating many genes ("hypoxia responsive elements" and "antioxidant responsive elements") [6]. Alongside other mechanisms (see Chapter 2), they contribute to improved mitochondrial integrity and function as well as anti-oxidative and anti-inflammatory processes, which may be altered in aging and due to mitochondrial dysfunction. On the other hand, oxidative stress [7] and chronic inflammation [8] possibly drive aging processes. Hypoxia conditioning thus may attenuate age-related functional decline by improving antioxidant and anti-inflammatory defenses, thereby increasing cellular and systemic resilience.

14.2.1 Severe hypoxia promotes aging

Severe or pathological hypoxia can induce mitochondrial damage, trigger oxidative insults, and modulate immune system function and inflammation. This is well known for obstructive sleep apnea, in which impaired breathing (i.e., repeated episodes of complete [apnea] or partial [hypopnea] obstruction of the upper airway) causes severe intermittent hypoxia during sleep [9]. The anticipated consequences of obstructive sleep apnea include oxidative stress and chronic inflammation, contributing to an elevated risk for the development of many diseases (e.g., cardiovascular, metabolic, and neurological diseases) and accelerated aging [9]. It is therefore plausible that severe hypoxia induces senescence.

This hypothesis finds support in laboratory studies. For example, cultured human white preadipocytes exposed to severe intermittent hypoxia (nine daily cycles consisting of 30 minutes of 0.1% oxygen followed by 30 minutes of normoxia for one week) showed accelerated senescence [10]. Another intermittent hypoxia protocol (5-min episodes of 10% oxygen interspersed with 3 min normoxia during 12 hours per day for 7 days) accelerated aging of the reproductive system in young male rats, manifested by decreased testosterone levels and increased oxidative stress and sexual dysfunction [11]. HIF-1 stabilization by severe hypoxia can further perturb gene expression by altering chromatin and epigenetic regulation in affected cells, leading to cellular senescence [12].

Not only can hypoxia modulate aging, but aging also affects physiological responses to hypoxia. While hypoxia conditioning can efficiently protect heart function, as demonstrated extensively in animal models, this potential has been found to be reduced in old rats [13]. These results align with observations that older age is associated with less efficient molecular pathways that control hypoxia adaptation, including those involving HIF [14]. HIF activity, and thus the capacity to regulate hypoxia-inducible gene expression (e.g., genes related to angiogenic factors or erythropoiesis) and to adapt to hypoxia, has been shown to be reduced in old versus young human fibroblasts [15] and in mice [16].

The interplay of age-related parameters and adaptations to hypoxia are illustrated in Figure 14.1.

14.2.2 Anti-aging effects of mild chronic and intermittent hypoxia?

Illustrating the Janus-faced consequences of hypoxia on health, other results highlight that specific hypoxia interventions might counteract aging and potentially extend lifespan and health-span (the time of our life during which we remain free of age-related diseases). The varied outcomes of hypoxia on aging and longevity stem from factors like the hypoxic dose and individual

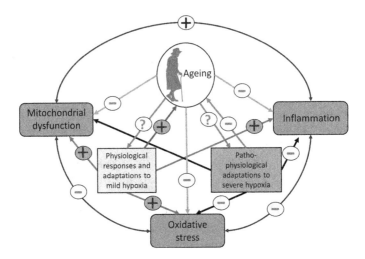

FIGURE 14.1 Crosstalk between aging and adaptations to hypoxia. Aging and severe hypoxia promote mitochondrial dysfunction, oxidative stress, and inflammation, while hypoxia conditioning may have opposing effects. Aging may further impair adaptations to hypoxia. Pluses indicate beneficial, minuses negative effects.

vulnerabilities. Severe hypoxia, with FiO_2 lower than 11%, or prolonged and frequent hypoxic episodes, represents models for pathological hypoxia and can promote aging. Conversely, mild continuous hypoxia, such as experienced at moderate altitudes (1,500–2,500 m, equivalent to an FiO_2 of about 18–15%) or calibrated hypoxia conditioning protocols, usually FiO_2 of ≥10% during a few cycles per day (3–15) with short hypoxic periods (1–10 min) and sufficient normoxic rest (at least 1–5 min) between each exposure, may induce protective adaptations supporting healthy aging.

Chronic hypoxia can substantially alter an organism's metabolism and thereby extend lifespan. Longevity-promoting metabolic regulation may explain increased lifespans observed in cells and some invertebrates (like the model-organism worm *Caenorhabditis elegans*) in environments of permanently reduced oxygen availability [17, 18]. The level of oxygen utilization appears crucial, since artificially induced mild impairments of mitochondrial respiration also extend lifespan in *Caenorhabditis elegans* [19], the fruit fly *Drosophila melanogaster* [20], and also in mice, demonstrating the relevance of this phenomenon for mammals [21, 22].

Moreover, animals such as the naked mole rat or the bowhead whale, which inhabit hypoxic environments and exhibit unusually long lives, are sometimes used as arguments for potential anti-aging effects of hypoxia. However, whether hypoxia exposures are the primary cause for their exceptional longevity and whether these findings are relevant for the aging-process in humans remain unclear.

There is limited direct evidence for effects of hypoxia exposure on aging in humans. However, several studies have explored the effects of long-term altitude exposure on mortality and the development of (often age-related) chronic diseases. The role of hypoxia in these studies must be interpreted with caution. Although people living in moderate to high altitudes are exposed to moderately hypoxic conditions due to lower atmospheric pressure and reduced oxygen availability, other factors such as differences in ultraviolet radiation, socioeconomic status, living conditions and lifestyle, access to commodities, and healthcare may also contribute to differences in vulnerability to diseases and life expectancy [23].

Several studies conducted in different countries demonstrate reduced mortality from various diseases among people residing at moderate altitudes. Lower numbers of deaths from cardiovascular diseases have been observed among people living at higher altitudes, both in the United States [24] and in the European Alps [25, 26]. The overall life expectancy, however, did not change with an increasing altitude of residence. While moderate altitude may reduce the risk for some chronic diseases, it may not affect or even increase the probability of dying from other causes. Certain types of cancer may be more prevalent at higher altitudes, possibly linked to higher irradiation levels, but mortality from some cancer types, including colorectal and breast cancer, seems to be lower [27, 28].

For some high-altitude populations, such as those in the South American Andes or Tibet, living at high altitude has been suggested to effectively extend lifespan. It is important to note that these studies compared different ethnicities, which could confound the results.

Taken together, while some observations suggest increased longevity in some animal species frequently exposed to hypoxia or in some humans living at moderate or high altitude, these results may be heavily confounded. Although some studies controlled for living conditions, access to healthcare, rate of agriculture, or size of residential area, much better-controlled longitudinal studies will be required to derive clear evidence for potential effects of altitude (or hypoxia) on longevity and aging. To investigate the influence of hypoxia on isolated aging parameters and to assess the influence of age on responses and adaptations following hypoxia exposure, interventional studies can be informative.

14.2.3 Exposing older people to hypoxia: Risks and opportunities

Individual differences in responses to hypoxia are crucial determinants for the quality and safety of outcomes following hypoxia exposure. These differences can be hereditary or modulated by preexisting vulnerabilities, such as diseases or age, and previous adaptations to hypoxic or other types of stress. It has been observed that acute erythropoietin expression is lower in older compared to younger individuals when adjusting the internal intensity of hypoxia to an peripheral oxygen saturation of 80% [29]. Although the exact mechanisms are not yet known, reduced stabilization of HIF and/or decreased renal function could explain this age-related phenomenon. Accordingly, older people are often more prone to hypoxemia and may have reduced cardiovascular and respiratory plasticity to manage hypoxic stress [30]. In addition, exposure to severe or prolonged hypoxia is associated with oxidative stress and DNA damage, which might be exacerbated at older age.

Despite reported changes in molecular responses to hypoxia, older people do not appear to be at increased risk for high-altitude illnesses like acute mountain sickness and pulmonary or cerebral edema [31]. Moreover, they remain responsive to hypoxia-based interventions. Intermittent hypoxia has been reported to have various beneficial effects on physiological systems and processes relevant for healthy aging. However, its efficacy may be more pronounced in diseased than in healthy populations. Current evidence shows no clear benefit of intermittent hypoxia interventions, alone or in combination with other treatments (e.g., exercise), for cardiometabolic, inflammatory, hematological, skeletal, cognitive, or body composition parameters in healthy older adults compared with similar interventions in normoxia [32]. This lack of clear benefits is likely not due to a general inefficacy of intermittent hypoxia in older people but rather to an insufficient hypoxic dose and/or type of intervention [33]. In particular, intermittent hypoxia protocols with higher inter-session density have shown some beneficial effects on hemodynamics, microvascular endothelial function, and work capacity, especially in untrained healthy older men [34]. In older people with chronic diseases or illnesses, such as coronary artery disease or chronic obstructive pulmonary disease, intermittent hypoxia interventions can improve aerobic capacity and exercise tolerance [35, 36], effects not necessarily observed in healthy older people [37]. Furthermore, appropriate protocols can provide cardioprotection and profoundly benefit cardiovascular functions [38, 39]. Mild intermittent hypoxia can also be neuroprotective [40] and improve glucose homeostasis [41], suggesting therapeutic value for several age-related diseases (see Table 14.1).

Although intermittent hypoxia interventions have been suggested as promising nonpharmacological strategies in older individuals for treating disease-specific symptoms and improving general health outcomes, the results must be interpreted with caution. Frequent limitations regarding the available studies include: (1) small sample sizes, (2) study heterogeneity (especially related to hypoxia dose, outcomes, and study design), (3) lack of adequate control groups, (4) incompletely described procedures (e.g., intervention and outcome measures), and (5) short duration of the intervention.

TABLE 14.1 Hypoxia conditioning benefits in age-related diseases

Disease	Main benefits	Literature
Neurological		
Mild cognitive impairment	**IHE** enhanced cerebral oxygenation and hypoxia-induced cerebrovasodilation and improved MMSE and total digit span score. **IHHE** improved MoCA score and reduces amyloid β and NET formation. Effects on ERP are inconclusive.	[42–44]
Respiratory		
Chronic obstructive pulmonary disease	**IHE** improved physical function (i.e., ↑ time to exhaustion and ↑ anaerobic threshold [CPET], ↓ heart rate and ↓ blood lactate concentration [6-MWT]), lung function (↑ FEV1, ↑ FEV1/FVC, ↑ DLCO, ↑ hypercapnic ventilatory response), cardiovascular function (↑ baroreflex sensitivity, ↑ HRV), increased tHb, and reduced plasma triglycerides.	[36, 45]
Cardiovascular		
Hypertension	**IHE** (passive or active) reduced systolic and diastolic blood pressure as well as malondialdehyde concentration. It increased nitric oxide metabolites, HIF-1α concentration, and 6-MWT distance.	[46, 47]
Heart failure with reduced ejection fraction	**PHE** improved physical function (i.e., ↑ peak VO2, ↑ time to exhaustion [CPET], ↑ 6-MWT distance, ↑ arm flexion MVC) and MLHFQ score. There was a trend for increased left ventricular ejection fraction after 4 weeks of PHE.	[48]
Coronary heart disease	**PHE** improved plasma lipid and lipoprotein concentration (i.e., ↓ total cholesterol, ↑ HDL cholesterol, ↓ VLDL cholesterol, ↓ LDL cholesterol, ↓ triglycerides) and myocardial perfusion. **IHE** increased red blood cell count and hemoglobin concentration (via blood gas analyses), improves aerobic capacity (i.e., ↓ perceived and ↓ physiological response to submaximal cycling) and exercise tolerance (i.e., ↑ peak VO2, ↑ minute ventilation, ↑ SaO2, ↓ blood lactate concentration at maximal exercise) **IHHE** improved physical function (i.e., ↑ time to exhaustion [CPET]), increased subscales of the MOS SF-36 score. Effects on peak VO2, plasma lipid and lipoprotein concentration, and Seattle Angina Questionnaire score are inconclusive.	[35, 49–52]

Table 14.1 (Continued)

Disease	Main benefits	Literature
Metabolic		
Metabolic syndrome	**Training and living at moderate altitude** reduced triglyceride concentration. Aerobic exercise under moderate hypoxia showed no additional benefits for men with metabolic syndrome. **IHHE** improved body composition (i.e., ↓ BMI, ↓ waist and ↓ hip circumference) as well as lipid and lipoprotein concentration (i.e., ↓ total cholesterol, ↓ LDL cholesterol, ↓ triglycerides) and reduced alanine aminotransferase and NTproBNP serum concentration.	[53–56]
Prediabetes and type 2 diabetes	In prediabetic patients, **IHE** and **IHHE** reduced fasting glucose and 2 h post-OGTT glycose concentration while **IHE** also reduced serum total cholesterol. In patients with type 2 diabetes, **PHE** can reduce 2 h post-OGTT while HbA1c, fasting glycose and insulin, free-fatty acids, and 2 h post-OGTT insulin were unaffected. When combining moderate hypoxia with aerobic exercise, no additive effect on physical function, vascular function, or glucose homeostasis was observed.	[57–59]
Geriatric patients	**IHHE** in addition to a multimodal training program improved global cognitive function (i.e., ↑ DemTect and ↑ CDT score) and increased 6-MWT distance more than a multimodal training program alone. **IHHE** prior to aerobic exercise increased CDT score and SPPB performance, reduced systolic blood pressure, and preserved TUG performance in comparison to aerobic exercise alone.	[60–64]
Cardiology outpatients	**IHHE** reduced diastolic blood pressure and may increase peak VO$_2$.	[65]

Abbreviations: BMI, body mass index; CDT, Clock Drawing Test; CPET, cardiopulmonary exercise test; DemTect, Dementia-Detection Test; DLCO, lung diffusion capacity for carbon monoxide; ERP, event related potential; FEV$_1$, forced expiratory volume in 1 s; FVC, forced expiratory vital capacity; HbA1c, hemoglobin A1c; HDL, high-density lipoprotein; HIF-1α, hypoxia-inducible factors 1α; HRV, heart rate variability; IHE, intermittent hypoxic exposure; IHHE, intermittent hypoxic–hyperoxic exposure; LDL, low-density lipoprotein; MLHFQ, Minnesota Living with Heart Failure Questionnaire; MMSE, Mini-Mental State Examination; MoCA, Montreal Cognitive Assessment; MOS SF-36, Medical Outcome Study Short Form 36; MVC, maximum voluntary contraction; NET, neutrophil extracellular traps; NTproBNP, N-terminal prohormone brain natriuretic peptide; PHE, passive hypoxic exposure; S$_a$O$_2$, arterial oxygen saturation; tHb, total hemoglobin; TUG, Timed « Up and Go » Test, VLDL, very low-density lipoprotein; VO$_2$, oxygen consumption, 2 h post-OGTT, 2 h post oral glucose tolerance test; 6-MWT, Six-minute Walk Test

Therefore, further randomized controlled trials with adequate sample sizes and intervention design are needed to confirm and extend the current evidence. Additionally, understanding the dose-response relationship of passive and/or active intermittent hypoxia interventions and explaining individual responses in older and/or diseased individuals is crucial.

Abbreviations

FiO_2 fractional inspired oxygen concentration
HIF   hypoxia-inducible factor

References

1. Hubbard, C.D., et al., *Consequences of preterm birth: Knowns, unknowns, and barriers to advancing cardiopulmonary health*. Integr Comp Biol, 2023. **62**(3): p. 693–704.
2. Debevec, T., et al., *Premature birth: A neglected consideration for altitude adaptation*. J Appl Physiol (1985), 2022. **133**(4): p. 975–978.
3. Jain, I.H., et al., *Hypoxia as a therapy for mitochondrial disease*. Science, 2016. **352**(6281): p. 54–61.
4. Ferrari, M., et al., *Hypoxia treatment reverses neurodegenerative disease in a mouse model of Leigh syndrome*. Proc Natl Acad Sci U S A, 2017. **114**(21): p. E4241–E4250.
5. Jain, I.H., et al., *Leigh syndrome mouse model can be rescued by interventions that normalize brain hyperoxia, but not HIF activation*. Cell Metabolism, 2019. **30**(4): p. 824–832. e3.
6. Almohanna, A.M. and S. Wray, *Hypoxic conditioning in blood vessels and smooth muscle tissues: Effects on function, mechanisms, and unknowns*. Am J Physiol Heart Circ Physiol, 2018. **315**(4): p. H756–H770.
7. Harman, D., *Aging: a theory based on free radical and radiation chemistry*. Science's SAGE KE, 2002. **2002**(37): p. 14.
8. Franceschi, C., et al., *Inflammaging and 'Garb-aging'*. Trends Endocrinol Metab, 2017. **28**(3): p. 199–212.
9. Arnardottir, E.S., et al., *Molecular signatures of obstructive sleep apnea in adults: A review and perspective*. Sleep, 2009. **32**(4): p. 447–470.
10. Polonis, K., et al., *Chronic intermittent hypoxia triggers a senescence-like phenotype in human white preadipocytes*. Sci Rep, 2020. **10**(1): p. 6846.
11. Wilson, E.N., et al., *Chronic intermittent hypoxia induces hormonal and male sexual behavioral changes: Hypoxia as an advancer of aging*. Physiol Behav, 2018. **189**: p. 64–73.
12. Salminen, A., K. Kaarniranta, and A. Kauppinen, *Hypoxia-inducible histone lysine demethylases: Impact on the aging process and age-related diseases*. Aging Dis, 2016. **7**(2): p. 180–200.
13. Honma, Y., et al., *Aging abolishes the cardioprotective effect of combination heat shock and hypoxic preconditioning in reperfused rat hearts*. Basic Res Cardiol, 2002. **97**(6): p. 489–495.
14. Katschinski, D.M., *Is there a molecular connection between hypoxia and aging?* Exp Gerontol, 2006. **41**(5): p. 482–484.

15. Kim, H., et al., *Analysis of the effect of aging on the response to hypoxia by cDNA microarray.* Mech Ageing Dev, 2003. **124**(8–9): p. 941–949.

16. Frenkel-Denkberg, G., D. Gershon, and A.P. Levy, *The function of hypoxia-inducible factor 1 (HIF-1) is impaired in senescent mice.* FEBS Lett, 1999. **462**(3): p. 341–344.

17. Packer, L. and K. Fuehr, *Low oxygen concentration extends the lifespan of cultured human diploid cells.* Nature, 1977. **267**(5610): p. 423–425.

18. Mehta, R., et al., *Proteasomal regulation of the hypoxic response modulates aging in C. elegans.* Science (New York, N.Y.), 2009. **324**(5931): p. 1196–1198.

19. Feng, J., F. Bussière, and S. Hekimi, *Mitochondrial electron transport is a key determinant of life span in Caenorhabditis elegans.* Developmental Cell, 2001. **1**(5): p. 633–644.

20. Copeland, J.M., et al., *Extension of Drosophila life span by RNAi of the mitochondrial respiratory chain.* Current Biology, 2009. **19**(19): p. 1591–1598.

21. Lapointe, J. and S. Hekimi, *Early mitochondrial dysfunction in long-lived Mclk1+/-mice.* Journal of Biological Chemistry, 2008. **283**(38): p. 26217–26227.

22. Dell'agnello, C., et al., *Increased longevity and refractoriness to Ca(2+)-dependent neurodegeneration in Surf1 knockout mice.* Human Molecular Genetics, 2007. **16**(4): p. 431–444.

23. Burtscher, M., *Effects of living at higher altitudes on mortality: A narrative review.* Aging and Disease, 2014. **5**(4): p. 274.

24. Ezzati, M., et al., *Altitude, life expectancy and mortality from ischaemic heart disease, stroke, COPD and cancers: National population-based analysis of US counties.* J Epidemiol Community Health, 2012. **66**(7): p. e17–e17.

25. Faeh, D., et al., *Lower mortality from coronary heart disease and stroke at higher altitudes in Switzerland.* Circulation, 2009. **120**(6): p. 495–501.

26. Burtscher, J., G.P. Millet, and M. Burtscher, *Does living at moderate altitudes in Austria affect mortality rates of various causes? An ecological study.* BMJ Open, 2021. **11**(6): p. e048520.

27. Youk, A.O., et al., *An ecological study of cancer mortality rates in high altitude counties of the United States.* High Alt Med Biol, 2012. **13**(2): p. 98–104.

28. Burtscher, J., et al., *Moderate altitude residence reduces male colorectal and female breast cancer mortality more than incidence: Therapeutic implications?* Cancers (Basel), 2021. **13**(17): p. 4420.

29. Törpel, A., et al., *Dose-response relationship of intermittent normobaric hypoxia to stimulate erythropoietin in the context of health promotion in young and old people.* Eur J Appl Physiol, 2019. **119**(5): p. 1065–1074.

30. Millet, G.P., et al., *Therapeutic use of exercising in hypoxia: Promises and limitations.* Frontiers in Physiology, 2016. **7**: 224.

31. Gianfredi, V., et al., *Does age have an impact on acute mountain sickness? A systematic review.* J Travel Med, 2020. **27**(6): p. taz104.

32. Timon, R., I. Martinez-Guardado, and F. Brocherie, *Effects of intermittent normobaric hypoxia on health-related outcomes in healthy older adults: A systematic review.* Sports Med Open, 2023. **9**(1): p. 19.

33. Schega, L., et al., *Effects of intermittent hypoxia on cognitive performance and quality of life in elderly adults: pilot study.* Gerontology, 2013. **59**(4): p. 316–323.

34. Shatilo, V.B., et al., *Effects of intermittent hypoxia training on exercise performance, hemodynamics, and ventilation in healthy senior men.* High Alt Med Biol, 2008. **9**(1): p. 43–52.

35. Burtscher, M., et al., *Intermittent hypoxia increases exercise tolerance in elderly men with and without coronary artery disease*. Int J Cardiol, 2004. **96**(2): p. 247–254.

36. Burtscher, M., et al., *Intermittent hypoxia increases exercise tolerance in patients at risk for or with mild COPD*. Respir Physiol Neurobiol, 2009. **165**(1): p. 97–103.

37. Burtscher, M., et al., *Effects of interval hypoxia on exercise tolerance: Special focus on patients with CAD or COPD*. Sleep and Breathing, 2010. **14**(3): p. 209–220.

38. Lizamore, C.A. and M.J. Hamlin, *The use of simulated altitude techniques for beneficial cardiovascular health outcomes in nonathletic, sedentary, and clinical populations: A literature review*. High Alt Med Biol, 2017. **18**(4): p. 305–321.

39. Mallet, R.T., et al., *Cardioprotection by intermittent hypoxia conditioning: Evidence, mechanisms and therapeutic potential*. Am J Physiol Heart Circ Physiol, 2018. **315**(2): p. H216–H232.

40. Burtscher, J., et al., *Hypoxia and brain aging: Neurodegeneration or neuroprotection?* Ageing Res Rev, 2021. **68**: p. 101343.

41. van Hulten, V., R.L.J. van Meijel, and G.H. Goossens, *The impact of hypoxia exposure on glucose homeostasis in metabolically compromised humans: A systematic review*. Rev Endocr Metab Disord, 2021. **22**(2): p. 471–483.

42. Serebrovska, Z.O., et al., *Intermittent hypoxia-hyperoxia training improves cognitive function and decreases circulating biomarkers of Alzheimer's disease in patients with mild cognitive impairment: A pilot study*. Int J Mol Sci, 2019. **20**(21): p. 5405.

43. Serebrovska, Z.O., et al., *Response of circulating inflammatory markers to intermittent hypoxia-hyperoxia training in healthy elderly people and patients with mild cognitive impairment*. Life (Basel), 2022. **12**(3): p. 432.

44. Wang, H., et al., *Intermittent hypoxia training for treating mild cognitive impairment: A pilot study*. Am J Alzheimers Dis Other Demen, 2020. **35**: p. 1533317519896725.

45. Haider, T., et al., *Interval hypoxic training improves autonomic cardiovascular and respiratory control in patients with mild chronic obstructive pulmonary disease*. J Hypertens, 2009. **27**(8): p. 1648–1654.

46. Muangritdech, N., et al., *Hypoxic training improves blood pressure, nitric oxide and hypoxia-inducible factor-1 alpha in hypertensive patients*. Eur J Appl Physiol, 2020. **120**(8): p. 1815–1826.

47. Lyamina, N.P., et al., *Normobaric hypoxia conditioning reduces blood pressure and normalizes nitric oxide synthesis in patients with arterial hypertension*. J Hypertens, 2011. **29**(11): p. 2265–2272.

48. Saeed, O., et al., *Improved exercise performance and skeletal muscle strength after simulated altitude exposure: A novel approach for patients with chronic heart failure*. J Cardiac Fail, 2012. **18**(5): p. 387–391.

49. Glazachev, O., et al., *Adaptations following an intermittent hypoxia-hyperoxia training in coronary artery disease patients: A controlled study*. Clin Cardiol, 2017. **40**(6): p. 370–376.

50. Glazachev, O.S., et al., *[Adaptation to dosed hypoxia–hyperoxia as a factor in improving the quality of life of elderly patients with cardiac pathology.]*. Adv Gerontol, 2019. **32**(1–2): p. 145–151.

51. Tin'kov, A.N. and V.A. Aksenov, *Effects of intermittent hypobaric hypoxia on blood lipid concentrations in male coronary heart disease patients*. High Alt Med Biol, 2002. **3**(3): p. 277–282.
52. del Pilar Valle, M., et al., *Improvement of myocardial perfusion in coronary patients after intermittent hypobaric hypoxia*. J Nucl Cardiol, 2006. **13**(1): p. 69–74.
53. Bestavashvili, A., et al., *The effects of intermittent hypoxic–hyperoxic exposures on lipid profile and inflammation in patients with metabolic syndrome*. Front Cardiovasc Med. 2021. **8**: 700826.
54. Bestavashvili, A., et al., *Intermittent hypoxic-hyperoxic exposures effects in patients with metabolic syndrome: Correction of cardiovascular and metabolic profile*. Biomedicines, 2022. **10**(3): p. 566.
55. Klug, L., et al., *Normobaric hypoxic conditioning in men with metabolic syndrome*. Physiological Reports, 2018. **6**(24): p. e13949.
56. Gutwenger, I., et al., *Pilot study on the effects of a 2-week hiking vacation at moderate versus low altitude on plasma parameters of carbohydrate and lipid metabolism in patients with metabolic syndrome*. BMC Research Notes, 2015. **8**: p. 103–103.
57. Serebrovska, T.V., et al., *Intermittent hypoxia/hyperoxia versus intermittent hypoxia/normoxia: Comparative study in prediabetes*. High Alt Med Biol, 2019. **20**(4): p. 383–391.
58. Schreuder, T.H., et al., *Impact of hypoxic versus normoxic training on physical fitness and vasculature in diabetes*. High Alt Med Biol, 2014. **15**(3): p. 349–355.
59. Marlatt, K.L., et al., *Two weeks of moderate hypoxia improves glucose tolerance in individuals with type 2 diabetes*. Int J Obes (Lond), 2020. **44**(3): p. 744–747.
60. Behrendt, T., et al., *Effects of intermittent hypoxia-hyperoxia exposure prior to aerobic cycling exercise on physical and cognitive performance in geriatric patients: A randomized controlled trial*. Front Physiol, 2022. **13**: p. 899096.
61. Behrendt, T., et al., *Influence of acute and chronic intermittent hypoxic–hyperoxic exposure prior to aerobic exercise on cardiovascular risk factors in geriatric patients: A randomized controlled trial*. Front Physiol, 2022. **13**: p. 1043536.
62. Bayer, U., et al., *Effects of intermittent hypoxia–hyperoxia on mobility and perceived health in geriatric patients performing a multimodal training intervention: A randomized controlled trial*. BMC Geriatrics, 2019. **19**(1): p. 167.
63. Bayer, U., et al., *Intermittent hypoxic-hyperoxic training on cognitive performance in geriatric patients*. Alzheimers Dement (N Y), 2017. **3**(1): p. 114–122.
64. Bayer, U., et al., *[Adaptation to intermittent hypoxia-hyperoxia improves cognitive performance and exercise tolerance in elderly]*. Adv Gerontol, 2017. **30**(2): p. 255–261.
65. Dudnik, E., et al., *Intermittent hypoxia-hyperoxia conditioning improves cardiorespiratory fitness in older comorbid cardiac outpatients without hematological changes: A randomized controlled trial*. High Alt Med Biol, 2018. **19**(4): p. 339–343.

SECTION 8

15

HYPOXIA CONDITIONING FOR PRE-ACCLIMATIZATION BEFORE GOING TO HIGH ALTITUDE

Martin Burtscher and Markus Tannheimer

15.1 Introduction

Terrestrial altitude ranges from sea level (0 m) to the top of Mount Everest (8,849 m). Height areas are usually defined as moderate (1,500–2,500 m), high (2,500–3,500 m), very high (3,500–5,500 m), and extreme altitude (>5,500 m) [1, 2]. Worldwide, about 400 million people permanently live above 1,500 m, and more than 100 million lowlanders annually visit regions higher than 2,500 m [3, 4]. While high-altitude dwellers are well adapted to the lower barometric pressure and related lower partial pressure of inspired oxygen (O_2), the reduced O_2 availability may provoke the development of acute high-altitude illnesses in visitors without appropriate acclimatization [1, 5]. As acute (unaccustomed) hypoxia (and not hypobaria) is the primary cause for high-altitude illness, repeated exposures to real and/or simulated altitudes before going to high mountains, such as, for skiing, trekking, or climbing, can be used to induce acclimatization [6].

15.2 High-altitude illnesses

Acute mountain sickness (AMS) is the most frequent illness developing in high-altitude visitors (with an incidence of about 7% at 2,200 m to over 50% at 4,559 m), which usually follows a benign disease course, while high-altitude cerebral (HACE) and pulmonary edema (HAPE) occur rather rarely (about 1% for HACE and up to 6% for HAPE) but are life-threatening [1, 5, 7]. In unacclimatized individuals, AMS develops typically within the first 6 to 12 h of acute high-altitude exposure, with headache as the cardinal symptom often accompanied by nausea, vomiting, dizziness, and fatigue [5].

DOI: 10.4324/9781003402879-24

If AMS progresses to HACE, this is indicated by additionally altered mental status and ataxia [8–10].

Concerning pathophysiological mechanisms responsible for high-altitude illnesses, elevation of intracranial pressure, brain swelling, and edema formation may play important roles [11]. The consequently activated and sensitized trigemino-vascular system via mechanical and/or biochemical (e.g., reactive oxygen species (ROS), nitric oxide (NO), and inflammatory molecules) may explain AMS symptoms [6, 12].

The second life-threatening high-altitude illness is HAPE, noncardiogenic pulmonary edema, which is a consequence of profound hypoxic pulmonary vasoconstriction [13]. The associated increase in pulmonary-artery and capillary pressures results in a noninflammatory and hemorrhagic alveolar–capillary leak [13, 14]. Thus, pronounced dyspnea and exercise intolerance are characteristic symptoms of HAPE (which may be followed by orthopnea, drowsiness, cough, and pink frothy sputum) [15, 16]. Genetic predisposition with exaggerated pulmonary vascular responses to hypoxia, possibly attributed to insufficient bioavailability of NO and high ROS levels in hypoxia or at altitude seem to be of pathophysiological relevance [6, 17].

It is important to mention that AMS symptoms are much more likely to occur when rapidly ascending to high altitude (and without acclimatization) [18], but typically the symptoms resolve over a few days of acclimatization [19, 20]. Moreover, it was demonstrated in mountaineers with unknown HAPE history that the HAPE incidence was only 0.2% when slowly ascending over 4 days to an altitude of 4,500 m, but the incidence increased to 6% with rapid ascent (1–2 days) [7]. It is not only the risk of high-altitude illness that is reduced by slow ascent and/or pre-acclimatization, but also the considerably reduced physical performance when acutely exposed to high altitude is much less affected when (pre)acclimatized [20, 21]. As repeated hypoxia/altitude exposures (hypoxia conditioning) before going to high altitude induce several adaptive physiological and molecular processes, such as increased pulmonary ventilation (ventilatory acclimatization), and activation of the hypoxia-inducible family of transcription factors (HIFs) and nuclear factor erythroid 2-related factor 2 (Nrf2) [6], the clinical and practical relevance of hypoxia conditioning becomes obvious.

15.3 Hypoxia conditioning by exposure to real altitude

Pre-acclimatization (by hypoxia conditioning) at moderate and higher altitudes in the surrounding area to individual locations of residence, such as mountainous areas of the Rocky Mountains or the Alps, the utilization of "staging" (staying at altitudes of about 2,000–3,000 m for several days before climbing to higher altitudes), and that of slow, graded ascents are known as traditional (pre)acclimatization strategies [20, 21]. Although these strategies have been known and practiced for decades, only a few studies have evaluated their efficacy in a controlled manner [22].

One of the major beneficial responses to high-altitude exposure is the increased alveolar minute ventilation (ventilatory acclimatization) and the associated recovery of the initially pronounced decrease of arterial oxygen-ation (SaO_2), which was shown to progressively increase and to reach a pla-teau after about 8–10 days at altitudes up to about 4,500 m [23]. Ventilatory acclimatization is accompanied by other physiological changes, such as increased heart rate and systemic blood pressure (in particular of the pulmo-nary artery), elevated diuresis and hemoconcentration [6]. Both improved SaO_2 and hemoglobin (Hb) concentration (initially due to hemoconcentra-tion and later because of the elevated erythropoiesis) contribute to the recov-ery of the initially lowered arterial oxygen content ($CaO_2 = Hb \times SaO_2$) [24]. While 8–10 days (a total of about 240 hours) of altitude/hypoxia exposure would be optimal for (pre)acclimatization (at least concerning ventilatory acclimatization), each single hour of staying at altitude/in hypoxia will induce some hypoxia conditioning. Beidleman et al., for instance, prevented AMS development completely at 4,300 m in individuals with 15 preceding 4-h daily exposures to 4,300 m [25].

Hypoxia conditioning is also induced by staging, subsequently allowing a more rapid ascent to higher altitudes associated with a lower risk of develop-ing high-altitude illnesses and partial preservation of physical performance [26]. A 6-day stay at 2,200 m effectively reduced the AMS incidence by about 50% [26], and the increase in pulmonary arterial pressure (and likely also the associated risk of HAPE) during the following rapid ascent to 4,300 m [27]. Figure 15.1. (modified from [28]) demonstrates hypoxia conditioning by com-bining pre-acclimatization at home and staging at 3,500 m before rapidly climbing an almost 7,000 m peak. Although the total time of hypoxia condi-tioning to climb this altitude at low risk for high-altitude illness does not essentially differ from that when ascending slowly, the number of days on the mountain (associated with natural hazards, changing weather conditions, and boring waiting times in camps) can be considerably reduced.

Hypoxia conditioning is also induced by slow ascent to high altitude. As a common rule, a daily ascent rate of 400–500 m (sleeping elevation) above 2,500 m should not be exceeded, with an additional resting day for every additional gain in altitude of 1,000–1,500 m or in the case of health com-plaints [1, 7, 20]. Richalet and colleagues demonstrated a reduced preva-lence of severe high-altitude illness (from 27% to 12%) when respecting this rule (plus taking acetazolamide for AMS prophylaxis) [29]. Optimally, pre-acclimatization is performed as close as possible before the main high-altitude sojourn, but there is some evidence that five or more days above 3,000 m within the previous 2 months will reduce the AMS risk during a following rapid ascent to 4,500 m [30]. Faster acclimatization after previous

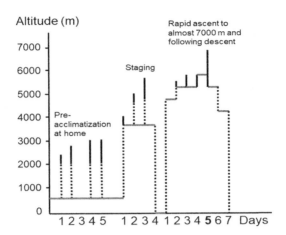

FIGURE 15.1 Example of climbing to an altitude of almost 7,000 m within 5 days (without any symptoms of AMS) after some pre-acclimatization at home and staging at a high-altitude village (4 days at about 3,500 m) with three ascents to 4,000–5,500 m. Dotted vertical lines are passive ascents (by car), solid vertical lines are active ascent, and red horizontal lines indicate sleeping altitude.

Modified according to Burtscher and Koch [28].

high-altitude sojourn has been reported [31], and may at least partially be due to the hypoxia adenosine response (erythrocyte hypoxic memory) in order to counteract hypoxia-induced maladaptation [32].

Taken together, beside the slow ascent at the target mountain, all types of pre-exposure including staging initiate the acclimatization process and are capable to reduce the risk of the development of high-altitude illness.

15.4 Hypoxia conditioning by exposure to simulated altitude

Another way to prepare the body for upcoming high-altitude exposure (hypoxia conditioning) is to use "artificial altitude," for which two options are available: hypobaric hypoxia (HH) and normobaric hypoxia (NH). The main motivation for conducting pre-acclimatization is to save time later at the mountain. Therefore, pre-acclimatization must be organized in a way that it can be carried out at home alongside one's daily work routine. For this purpose, the proximity to the place of residence is crucial.

When using a hypobaric chamber, as done, for example, in the "Operation Everest Studies" [33–35], it involves HH, which is similar to the natural reduced barometric pressure at altitude but without other influencing factors like weather, UV radiation, and cold. However, the use of hypobaric chambers for pre-acclimatization is limited by their low availability and high costs.

The second option involves NH (Figure 15.2), where the percentage of O_2 in the air is reduced from the normal 20.9% to the desired target altitude's pO_2 (e.g., 15.4% O_2: pO_2 = 117.0 mmHg $\triangleq$ 2,500 m) [36]. NH is an established technique in fire protection because an open flame is nearly impossible below 15% O_2, and even explosive substances like gasoline won't burn below 13% O_2 [36, 37]. A generator produces the hypoxic gas mixture used for NH exposure (NHE). Since the construction requirements for an NH-room are much simpler than for a hypobaric chamber, NH is much more cost-effective than HH, and an NH-room can be easily accessed or exited through a normal door. NH is available in a tent version with a mobile generator, making it practical to use anywhere [38]. For years, it has been used for altitude training of elite athletes [39, 40], pre-acclimatization of professional mountaineers [41–43], or in military applications [44, 45]. Nowadays NH is increasingly

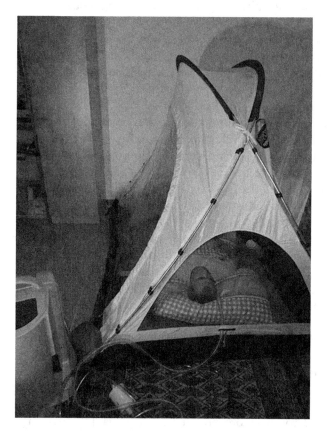

FIGURE 15.2　Sleeping in normobaric hypoxia for pre-acclimatization before climbing a high mountain.

utilized in commercial expedition mountaineering [46, 47], and in some cases, it is even required by expedition companies [48].

From a scientific perspective, different hypoxia conditioning effects of NH and HH are being discussed [49, 50]. The two main influencing factors are the water vapor pressure (pH_2O) [51] and the respiratory resistance [52]. Since the pH_2O remains constant at 47 mmHg at body temperature, its influence increases with increasing "altitude" in HH compared to NH. Even if the pO_2 is set to the same "altitude" in both cases, the perceived altitude in NH is lower, and therefore, its physiological effect is also reduced. For instance, at an altitude of 4,559 m (Capanna Margherita), the inspiratory pO_2 is 80 mmHg in HH and 85 mmHg in NH [51]. The respiratory resistance is lower in HH due to the reduced air density compared to NH. This reduces the necessary respiratory effort in HH, especially in cases of high respiratory volumes during intense physical activity. For example, at an altitude of 3,000 m, Laymon et al. calculated a 72% increased respiratory effort (153 ml O_2/min) for NH compared to HH during moderate physical activity [52]. Since these two effects behave oppositely, depending on the chosen altitude and exercise intensity, there may be significantly different effects between NH and HH [53]. However, these differences play a minor role in pre-acclimatization for expedition mountaineering because the primary focus is on implementing pre-acclimatization into the normal daily work routine. In most cases, this is only feasible with NH. Therefore, the following discussion will concentrate on pre-acclimatization using NH, although the recommendations would generally apply to HH as well. However, HH might be much more challenging to implement not only due to its availability but also due to the complex compression and decompression issues when entering and leaving the hypobaric chamber.

A crucial point to consider is that achieving acclimatization doesn't require spending the entire day in hypoxia [44]. Acclimatization effects can already be observed with very short exposure times of just a few hours per day [44, 54, 55]. However, there are currently no studies determining the optimal duration of daily hypoxia exposure for the best possible acclimatization. This depends significantly on the desired target altitude for acclimatization, making individual studies necessary for each altitude. Case reports, personal experiences, and observations from commercial expedition companies indicate that 24 hours a day of exposure to NH are not necessary for achieving an optimal effect [42, 46, 56]. Nevertheless, longer exposure times lead to more pronounced acclimatization effects [30, 57].

The higher the target altitude for acclimatization, the greater the required hypoxic dose, and it seems that to some extent, a shorter exposure time can be compensated for by more pronounced hypoxia [19]. As an example, the accomplished alpinist Kilian Jornet spent 380 hours in NH during the two months before his record ascent to Mount Everest (8,848 m) in just 26.5 hours.

Additionally, he spent 100 hours at real altitudes going as high as 4,200 m in the Alps [42]. The hypoxic dose in NHE is determined by the degree of hypoxia, the duration, the number, and the timing of each NHE session, as well as whether NHE is conducted during sleep at night, resting during the day, or while performing physical exercise [25, 44, 57]. This results in a large number of possible NHE protocols [44, 45], and it remains unclear which combination constitutes the ideal protocol, considering the target altitude for acclimatization [46, 58]. In practical applications, NHE will mostly be carried out in a way that can be best integrated into the daily work routine. Therefore, NHE is predominantly performed during sleep at night to accommodate this need.

NHE has the fundamental advantage that the development of AMS is practically excluded due to its latency [46, 59]. Unlike real high-altitude environments, the hypoxic environment in NHE can be easily and immediately exited, allowing for a much more ambitious acclimatization profile. Therefore, the recommendations from companies renting out NHE equipment, which suggest a 6-day sleep height increment until sleeping above 2,500 m, are not justifiable [59]. Typical acclimatization recommendations limit the increase in sleeping altitude to 300–500 m per day only above 2,500 m [5, 60–62]. In the case of healthy, athletic individuals, NHE has been initiated at a sleeping altitude of 2,800 m and incrementally increased to 5,400 m within 10 days, depending on the quality of sleep [46]. Since NHE is usually conducted alongside regular daily activities, restful sleep is necessary for optimal professional performance. Therefore, sleep quality becomes the limiting factor for increasing sleeping altitude. If the sleep quality is good, the altitude is further increased for the next night, while in cases of poor sleep, the current altitude might be maintained, or even reduced during the night if needed, selecting a lower "altitude" at the generator. It is advisable to use a pulse oximeter for monitoring SaO_2 during NHE. For sleep measurements, the alarm threshold should not be set too high, as this may lead to frequent false alarms due to the circadian rhythm of SaO_2 with a nightly minimum shortly before midnight [63] and the periodic breathing that typically occurs during sleep [64], which can, in turn, disturb sleep. Therefore, alarm thresholds of $SaO_2 = 70\%$ are recommended up to altitudes of 4,000 m, and 60% between 4,000 and 6,000 m during NHE [46]. During NHE with a mask in the awake state (at rest or during active training), it is permissible to achieve SaO_2 levels <70% if the individual feels comfortable, as the mask can be easily removed in case of discomfort.

In summary, pre-acclimatization using NHE allows for a significant reduction in time spent at targeted mountain, potentially leading to improved chances to reach the summit due to reduced risks of travel-related illnesses like traveler's diarrhea and better rest conditions for the final ascent. NHE can be performed independent of weather conditions, and the risk of developing

AMS is negligible, allowing for more progressive acclimatization protocols. Depending on the planned expedition and the participants' level of experience, as well as the desire to not only summit the peak but also experience the mountain's surroundings, traditional acclimatization methods on the mountain remain important.

15.5 Conclusions

All pre-exposures to real and/or simulated altitude offer valuable benefits, but the choice between pre-acclimatization using NHE and traditional acclimatization on the mountain depends on the specific expedition goals, the participants' skills, and the desire for a comprehensive mountain experience beyond just reaching the summit.

Abbreviations

AMS	acute mountain sickness
CaO_2	arterial oxygen content
HACE	high-altitude cerebral edema
HAPE	high-altitude pulmonary edema
Hb	hemoglobin
HH	hypobaric hypoxia
HIF	hypoxia inducible factor
NH	normobaric hypoxia
NO	nitric oxide
Nrf2	nuclear factor erythroid 2-related factor
O_2	oxygen
pH_2O	water vapor pressure
pO_2	partial pressure of oxygen
ROS	reactive oxygen species
SaO_2	arterial oxygen saturation.

References

1. Netzer, N., et al., *Hypoxia-related altitude illnesses.* J Travel Med, 2013. 20(4): p. 247–55.
2. Schobersberger, W., et al., *Austrian Moderate Altitude Studies (AMAS): Benefits of exposure to moderate altitudes (1,500–2,500 m).* Sleep Breath, 2010. 14(3): p. 201–7.
3. Cohen, J.E. and C. Small, *Hypsographic demography: The distribution of human population by altitude.* Proc Natl Acad Sci U S A, 1998. 95(24): p. 14009–14.
4. Mallet, R.T., et al., *Impact of high altitude on cardiovascular health: Current perspectives.* Vasc Health Risk Manag, 2021. 17: p. 317–35.
5. Hackett, P.H. and R.C. Roach, *High-altitude illness.* N Engl J Med, 2001. 345(2): p. 107–14.

6. Mallet, R.T., et al., *Molecular mechanisms of high-altitude acclimatization.* Int J Mol Sci, 2023. **24**(2).

7. Bärtsch, P. and E.R. Swenson, *Clinical practice: Acute high-altitude illnesses.* N Engl J Med, 2013. **368**(24): p. 2294–302.

8. Gallagher, S.A. and P.H. Hackett, *High-altitude illness.* Emerg Med Clin North Am, 2004. **22**(2): p. 329–55, viii.

9. Roach, R.C., et al., *The 2018 Lake Louise acute mountain sickness score.* High Alt Med Biol, 2018. **19**(1): p. 4–6.

10. Wu, T., et al., *Ataxia: an early indicator in high altitude cerebral edema.* High Alt Med Biol, 2006. **7**(4): p. 275–80.

11. Sagoo, R.S., et al., *Magnetic Resonance investigation into the mechanisms involved in the development of high-altitude cerebral edema.* J Cereb Blood Flow Metab, 2017. **37**(1): p. 319–31.

12. Burtscher, M., et al., *Aspirin for prophylaxis against headache at high altitudes: randomised, double blind, placebo controlled trial.* BMJ, 1998. **316**(7137): p. 1057–8.

13. Swenson, E.R. and P. Bärtsch, *High-altitude pulmonary edema.* Compr Physiol, 2012. **2**(4): p. 2753–73.

14. Maggiorini, M., et al., *High-altitude pulmonary edema is initially caused by an increase in capillary pressure.* Circulation, 2001. **103**(16): p. 2078–83.

15. Bärtsch, P., et al., *High altitude pulmonary oedema.* Swiss Med Wkly, 2003. **133**(27–28): p. 377–84.

16. Schoene, R.B., *Pulmonary edema at high altitude. Review, pathophysiology, and update.* Clin Chest Med, 1985. **6**(3): p. 491–507.

17. Eichstaedt, C.A., et al., *Genetic predisposition to high-altitude pulmonary edema.* High Alt Med Biol, 2020. **21**(1): p. 28–36.

18. Burtscher, J., et al., *Flying to high-altitude destinations: Is the risk of acute mountain sickness greater?* J Travel Med, 2023. 30: p. .taad011.

19. Fulco, C.S., B.A. Beidleman, and S.R. Muza, *Effectiveness of preacclimatization strategies for high-altitude exposure.* Exerc Sport Sci Rev, 2013. **41**(1): p. 55–63.

20. Burtscher, M., U. Hefti, and J.P. Hefti, *High-altitude illnesses: Old stories and new insights into the pathophysiology, treatment and prevention.* Sports Med Health Sci, 2021. **3**(2): p. 59–69.

21. Burtscher, M., G.P. Millet, and J. Burtscher, *Hypoxia conditioning for high-altitude pre-acclimatization.* J Sci Sport Exer, 2022. 4: p. 331–45.

22. Bloch, K.E., et al., *Effect of ascent protocol on acute mountain sickness and success at Muztagh Ata, 7546 m.* High Alt Med Biol, 2009. **10**(1): p. 25–32.

23. Sato, M., J.W. Severinghaus, and P. Bickler, *Time course of augmentation and depression of hypoxic ventilatory responses at altitude.* J Appl Physiol (1985), 1994. **77**(1): p. 313–6.

24. Calbet, J.A., et al., *Why is VO2 max after altitude acclimatization still reduced despite normalization of arterial O2 content?* Am J Physiol Regul Integr Comp Physiol, 2003. **284**(2): p. R304–16.

25. Beidleman, B.A., et al., *Intermittent altitude exposures reduce acute mountain sickness at 4300 m.* Clin Sci (Lond), 2004. **106**(3): p. 321–8.

26. Beidleman, B.A., et al., *Effect of six days of staging on physiologic adjustments and acute mountain sickness during ascent to 4300 meters.* High Alt Med Biol, 2009. **10**(3): p. 253–60.

27. Baggish, A.L., et al., *The impact of moderate-altitude staging on pulmonary arterial hemodynamics after ascent to high altitude*. High Alt Med Biol, 2010. **11**(2): p. 139–45.

28. Burtscher, M. and R. Koch, *Effects of pre-acclimatization applying the "climb high and sleep low"maxim: An example of rapid but safe ascent to extreme altitude*. J Human Perform Extreme Envir, 2016. **12**(2): p. 2.

29. Richalet, J.P., et al., *Validation of a score for the detection of subjects with high risk for severe high-altitude illness*. Med Sci Sports Exerc, 2020. 53: p. 1294–1302. Publish Ahead of Print.

30. Muza, S.R., B.A. Beidleman, and C.S. Fulco, *Altitude preexposure recommendations for inducing acclimatization*. High Alt Med Biol, 2010. **11**(2): p. 87–92.

31. Beidleman, B.A., et al., *Exercise responses after altitude acclimatization are retained during reintroduction to altitude*. Med Sci Sports Exerc, 1997. **29**(12): p. 1588–95.

32. Song, A., et al., *Erythrocytes retain hypoxic adenosine response for faster acclimatization upon re-ascent*. Nat Commun, 2017. **8**: p. 14108.

33. Houston, C.S., *Operation Everest one and two. Studies of acclimatization to simulated high altitude*. Respiration, 1997. **64**(6): p. 398–406.

34. Houston, C.S., et al., *Operation Everest II: man at extreme altitude*. J Appl Physiol (1985), 1987. **63**(2): p. 877–82.

35. Richalet, J.-P., *Operation Everest III: COMEX'97*. High Alt Med Biol, 2010. **11**(2): p. 121–32.

36. Küpper, T., et al., *Work in hypoxic conditions-consensus statement of the medical commission of the Union Internationale des Associations d'Alpinisme (UIAA MedCom)*. Ann Occup Hyg, 2011. **55**(4): p. 369–86.

37. Angerer, P. and D. Nowak, *Working in permanent hypoxia for fire protection—impact on health*. Int Arch Occup Environ Health, 2003. **76**(2): p. 87–102.

38. Bhaumik, G., et al., Rapid acclimatization strategies for high-altitude induction, in *Translational Research in Environmental and Occupational Stress*, S.A. Singh, N.R. Prabhakar, and S.N. Pentyala, Editors. 2014, Springer: New Delhi. p. 135–54.

39. Richalet, J.P. and C.J. Gore, *Live and/or sleep high: Train low, using normobaric hypoxia*. Scand J Med Sci Sports, 2008. **18**(1): p. 29–37.

40. Mekjavic, I.B., et al., *Intermittent normobaric hypoxic exposures at rest: Effects on performance in normoxia and hypoxia*. Aviat Space Environ Med, 2012. **83**(10): p. 942–50.

41. Harrington, E. *Emily Harrington on her rapid ascent of Cho Oyu*. 2016 [cited 2020 06.08.2023].

42. Millet, G.P. and K. Jornet, *On top to the top-acclimatization strategy for the "fastest known time" to Everest*. Int J Sport Physiol Perform, 2019. **1**: p. 1–12.

43. Lozancich, K. *Woman climbs Everest in two weeks, breaks round trip record*. 2019 [cited 2020 06.08.2023].

44. Muza, S.R., *Military applications of hypoxic training for high-altitude operations*. Med Sci Sports Exerc, 2007. **39**(9): p. 1625–31.

45. Bhaumik, G., et al., *Effect of intermittent normobaric hypoxia exposures on acute mountain sickness during acute ascent to 3500 m in Indian military personnel*. Def Life Sci J 2018. **3**(3): p. 209–15.

46. Tannheimer, M. and R. Lechner, *Rapid ascents of Mt Everest: Normobaric hypoxic preacclimatization*. J Travel Med, 2020. **27**(6): p. 1–7.

47. Furtenbach, L. 2019 [cited 2020 06.08.2023].

48. Tannheimer, M., *Intermittent simulated hypoxia for pre-acclimatization.* Sleep Breath, 2010. **14**(3): p. 185–6.

49. Richard, N.A. and M.S. Koehle, *Differences in cardio-ventilatory responses to hypobaric and normobaric hypoxia: A review.* Aviat Space Environ Med, 2012. **83**(7): p. 677–84.

50. Millet, G.P., R. Faiss, and V. Pialoux, *Evidence for differences between hypobaric and normobaric hypoxia is conclusive.* Exerc Sport Sci Rev, 2013. **41**(2): p. 133.

51. Koehle, M.S. and M.J. MacInnis, *Correct hypoxic dose and exhaled no clarification.* J Appl Physiol, 2012. **112**(10): p. 1788–9.

52. Laymon, A.S., J.L. Stickford, and J.C. Weavil, *Differences in respiratory muscle metabolic cost between normobaric and hypobaric hypoxia.* J Appl Physiol, 2012. **112**(10): p. 1792.

53. Savourey, G., et al., *Normo- and hypobaric hypoxia: Are there any physiological differences?* Eur J Appl Physiol, 2003. **89**(2): p. 122–6.

54. Katayama, K., et al., *Effect of a repeated series of intermittent hypoxic exposures on ventilatory response in humans.* High Alt Med Biol, 2005. **6**(1): p. 50–9.

55. Burtscher, M., E. Brandstatter, and H. Gatterer, *Preacclimatization in simulated altitudes.* Sleep Breath, 2008. **12**(2): p. 109–14.

56. Furtenbach, L., *Complete bloody hogwash.* Berg & Steigen, 2018. **104**(4): p. 28–35.

57. Fulco, C.S., et al., *Effect of repeated normobaric hypoxia exposures during sleep on acute mountain sickness, exercise performance, and sleep during exposure to terrestrial altitude.* Am J Physiol Regul Integr Comp Physiol, 2011. **300**(2): p. 428–36.

58. Jones, J.E., et al., *Intermittent hypoxic exposure does not improve sleep at 4300 m.* High Alt Med Biol, 2008. **9**(4): p. 281–7.

59. Tannheimer, M. and R. Lechner, *An analysis of commercially recommended profiles for normobaric preacclimatization.* Health Prmot Phys Act, 2021. **14**(1): p. 25–9.

60. Bärtsch, P. and B. Saltin, *General introduction to altitude adaptation and mountain sickness.* Scand J Med Sci Sports, 2008. **18**(s1): p. 1–10.

61. Luks, A.M., E.R. Swenson, and P. Bärtsch, *Acute high-altitude sickness.* Eur Respir Rev, 2017. **26**(143): p. 1–14.

62. West, J.B., *High-altitude medicine.* Am J Respir Crit Care Med, 2012. **186**(12): p. 1229–37.

63. Tannheimer, M., et al., *Oxygen saturation increases over the course of the night in mountaineers at high altitude (3050–6354 m).* J Travel Med, 2017. **24**(5): p. 1–6.

64. Tannheimer, M. and R. Lechner, *The correct measurement of oxygen saturation at high altitude.* Sleep Breath, 2019. **23**(4): p. 1101–6.

16

ALTITUDE/HYPOXIC TRAINING FOR ENDURANCE ATHLETES

Grégoire Millet and Franck Brocherie

16.1 Introduction

Since the early overview article of Randall Wilber [1] and the characterization of three main types of altitude/hypoxic training (live high–train high, LHTH; live high–train low, LHTL; and live low–train high LLTH), many variations of these types have been described in the last 15 years: First, we proposed a new combination of hypoxic methods (live high–train low and high; LHTLH) associating LHTL (sleeping between 2,500 and 3,000 m) with training near sea-level except for a few (2–3 per week) LLTH high-intensity sessions at altitude [2]; second, the development of different types of LLTH methods (e.g., RSH, repeated sprint training in hypoxia or RTH, resistance training in hypoxia originally dedicated for team- or racket sports [3, 4]—see Chapter 17) led to a widening (or maybe a sophistication) of the available methods (see Figure 16.1 for the panorama of all methods currently proposed).

As a consequence, several important questions arise for the endurance athletes and for their support staff.

1. What are the benefits for each method of altitude training for endurance athletes?
2. What are the potential risks and drawbacks for each method of altitude training for endurance athletes?
3. How can the beneficial effects be optimized and potential deleterious ones be mitigated?
4. Which are the consequences in term of periodization?

DOI: 10.4324/9781003402879-25

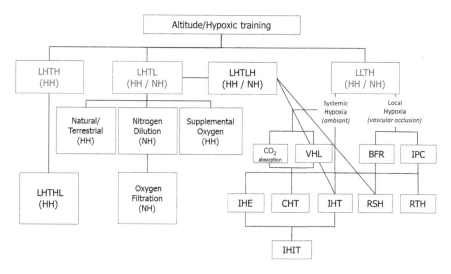

FIGURE 16.1   Current panorama of all attitude training methods.

LHTH, live high–train high; **LHTL**, live high–train low; **LLTH**, live low–train high; **LHTLH**, live high–train low and high; **LHTHL**, live high–train high and low; **CO_2 absorption**, rebreathing with a mask; **VHL**, voluntary hypoventilation at low lung volume; **IPC**, ischemic pre-conditioning; **BFR**, blood flow restriction; **IHE**, intermittent hypoxic exposure; **CHT**, continuous hypoxic training; **IHT**, interval hypoxic training; **RSH**, repeated sprint training in hypoxia; **RTH**, resistance training in hypoxia; **IHE** during interval-training; **IHIT**, intermittent hypoxic interval-training; **NH**, normobaric hypoxia; **HH**, hypobaric hypoxia.

Adapted from [4].

16.2 Pros and cons of altitude/hypoxic training for endurance athletes

16.2.1 Benefits of altitude training for endurance athletes

The primary—and historically first investigated—mechanism assumes that altitude training is effective for increasing the aerobic capacity of the athletes, mainly by improving the oxygen transport capacity (e.g., the convective component of VO_2max [5]). Prolonged exposure to optimal altitude levels (i.e., 2,200 to 2,800 m) induces positive hematological effects [6], as long as the hypoxic dose is high enough. Both LHTH or LHTL can lead to an estimated increase in total hemoglobin mass (Hb_{mass}) of 1.0–1.1% per 100 h of exposure in both NH and HH [7–9]. An alternative point of view that "altitude training does not convincingly increase exercise performance and should not be recommended to elite (endurance) athletes" [10] was based on the belief that athletes with a high pre-altitude (LHTH or LHTL) Hb_{mass} value may have reached a "ceiling" level and would therefore not increase Hb_{mass} and VO_2max [11]. This viewpoint supporting a noneffectiveness of LHTL (or LHTH) may arise from inaccurate data coming from "noisy" (poor signal-to-noise ratio) data [12]. It is now well-established that even athletes with high Hb_{mass} or VO_2max values would benefit from altitude training (3–4% increase in both Hb_{mass} and VO_2max)max with a high enough hypoxic dose and an adequate monitoring [13]. Confirmation comes from the practitioners; for example, a majority of British distance runners and support staff utilized altitude training and considered hypoxia as a "very important" training factor [14]. Moreover, case studies in world-class endurance athletes—for instance, in swimming [15], biathlon [16], mountaineering [17], running [18] or cycling [19]—have been published and confirm the wide use and the effectiveness of altitude training by the most successful endurance athletes of their respective sports. Finally, it is of interest to observe that athletes are pushing for an access to hypoxic facilities in countries where it was until now limited (e.g., Norway) with subsequent sport success. A remaining point of discussion regarding the hematological benefits is on the potential differences between LHTL and LHTH—when hypoxic dose is matched—[20], pointing out the significance of the intermittent pattern of exposure to hypoxia.

Beyond the well-described hematological benefits, several peripheral adaptations of LHTH and LHTL (i.e., angiogenesis, glucose transport, glycolysis, and pH regulation) were early reported [21], independent of the Hb_{mass} increase. The beneficial nonhematological factors may include improved muscle and mitochondrial efficiency, greater muscle buffering capacity, and a better lactate regulation. Future research should examine both hematological and nonhematological mechanisms of adaptation to hypoxia that might enhance the performance of elite athletes at sea level [2]. Moreover, even for endurance athletes, hypoxic training is not limited to methods based on prolonged exposure to hypoxia (LHTH, LHTL, or LHTLH) anymore. Recent innovative methods such as RSH [22, 23] have been shown to be effective for improving repeated-sprint ability in intermittent [team (rugby, football, field hockey) and racket (tennis)]; (see Chapter 17) sports and are also used by endurance (cycling, cross-country ski) athletes. For an updated review, see [24]. The influence of integrating high-intensity exercises during altitude exposure—which was originally not recommended—on the physiological responses remains poorly understood [25]: even if combining prolonged altitude exposure and high(er)-intensity exercises (i.e., LHTLH) was shown to be similarly effective to LHTL on the erythropoietic responses [26], further research is requested to confirm if the observed peripheral molecular adaptation [27] may lead to an improved muscle oxygen diffusion capacity and subsequently to a larger increase in VO_{2max}. Some mechanisms (e.g., improved muscle resistance to fatigue) are specific to RSH and therefore independent to the magnitude of the hypoxic dose and are not observed either with passive exposure to hypoxia or in the other hypoxic methods utilizing lower training intensities.

16.2.2 Potential risks and maladaptation of altitude training for endurance athletes

Several factors may limit the Hb_{mass} increase. There is still a need for better understanding of the mechanistic relationships with erythropoiesis. The health status of the athlete (illness/injuries/mental health) [28]; an insufficient iron store or supplementation, particularly in female athletes [29]; insufficient hydration to counterbalance the increased respiratory water loss due to hyperventilation and increased diuresis as a consequence of the respiratory alkalosis [30]; and insufficient energy (particularly carbohydrate and amino acids) availability [31] may all lead to altitude-related maladaptation [32]. Of practical importance is that the effect of all these factors can be minimized—or at least controlled—with an effective monitoring by the support staff during altitude training camps (Table 16.1) [33]. Such monitoring is particularly important in endurance athletes since they can be subjected to a large exercise-induced arterial hypoxemia [34] leading to a larger decrease in VO_{2max} and aerobic endurance than their less-performant counterparts [35]. Among the various complementary monitoring means (Table 16.1), we recommend heart rate variability guided training for limiting the perceived fatigue as well as the increased sympathetic activation and associated sleep deterioration during LHTL [36].

16.2.3 How to optimize the beneficial effects of "classical" altitude training methods and mitigate the deleterious ones?

One important criterion for optimizing hematological responses is the hypoxic dose that is the combination of the altitude level, the exposure duration, and the intermittent pattern. It is generally recommended to stay at altitudes between 2,200 and 2,500 m (in HH) [37], but it can be higher for experienced athletes and/or highlanders. In NH (i.e., sleeping in hypoxic rooms), F_iO_2 has to be set as if the altitude is 200–300 m higher since there is an additional hypobaric effect (i.e., differences in water vapor pressure and the respiratory resistance; see Chapter 15); such as shown by a lower (~1–3%) oxygen saturation and more periodic breathing during sleep in HH than in NH [38, 39].

The exposure duration has to be at least 3 weeks, but it is recommended optimally to last 4 weeks for inducing a significant (3–4%) Hb_{mass} increase [33]. If mainly peripheral adaptation is targeted, particularly pH regulation and buffering capacity [40], a shorter exposure is acceptable. This is of interest for endurance sports with repeated maximal-intensity bouts (e.g., cycling, cross-country skiing).

When performing "classical" altitude training camps (i.e., LHTH and LHTL), endurance athletes have to focus on the ventilatory acclimatization, a process that starts immediately after arrival and that will impact the overall

TABLE 16.1 Health risks and mitigation strategies during LHTH or LHTL altitude training in endurance athletes

Risks	Mitigation	Usefulness
Dehydration	Refractometer (urine specific gravity)	***
	Bioimpedance (intra- and extracellular water)	**
	Measurement of fluid intake	*
	Acute change in body weight	*
Desaturation	Oximeter (during sleep): Progressive SpO_2 increase expected during the first 4–6 nights	***
		*
	Oximeter (during exercise): Values maintained > 80% during the first days	**
	NIRS (during exercise)	**
Sympathetic overactivation	Daily measurement of heart rate variability at rest	***
Infection (URTI)	Adapted clothing (gloves, hat, etc.)	***
	Supplementation (e.g., glutamine)	*
Recovery—Sleep quality	Daily questionnaire (e.g., GSQS)	**
	Use of wearables for tracking sleep quality	*
General fatigue	Daily measurement of heart rate variability at rest	***
		***
	RPE post-training sessions	*
	Daily questionnaire at rest (e.g., DALDA)	**
	Change of periodization if needed	***
	Longer recovery periods during interval-training	
Muscle fatigue	Increased intake of carbohydrates and amino acids	***
		**
	Daily massage	**
Ventilatory acclimatization	Monitoring of breathing frequency during sleep (wearables)	*
		*
	Pre-altitude respiratory muscle training (e.g., Powerbreath)	*

URTI: Upper respiratory tract infection; NIRS: near infrared spectroscopy; GSQS: Groningen sleep quality scale; DALDA: daily analysis of life demands for athletes.

post-altitude benefits. This phase lasts usually 7–10 days but can be shorter depending on the frequency of hypoxic exposure of the athlete, for example, in athletes who are very experienced to altitude [18]. In this phase the athletes acclimatize to the reduced ambient oxygen pressure at altitude. High-intensity exercises such as interval training are not recommended. Longer recovery periods and larger fluid intake are necessary [31].

The primary training phase follows the acclimatization phase and lasts between two to three weeks. A key factor is to perform interval-training exercises at progressively increased training intensities. The altitude-induced normoxia-to-hypoxia decrease in VO_{2max} has been estimated to be of 6–7% (range 4.6–7.5%) decrease per 1,000 m increasing altitude immediately after arrival [41]. Even with the adaptive acclimatization process that will progressively reduce the gap between normoxic and hypoxic exercise capacities, maintaining slower training intensities until the end of the altitude camp is recommended (e.g., <6–10% after 3 weeks at 2,200–2,500 m, when compared to sea level) [8].

The time course of the different physiological responses explains the post-altitude adaptations, but the optimal timing for the competition remains unclear. However, the immediate positive phase (2–5 days after return to sea level) may be mainly due to hemodilution combined with the persistence of ventilatory adaptations. A second negative (i.e., where the likelihood of good performance is lower) phase (5–12 days) might be related to the altered energy cost, while the third phase (i.e., days 13–28) consists in a plateau of enhanced performance. Among the primary benefits of altitude training explaining this positive plateau, 3–10% improvement in exercise economy [21] is probably one of the most important—and least understood—benefits for endurance athletes [42]. A decreased cost of ventilation, greater carbohydrate use for oxidative phosphorylation, and improved mitochondrial efficiency are likely among the main mechanisms. Overall, the time course of de-acclimatization responses of hematological and ventilatory factors are likely the main triggers of the post-altitude responses, while the need for a biomechanical "recalibration" of locomotion pattern that was first hypothesized [42] is not valid anymore, at least in middle-distance runners [43].

We propose an updated list of various potential risks and mitigation strategies during LHTH or LHTL altitude training in endurance athletes (Table 16.1). Figure 16.2 displays the most useful devices and tools for effective daily monitoring of the athletes. Monitoring hydration, desaturation/deoxygenation, fatigue by heart rate variability and/or questionnaires, and training intensities is fundamental. The support staff has to ensure also that the athletes do not get sick (adapted clothing; supplementation).

16.2.4 How to organize the different training methods? Yearly periodization

The general organization of the different altitude training methods over the yearly program or the multi-year sport career depends on many factors such as the level and experience of the athletes and the targeted competition and the characteristics of the sport (e.g., the oxidative versus glycolytic balance). For endurance athletes, the hematological factors are of primary importance. Therefore, a succession of LHTH camps interspersed with LLTH blocks may be the optimal option to improve both central and peripheral adaptations.

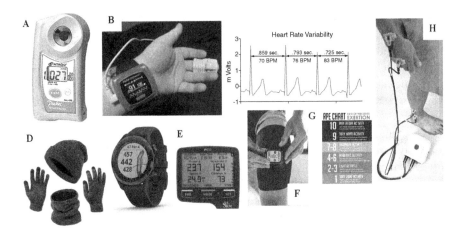

FIGURE 16.2 The most important devices for monitoring altitude adaptations in endurance athletes (ranked by practical importance). A. Refractometer (urine specific gravity); B. Oximeter (pulse O_2 saturation); C. heart rate variability (fatigue; sympathetic activation); D. Adapted clothing; E. GPS (training velocity) or Powermeter (power output); F. NIRS (near infrared spectroscopy); G. RPE (ratings of perceived exertion) scale; H. Bioimpedance (body composition, body water status).

Moreover, even if questions still exist, at the moment, we believe that there is enough evidence to support the idea that LHTLH is the best option in the final preparation prior to an important competition [2] (Figure 16.3).

16.3 Conclusion

Many qualified researchers with long experience of working in elite sport [1, 2, 8, 26, 31, 44] provided a large body of robust data that support the effectiveness of altitude training for endurance athletes. This is also supported by the increasing number of elite athletes who perform different types of altitude or hypoxic training. However, many questions remain for understanding the mechanisms and improving the way altitude training methods are performed.

In our opinion, the optimal combination of the different hypoxic training methods depending on the training phases and athlete and sport characteristics [2, 26] as well as with other physiological stressors (e.g., environmental conditions such as heat or cold, strength methods such as eccentric training, nutritional supplementation such as nitrate or ketone) are important avenues for future research.

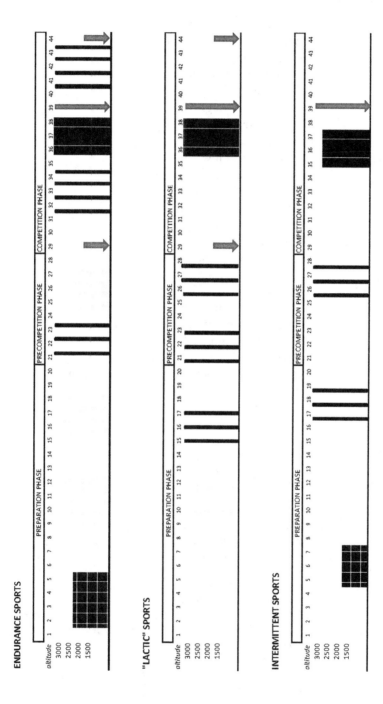

FIGURE 16.3 Schematic view of periodization of hypoxic methods in endurance, glycolytic, and intermittent sports. Adapted from [2].

Abbreviations

BFR	blood flow restriction
CHT	continuous hypoxic training
CO_2 absorption	rebreathing with a mask
DALDA	Daily Analysis of Life Demands for Athletes
GSQS	Groningen Sleep Quality Scale
LHTH	live high–train high
LHTL	live high–train low
LLTH	live low–train high
LHTLH	live high–train low and high
LHTHL	live high–train high and low
NH	normobaric hypoxia
NIRS	near infrared spectroscopy
Hbmass	hemoglobin mass
HH	hypobaric hypoxia
IPC	ischemic pre-conditioning
IHE	intermittent hypoxic exposure
IHT	interval hypoxic training
IHIT	intermittent hypoxic interval-training
RSH	repeated sprint training in hypoxia
RTH	resistance training in hypoxia
URTI	upper respiratory tract infection
VHL	voluntary hypoventilation at low lung volume
VO_{2max}	maximal oxygen consumption.

References

1. Wilber, R.L., *Application of altitude/hypoxic training by elite athletes.* Med Sci Sports Exerc, 2007. **39**(9): p. 1610–24.
2. Millet, G.P., et al., *Combining hypoxic methods for peak performance.* Sports Med, 2010. **40**(1): p. 1–25.
3. Millet, G.P., et al., *Hypoxic training and team sports: A challenge to traditional methods?* Br J Sports Med, 2013. **47 Suppl 1**: p. i6–i7.
4. Girard, O., F. Brocherie, and G.P. Millet, *Effects of altitude/hypoxia on single- and multiple-sprint performance: A comprehensive review.* Sports Med, 2017. **47**(10): p. 1931–49.
5. Wagner, P.D., *A theoretical analysis of factors determining VO2 MAX at sea level and altitude.* Respir Physiol, 1996. **106**(3): p. 329–43.
6. Levine, B.D. and J. Stray-Gundersen, *Point: Positive effects of intermittent hypoxia (live high:train low) on exercise performance are mediated primarily by augmented red cell volume.* J Appl Physiol, 2005. **99**(5): p. 2053–5.
7. Gore, C.J., et al., *Altitude training and haemoglobin mass from the optimised carbon monoxide rebreathing method determined by a meta-analysis.* Br J Sports Med, 2013. **47 Suppl 1**: p. i31–9.

8. Wehrlin, J.P., B. Marti, and J. Hallen, *Hemoglobin Mass and Aerobic Performance at Moderate Altitude in Elite Athletes.* Adv Exp Med Biol, 2016. **903**: p. 357–74.
9. Hauser, A., et al., *Individual hemoglobin mass response to normobaric and hypobaric "live high-train low": A one-year crossover study.* J Appl Physiol, 2017. **123**(2): p. 387–93.
10. Lundby, C. and P. Robach, *Does "altitude training" increase exercise performance in elite athletes?* Exp Physiol, 2016. **46**: p. 792–795.
11. Robach, P. and C. Lundby, *Is live high-train low altitude training relevant for elite athletes with already high total hemoglobin mass?* Scand J Med Sci Sports, 2012. **22**(3): p. 303–5.
12. Millet, G.P., et al., *Is live high-train low altitude training relevant for elite athletes? Flawed analysis from inaccurate data.* Br J Sports Med, 2017. **53**: p. 923–925.
13. Hauser, A., et al., *Do male athletes with already high initial haemoglobin mass benefit from "live high-train low" altitude training?* Exp Physiol, 2018. **103**(1): p. 68–76.
14. Turner, G., et al., *Altitude training in endurance running: Perceptions of elite athletes and support staff.* J Sports Sci, 2019. **37**(2): p. 163–72.
15. Schmitt, L., et al., *Monitoring training and fatigue status with heart rate variability: Case study in a swimming Olympic champion.* J Fitness Research, 2016. **5**(3): p. 38–45.
16. Schmitt, L., S. Bouthiaux, and G.P. Millet, *Eleven years' monitoring of the world's most successful male biathlete of the last decade.* Int J Sports Physiol Perform, 2021. **16**(6): p. 900–5.
17. Millet, G.P. and K. Jornet, *On top to the top-acclimatization strategy for the "fastest known time" to Mount Everest.* Int J Sports Physiol Perform, 2019. **14**(10): p. 1438–41.
18. Pugliese, L., et al., *Training diaries during altitude training camp in two Olympic champions: An observational case study.* J Sports Sci Med, 2014. **13**(3): p. 666–72.
19. Bourdillon, N., et al., *Daily cardiac autonomic responses during the Tour de France in a male professional cyclist.* Front Neurosci, 2023. **17**: p. 1221957.
20. Millet, G.P. and F. Brocherie, *Hypoxic training is beneficial in elite athletes.* Med Sci Sports Exerc, 2020. **52**(2): p. 515–18.
21. Gore, C.J., S.A. Clark, and P.U. Saunders, *Nonhematological mechanisms of improved sea-level performance after hypoxic exposure.* Med Sci Sports Exerc, 2007. **39**(9): p. 1600–9.
22. Faiss, R., O. Girard, and G.P. Millet, *Advancing hypoxic training in team sports: From intermittent hypoxic training to repeated sprint training in hypoxia.* Br J Sports Med, 2013. **47 Suppl 1**: p. i45–i50.
23. Faiss, R., et al., *Significant molecular and systemic adaptations after repeated sprint training in hypoxia.* PLoS One, 2013. **8**(2): p. e56522.
24. Millet, G.P., et al., *Repeated sprint training in hypoxia—An innovative method.* Deutsche Zeitschrift für Sportmedizin, 2019. **2019**: p. 115–122.
25. Rundqvist, H. and T. Gustafsson, *Hypoxic sprint exercise as a complement to the "live high-train low" regimen.* Acta Physiol (Oxf), 2018. **222**(1).
26. Brocherie, F., et al., *"Live high-train low and high" hypoxic training improves team-sport performance.* Med Sci Sports Exerc, 2015. **47**(10): p. 2140–9.

27. Brocherie, F., et al., *Repeated maximal-intensity hypoxic exercise superimposed to hypoxic residence boosts skeletal muscle transcriptional responses in elite team-sport athletes.* Acta Physiol (Oxf), 2018. **222**(1).
28. Wachsmuth, N.B., et al., *The effects of classic altitude training on hemoglobin mass in swimmers.* Eur J Appl Physiol, 2013. **113**(5): p. 1199–211.
29. Garvican-Lewis, L.A., et al., *Iron supplementation and altitude: Decision making using a regression tree.* J Sports Sci Med, 2016. **15**(1): p. 204–5.
30. Butterfield, G.E., *Nutrient requirements at high altitude.* Clin Sports Med, 1999. **18**(3): p. 607–21, viii.
31. Mujika, I., A.P. Sharma, and T. Stellingwerff, *Contemporary periodization of altitude training for elite endurance athletes: A narrative review.* Sports Med, 2019. **49**(11): p. 1651–1669.
32. Dempsey, J.A. and B.J. Morgan, *Humans in hypoxia: A conspiracy of maladaptation?!* Physiology (Bethesda), 2015. **30**(4): p. 304–16.
33. Constantini, K., D.P. Wilhite, and R.F. Chapman, *A clinician guide to altitude training for optimal endurance exercise performance at sea level.* High Alt Med Biol, 2017. **18**: p. 93–101.
34. Constantini, K., et al., *Prevalence of exercise-induced arterial hypoxemia in distance runners at sea level.* Med Sci Sports Exerc, 2017. **49**(5): p. 948–54.
35. Chapman, R.F., et al., *Impairment of 3000-m run time at altitude is influenced by arterial oxyhemoglobin saturation.* Med Sci Sports Exerc, 2011. **43**(9): p. 1649–56.
36. Schmitt, L., et al., *Live high-train low guided by daily heart rate variability in elite Nordic-skiers.* Eur J Appl Physiol, 2018. **118**(2): p. 419–28.
37. Chapman, R.F., et al., *Defining the "dose" of altitude training: how high to live for optimal sea level performance enhancement.* J Appl Physiol (1985), 2014. **116**(6): p. 595–603.
38. Saugy, J.J., et al., *Sleep Disordered Breathing During Live High-Train Low in Normobaric Versus Hypobaric Hypoxia.* High Alt Med Biol, 2016. **17**(3): p. 233–38.
39. Heinzer, R., et al., *Comparison of sleep disorders between real and simulated 3,450-m altitude.* Sleep, 2016. **39**(8): p. 1517–23.
40. Mizuno, M., et al., *Limb skeletal muscle adaptation in athletes after training at altitude.* J Appl Physiol, 1990. **68**(2): p. 496–502.
41. Wehrlin, J.P. and J. Hallen, *Linear decrease in .VO2max and performance with increasing altitude in endurance athletes.* Eur J Appl Physiol, 2006. **96**(4): p. 404–12.
42. Chapman, R.F., et al., *Timing of return from altitude training for optimal sea level performance.* J Appl Physiol (1985), 2014. **116**(7): p. 837–43.
43. Millet, G.P., et al., *Is altitude training bad for the running mechanics of middle-distance runners?* Int J Sports Physiol Perform, 2021. **16**: p. 1359–1362.
44. Garvican, L.A., et al., *Hemoglobin mass response to simulated hypoxia "blinded" by noisy measurement?* J Appl Physiol (1985), 2012. **112**(10): p. 1797–8; author reply 1799.

17

ALTITUDE TRAINING IN TEAM-SPORT ATHLETES

Franck Brocherie, Olivier Girard and Grégoire Millet

17.1 Introduction

Team-sports performance requires complex technical and motor skills, tactical proficiency, and highly developed specific physical capacities that encompass speed, agility, muscular strength, power, and endurance [1, 2]. Although outcomes in team sports hinge on technical and tactical actions, coaches and conditioning staffs are striving for innovative approaches to improve players' physical performance. Therefore, several altitude/hypoxic methods [3–5], developed over time (see Chapter 4), could offer benefits to team-sport specific physical capacities and their underlying physiological mechanisms.

Elevations as low as 600–1,200 m could already alter technical and tactical aspects (mainly due to a lower air resistance that affects ball flight characteristics) [6, 7] and compromise team-sport performance with some identified physical impairments [2, 6]. These physically deleterious effects include lower total distance covered, and high-velocity running and acceleration frequency that hinder players' capacity to repeat intense efforts [2, 7, 8]. This suggests that team-sport (pre-)acclimatization (natural altitude) or acclimation (simulated environment) is a prerequisite like in endurance-based sports (see Chapters 15 and 16). However, the challenge in team sports is to find a sufficient long time-window to follow the recommendations for succesfull "live high-train high" (LHTH) and "live high-train low" (LHTL) methods [9–11]. Because team-sport athletes possess an efficient combination of aerobic and anaerobic capacities [12], they can derive benefits from the latest altitude/ hypoxic training advancements, particularly emerging from new "live low–train high" (LLTH) interventions and combinations of methods. This chapter will therefore provide an overview of traditional and innovative altitude/

DOI: 10.4324/9781003402879-26

hypoxic training methods, with their respectives pros and cons in reference to team-sports requirements and constraints.

17.2 Traditional chronic altitude/hypoxic training approach

As presented in Chapter 16, the "traditional" LHTH and LHTL, recognized as the "gold standard" method (permitting to maintain high training intensity at or near sea level), are generally used for acclimatization before altitude competitions or for improving sea-level performance (Table 17.1). These methods primarily rely on the erythropoietic effect [i.e., the production of erythrocytes or red blood cells stimulated by erythropoietin (EPO)] and related hematological benefits [i.e., increased oxygen-carrying capacity measured through hemoglobin mass (Hb_{mass})]. Although debated [e.g., [13, 14]], these approaches may lead to performance enhancement including enhanced maximal oxygen consumption (VO_{2max}) following chronic terrestrial or simulated hypoxic exposure lasting 3–4 weeks [9, 15].

It is generally accepted that for 100 h of exposure to LHTH (>2,100 m) or LHTL (~3,000 m), Hb_{mass} increases by ~1% [16, 17]. Individual variability exists, influenced by factors like the magnitude of hypoxia-induced Hb_{mass} increase [18] while the influence of the initial Hb_{mass} levels is still debated and is likely minimal [19, 20]. Highly trained endurance athletes and elite field hockey players with high initial Hb_{mass} values (≤ 14 g.kg^{-1}) showed gains of 3–4% [20–22]. While the implementation of chronic hypoxic approaches, such as LHTH and LHTL, poses planning contraints, requires extended preparation periods (e.g., pre-season or winter break), or access to artificial normobaric hypoxic facilities to overcome geographical limitations, an increasing number of team-sport squads are incorporating these approaches [23]. However, there is limited published evidence showing improved team-sport performance following LHTH/LHTL camps. For instance, Australian footballers increased Hb_{mass} and aerobic performance after a 19–21-day LHTH camp during the preseason [24, 25]. With a shorter 10-day LHTL camp, water polo players showed a 3–4% increase in Hb_{mass} with performance gains on a specific swim test [26]. These findings suggest that a 2-week LHTL camp could effectively improve aerobic fitness in "realistic" conditions as part of a preseason team-sport preparation compared to the longer "traditionnal" LHTH/LHTL approach used in endurance-based sports.

17.3 Intermittent altitude/hypoxic training

Innovative LLTH methods have shown promise with advancements in normobaric hypoxia equipment [3–5, 10]. LLTH-induced peripheral adaptations and improvements in neuromuscular system efficiency align well with the team-sport specific requirements, as match performance relies not only

TABLE 17.1 Summary of the main altitude/hypoxic training method available for team-sports with their respective pros and cons

Altitude/hypoxic training method	Physiological adaptations	Practical implications	
		Pros	Cons
Live high–train high (LHTH)	Increased red blood cell production and oxygen-carrying capacity Improved oxygen utilization	Acclimatization/acclimation to hypoxia Improved aerobic performance at altitude and at sea-level	Periodization: (a) Temporary reduction in performance during the initial adaptation phase (b) length (3–4 weeks) Individual variability: need to carefully monitor training load with individual adjustments Lower resistance: negative effect on technical/tactical skills
Live high–train low (LHTL)	Idem LHTH	Idem LHTH + Train low component: (a) Maintenance of high-intensity training intensity, with potential improved aerobic and anaerobic performance (b) Counteract negative effect of air resistance	Idem LHTH (periodization) + Logistical challenges: Multiple travels to altitude residence and training facilities, possibly counteracted by the use of simulated facilities (that also permit individualization of hypoxic dose)
Repeated-sprint training in hypoxia (RSH)	Improved behavior of fast-twitch fibers Greater microvascular oxygen delivery Specific skeletal muscle tissue adaptations	Targets team-sport specific demands, in particular fatigue resistance (repeated-sprint ability), with primarily focus on anaerobic benefits (enhanced glycolytic and buffering capacities). Shock microcycle: time-efficient strategy to induce superior fitness improvements compared with usual training methods	Possible risk of overreaching/overtraining: need to consider exercise mode, exercise-to-rest ratio, accompanying training, etc. and to provide sufficient recovery period. Equipment and facility requirements which may not be widely accessible; possible alternative: the use of voluntary hypoventilation (RSH-VHL)
Live high–train low and high (LHTLH)	Idem LHTL + RSH without any blunting effect	Periodization: application in realistic calendar (2 weeks) Concomitant development of anaerobic and aerobic pathways	Idem LHTH/LHTL and RSH

on oxygen-carrying capacity but mainly on repeated-sprint ability. While adding a hypoxic stimulus during exercise training may not be sufficient to increase Hb_{mass} [27], it generally induces specific muscular adaptations (e.g., increase in the number of capillaries per fiber, mitochondrial density, and myoglobin concentration). These adaptations contribute to improved oxygen diffusion and increased enzymatic oxidative activity, which does not not occur, or occurs to a lesser extent, under normoxic conditions [28].

With limited costs and travel constraints for team-sport players, who can stay in their training environment and maintain their lifestyle, the LLTH paradigm offers a variety of training options using local or systemic hypoxia combined with passive or active modalities (Figure 17.1) [5, 29]. The following sections present relevant methods implemented in team sports.

17.3.1 High-intensity hypoxic training: From intermittent hypoxic training to repeated-sprint training in hypoxia

Exercise-induced physiological adaptation is influenced by several training variables such as volume and intensity [30, 31]. Intermittent hypoxic training (IHT; e.g., 3–5 sets of 2–5 min at intensities of 80–100% VO_{2max} with 2–4 min of recovery at simulated altitudes of 2,500–3,000 m) induces a higher increase in total mitochondrial volume density and capillary length density compared to low-intensity training in hypoxia [32, 33] and similar training in normoxia [34]. However, the analysis of the scientific literature is not as clear-cut [35] mainly due to limitations of a decreased intensity of hypoxic-induced training stimulus that did not exceed the maximal aerobic power or VO_{2max} [29]. For example, a 30-min IHT intervention for 2–3 days per week during 4 weeks with either moderately trained team sports players [36] or amateur Australian footbal players [37] was not more effective than equivalent sea-level training. Inness et al. [38] reported that a 2-week IHT intervention increased semi-professional Australian football players' performance in Yo-Yo intermittent recovery level 2, with no further increase after an additional two weeks of IHT. These divergent IHT-induced outcomes highlight the importance of both training intensity and the severity of the hypoxic stimulus in IHT design.

Given the use of shock microcycles, including high-intensity training in congested team-sport schedules [e.g., [39, 40], integrating maximal-intensity hypoxic training appears as a promising and time-efficient alternative to improve team sports-specific performance (Table 17.1). The repeated-sprint training in hypoxia (RSH) method fundamentally differs from IHT as it requires the completion of maximal short duration ($\leq$30 s) efforts—demanding a very high recruitment of fast-twitch fibers—interspersed with incomplete recovery periods in a hypoxic environment. Although still hypothetical, the underlying mechanisms of RSH rely on improved behavior of fast-twitch fibers

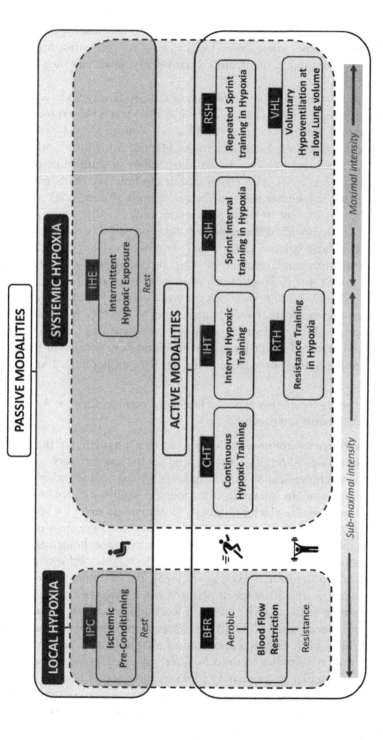

FIGURE 17.1 Schematic overview of "living low–training high" (LLTH) altitude/hypoxic methods. Modified from Girard et al. 2020 [5].

[through compensatory vasodilatation [41], greater microvascular oxygen delivery [42], and possible better phosphocreatine resynthesis] and specific skeletal muscle tissue adaptations (i.e., capillary-to-fiber ratio, fiber cross-section area, myoglobin content, and oxidative enzyme activity such as citrate synthase) [43–45].

Since a pioneering study [43] consisting of eight RSH sessions (3 × 10–20 s, 3,000 m) performed by cyclists over 4 weeks, several RSH protocols have been succesfully tested in soccer [46, 47], rugby union [48–51], rugby sevens[52], field hockey [44, 45, 53], lacrosse [54], and Australian football [55]. This provides relevant evidence-based information to team-sport practitioners [see Table 2 in [56]], with recent findings to fine-tune the hypoxic dose [indicating that the higher may not be better with altitude level as low as 2,000 m being sufficient in some population; [52, 57–60]], exercise-to-rest ratio [1–2 vs. 1–5 with different sprint durations to differently stress the oxidative-glycolytic balance [59, 61–63]] and microcycle length [2- versus 5-weeks RSH with similar outcomes [64]). In summary, 2–3 sport-specific RSH (3–4 sets of 4–7 5–20-s sprints; exercise-to-rest ratio 1–2 to 1–5; altitude level of 2,000–3,000 m) sessions per week over 2–3 weeks appears suitable for most team sports. Finally, alternatives to systemic hypoxia include repeated-sprint training induced by voluntary hypoventilation [65–68], lower load-induced repeated-sprint training with blood-flow restriction [69], and other promising options to explore in the future (see Chapters 21 and 22).

17.3.2 Resistance training in hypoxia: From low load localized to high-systemic approach

Blood flow–restricted training (BFR, aka "Kaatsu") has entered the toolbox of strength and conditioning coaches due to its low-intensity and time-efficient approach, replicating some benefits of typical high-intensity training. Briefly, by applying an inflatable cuff around a limb (i.e., proximal to the muscles to be trained), which produces a local hypoxic stress by limiting the blood supply to and from the contracted muscles) the performance of low-load resistance exercise training results in positive morphological adaptations and strength gains [70–72], with some transferable performance gains in single- and repeated-sprint exercises [73–75]. For example, netball players reported higher 5- and 10-m sprint performance improvements than control (similar training without BFR) after a 5-week low-load BFR training [74]. Further, endurance training [76], as well as team-sport specific training combined with BFR [77], targets a spectrum of adaptations in skeletal muscle, spanning from myofibrillar to mitochondrial adjustments that concurrently benefit both muscular strength and endurance qualities [72].

Similar to the historical BFR approach, resistance training in systemic hypoxia (RTH) could also enhance the metabolic stress (i.e., anaerobic system) and consequently the hypertrophic responses (e.g., increased endocrine responses, increased myokine production, accelerated recruitment of higher threshold motor units) [70]. The pionneering low-load RTH study [i.e., 6 sets of 25 repetitions at 30% of maximal repetition (1RM) combined with hypoxic exposure (~4,000 m), three times per week for 4 weeks) did not show additional gains in maximal strength compared to control [78]. Conversely, 5 weeks of RTH (20% 1RM at an oxygen saturation of ~80%) resulted in greater maximal strength and muscle hypertrophy and faster 5- and 10-m sprints performance than control in netball players [74]. Interestingly, although high-load resistance might not provide additional benefits over low- and moderate-load RTH [79, 80], 12 RTH sessions (85–92.5% 1RM) over 3 weeks improved strength in professional rugby players [81], calling for further investigation on the RTH's dose-response. Specific recommendations are available elsewhere [82], and more details in the BFR and RTH approaches are also available in Chapter 18.

17.3.3 Combining altitude/hypoxic training methods: A time-efficient alternative

Given the importance of both aerobic and anaerobic pathways in team sports, the combination of different altitude/hypoxic training methods [10] appears as a realistic and time-efficient option to optimize overall players fitness (Table 17.1). Assuming the usefulness of chronic altitude/hypoxic exposure (LHTH, LHTL methods) in enhancing aerobic qualities, its combination with RSH that improves fatigue resistance during team-sport specific tasks [43, 47, 55] should maximize the physiological benefits and mitigate some side effects (i.e., decreased plasma volume and ATP-asic Na^+/K^+ activity) observed when the methods are used in isolation [23]. Using such a combined approach mixing LHTL and RSH, 2 weeks of "live high–train low and high" (LHTLH) demonstrated larger improvements in Hb_{mass} (+3–4%, of similar magnitude that previous team-sport LHTL studies [24, 26]), as well as aerobic (+21–40% in Yo-Yo intermittent recovery test level 2) and anarobic fitness (–3/6% in repeated-sprint cumulated time), in elite field hockey players compared to LHTL combined with sea-level repeated-sprint training [83]. Of note, results persisted 3 weeks after intervention, with increase in Hb_{mass} not impaired by RSH-induced mechanisms. The superiority of LHTLH to LHTL advocates that peripheral adaptations are probably more robust than oxygen-carrying capacity to explain performance enhancement and/or maintenance after LHTLH.

Different combination options exist according to the altitude/hypoxic training methods used, the hypoxic dose, the exercise intensity. For example, an 8-week low-altitude LHTLH, with chronic exposure at 825 m and regular IHT sessions at 3,000 m, led to hematological adaptations and improvements in maximal sprint and aerobic performance in soccer players [84]. Conversely, 4 weeks of LHTLH (10 h per day normobaric LHTL at 2,500 m; with 2 × 30-min cycling exercise at 72% VO_{2max} per week) significantly improved erythropoiesis and hemoglobin production, with concomittant higher yo-yo intermittent endurance [85]. Recently, Bouten et al. [63] combined 3 weeks of LHTH (1,850 m) with RSH (exercise-to-rest ratios: 1:2 versus 1:5 at 3,000 m) in elite female rugby sevens players and showed improvements in repeated-sprint ability. While the higher exercise-to-rest ratio (1:2) was more effective than the lower ratio (1:5), both approaches successfully improved repeated-sprint performance without any negative effect from the LHTH component. This demonstrates the potential for more successful combined altitude/hypoxic stress-related interventions (see Chapters 21 and 22).

17.4 Conclusion

In summary, team-sport practitioners now have a multitude of altitude/hypoxic training methods, encompassing traditional chronic exposure and innovative intermittent approachs, as well as their combinations. These methods can target different team-sport performance determinants, either in isolation or concomittantly. While the implementation of hypoxic equipment in team-sport facilities is growing, the task lies in carefully considering the pros and cons of each method and integrating them into sport-specific periodization for best outcomes. Despite significant progress in improving physical performance and understanding underlying mechanisms, there is still room for further evidence-based recommendations, in particular regarding the choice of the "hypoxic dose" (i.e., level and duration) and the training load (i.e., content, volume, intensity).

Abbreviations

BFR   blood-flow restricted training
Hb_{mass} hemoglobin mass
IHT   high-intensity training in hypoxia
LHTH   "live high–train high"
LHTL   "live high–train low"
LHTLH   "live high–train low and high"
LLTH   "live low–train high"
RSH   repeated-sprint training in hypoxia
RTH   resistance training in hypoxia
VO_{2max} maximal oxygen consumption.

References

1. Bishop, D.J. and O. Girard, *Determinants of team-sport performance: Implications for altitude training by team-sport athletes.* Br J Sports Med, 2013. **47 Suppl 1:** p. i17–21.
2. Billaut, F., C.J. Gore, and R.J. Aughey, *Enhancing team-sport athlete performance: Is altitude training relevant?* Sports Med, 2012. **42**(9): p. 751–67.

3. Millet, G.P., et al., *Hypoxic training and team sports: a challenge to traditional methods?* Br J Sports Med, 2013. **47 Suppl 1**: p. i6–i7.
4. Girard, O., F. Brocherie, and G.P. Millet, *Effects of altitude/hypoxia on single- and multiple-sprint performance: A comprehensive review.* Sports Med, 2017. **47**(10): p. 1931–1949.
5. Girard, O., et al., *An updated panorama of "living low-training high" altitude/hypoxic methods.* Front. Sports Act. Living, 2020. **2**(26).
6. Levine, B.D., J. Stray-Gundersen, and R.D. Mehta, *Effect of altitude on football performance.* Scand J Med Sci Sports, 2008. **18 Suppl 1**: p. 76–84.
7. Nassis, G.P., *Effect of altitude on football performance: analysis of the 2010 FIFA World Cup Data.* J Strength Cond Res, 2013. **27**(3): p. 703–7.
8. McSharry, P.E., *Effect of altitude on physiological performance: a statistical analysis using results of international football games.* BMJ, 2007. **335**(7633): p. 1278–81.
9. Wilber, R.L., *Application of altitude/hypoxic training by elite athletes.* Med Sci Sports Exerc, 2007. **39**(9): p. 1610–24.
10. Millet, G.P., et al., *Combining hypoxic methods for peak performance.* Sports Med, 2010. **40**(1): p. 1–25.
11. Girard, O., et al., *"Living high-training low" for Olympic medal performance: What have we learned 25 years after implementation?* Int J Sports Physiol Perform, 2023. **18**(6): p. 563–72.
12. Bishop, D., O. Girard, and A. Mendez-Villanueva, *Repeated-sprint ability—part II: recommendations for training.* Sports Med, 2011. **41**(9): p. 741–56.
13. Millet, G.P. and F. Brocherie, *Hypoxic training is beneficial in elite athletes.* Med Sci Sports Exerc, 2020. **52**(2): p. 515–18.
14. Siebenmann, C. and J.A. Dempsey, *Hypoxic training is not beneficial in elite athletes.* Med Sci Sports Exerc, 2020. **52**(2): p. 519–22.
15. Bonetti, D.L. and W.G. Hopkins, *Sea-level exercise performance following adaptation to hypoxia: A meta-analysis.* Sports Med, 2009. **39**(2): p. 107–27.
16. Gore, C.J., et al., *Altitude training and haemoglobin mass from the optimised carbon monoxide rebreathing method determined by a meta-analysis.* Br J Sports Med, 2013. **47 Suppl 1**: p. i31–9.
17. Wehrlin, J.P., B. Marti, and J. Hallen, *Hemoglobin mass and aerobic performance at moderate altitude in elite athletes.* Adv Exp Med Biol, 2016. **903**: p. 357–74.
18. Levine, B.D. and J. Stray-Gundersen, *Dose-response of altitude training: how much altitude is enough?* Adv Exp Med Biol, 2006. **588**: p. 233–47.
19. Robach, P. and C. Lundby, *Is live high-train low altitude training relevant for elite athletes with already high total hemoglobin mass?* Scand J Med Sci Sports, 2012. **22**(3): p. 303–5.
20. Millet, G.P., et al., *Is live high-train low altitude training relevant for elite athletes? Flawed analysis from inaccurate data.* Br J Sports Med, 2019. **53**(15): p. 923–5.
21. Hauser, A., et al., *Do male athletes with already high initial haemoglobin mass benefit from "live high-train low" altitude training?* Exp Physiol, 2018. **103**(1): p. 68–76.
22. Saunders, P.U., et al., *Relationship between changes in haemoglobin mass and maximal oxygen uptake after hypoxic exposure.* Br J Sports Med, 2013. **47 Suppl 1**: p. i26–30.
23. Girard, O., et al., *Position statement—altitude training for improving team-sport players' performance: current knowledge and unresolved issues.* Br J Sports Med, 2013. **47 Suppl 1**: p. i8–16.
24. McLean, B.D., et al., *Physiological and performance responses to a preseason altitude-training camp in elite team-sport athletes.* Int J Sports Physiol Perform, 2013. **8**(4): p. 391–9.

25. Inness, M.W.H., F. Billaut, and R.J. Aughey, *Live-high train-low improves repeated time-trial and yo-yo IR2 performance in sub-elite team-sport athletes.* J Sci Med Sport, 2017. **20**(2): p. 190–195.
26. Garvican-Lewis, L.A., et al., *Ten days of simulated live high:train low altitude training increases Hbmass in elite water polo players.* Br J Sports Med, 2013. **47 Suppl 1**: p. i70–3.
27. Humberstone-Gough, C.E., et al., *Comparison of live high: train low altitude and intermittent hypoxic exposure.* J Sports Sci Med, 2013. **12**(3): p. 394–401.
28. Hoppeler, H. and M. Vogt, *Muscle tissue adaptations to hypoxia.* J Exp Biol, 2001. **204**(Pt 18): p. 3133–9.
29. McLean, B.D., C.J. Gore, and J. Kemp, *Application of "live low-train high" for enhancing normoxic exercise performance in team sport athletes.* Sports Med, 2014. **44**(9): p. 1275–87.
30. Bishop, D.J., J. Botella, and C. Granata, *CrossTalk opposing view: Exercise training volume is more important than training intensity to promote increases in mitochondrial content.* J Physiol, 2019. DOI: 10536/DRO/DU:30158133
31. MacInnis, M.J., L.E. Skelly, and M.J. Gibala, *CrossTalk proposal: Exercise training intensity is more important than volume to promote increases in human skeletal muscle mitochondrial content.* J Physiol, 2019. 597: p. 4111–4113.
32. Geiser, J., et al., *Training high—living low: Changes of aerobic performance and muscle structure with training at simulated altitude.* Int J Sports Med, 2001. **22**(8): p. 579–85.
33. Vogt, M., et al., *Molecular adaptations in human skeletal muscle to endurance training under simulated hypoxic conditions.* J Appl Physiol, 2001. **91**(1): p. 173–82.
34. Zoll, J., et al., *Exercise training in normobaric hypoxia in endurance runners. III. Muscular adjustments of selected gene transcripts.* J Appl Physiol, 2006. **100**(4): p. 1258–66.
35. Faiss, R., O. Girard, and G.P. Millet, *Advancing hypoxic training in team sports: From intermittent hypoxic training to repeated sprint training in hypoxia.* Br J Sports Med, 2013. **47 Suppl 1**: p. i45–i50.
36. Morton, J.P. and N.T. Cable, *Effects of intermittent hypoxic training on aerobic and anaerobic performance.* Ergonomics, 2005. **48**(11–14): p. 1535–46.
37. McLean, B.D., et al., *Changes in running performance after four weeks of interval hypoxic training in Australian footballers: A single-blind placebo-controlled study.* J Strength Cond Res, 2015. **29**(11): p. 3206–15.
38. Inness, M.W., F. Billaut, and R.J. Aughey, *Team-sport athletes' improvement of performance on the yo-yo intermittent recovery test level 2, but not of time-trial performance, with intermittent hypoxic training.* Int J Sports Physiol Perform, 2016. **11**(1): p. 15–21.
39. Brocherie, F., J. Perez, and G. Guilhem, *Effects of a 14-day high-intensity shock microcycle in high-level ice hockey players' fitness.* J Strength Cond Res, 2020.
40. Wahl, P., M. Guldner, and J. Mester, *Effects and sustainability of a 13-day high-intensity shock microcycle in soccer.* J Sports Sci Med, 2014. **13**(2): p. 259–65.
41. Casey, D.P. and M.J. Joyner, *Compensatory vasodilatation during hypoxic exercise: mechanisms responsible for matching oxygen supply to demand.* J Physiol, 2012. **590**(Pt 24): p. 6321–6.
42. Cleland, S.M., et al., *Effects of prior heavy-intensity exercise on oxygen uptake and muscle deoxygenation kinetics of a subsequent heavy-intensity cycling and knee-extension exercise.* Appl Physiol Nutr Metab, 2012. **37**(1): p. 138–48.
43. Faiss, R., et al., *Significant molecular and systemic adaptations after repeated sprint training in hypoxia.* PLoS One, 2013. **8**(2): p. e56522.
44. Brocherie, F., et al., *Repeated maximal-intensity hypoxic exercise superimposed to hypoxic residence boosts skeletal muscle transcriptional responses in elite team-sport athletes.* Acta Physiol (Oxf), 2018. **222**(1): p. e12851.

45. van der Zwaard, S., et al., *Adaptations in muscle oxidative capacity, fiber size, and oxygen supply capacity after repeated-sprint training in hypoxia combined with chronic hypoxic exposure.* J Appl Physiol (1985), 2018. **124**(6): p. 1403–12.
46. Gatterer, H., et al., *Shuttle-run sprint training in hypoxia for youth elite soccer players: A pilot study.* J Sports Sci Med, 2014. **13**(4): p. 731–5.
47. Brocherie, F., et al., *High-intensity intermittent training in hypoxia: a double-blinded, placebo-controlled field study in youth football players.* J Strength Cond Res, 2015. **29**(1): p. 226–37.
48. Galvin, H.M., et al., *Repeated sprint training in normobaric hypoxia.* Br J Sports Med, 2013. **47 Suppl 1**: p. i74–9.
49. Beard, A., et al., *Repeated-sprint training in hypoxia in International Rugby Union players.* Int J Sports Physiol Perform, 2019. **14**(6): p. 850–4.
50. Beard, A., et al., *Upper-body repeated-sprint training in hypoxia in international rugby union players.* Eur J Sport Sci, 2019. **19**(9): p. 1175–83.
51. Hamlin, M.J., et al., *Hypoxic repeat sprint training improves rugby player's repeated sprint but not endurance performance.* Front Physiol, 2017. **8**: p. 24.
52. Pramkratok W., T. Songsupap, and T. Yimlamai. *Repeated sprint training under hypoxia improves aerobic performance and repeated sprint ability by enhancing muscle deoxygenation and markers of angiogenesis in rugby sevens.* Eur J Appl Physiol, 2022 Mar. **122**(3): p. 611–22. doi: 10.1007/s00421-021-04861-8
53. James, C. and O. Girard, *In-season repeated-sprint training in hypoxia in international field hockey players.* Front Sports Act Living, 2020. **2**: p. 66.
54. Kasai, N., et al., *Effect of training in hypoxia on repeated sprint performance in female athletes.* Springerplus, 2015. **4**: p. 310.
55. Goods, P.S., et al., *No additional benefit of repeat-sprint training in hypoxia than in normoxia on sea-level repeat-sprint ability.* J Sports Sci Med, 2015. **14**(3): p. 681–8.
56. Brocherie, F., et al., *Effects of repeated-sprint training in hypoxia on sea-level performance: A meta-analysis.* Sports Med, 2017. **47**(8): p. 1651–60.
57. Goods, P.S., et al., *Effect of different simulated altitudes on repeat-sprint performance in team-sport athletes.* Int J Sports Physiol Perform, 2014. **9**(5): p. 857–62.
58. Camacho-Cardenosa, M., et al., *Effects of swimming-specific repeated-sprint training in hypoxia training in swimmers.* Front Sports Act Living, 2020. **2**: p. 100.
59. Tong, T.K., et al., *Acute performance responses to repeated treadmill sprints in hypoxia with varying inspired oxygen fractions, exercise-to-recovery ratios and recovery modalities.* Eur J Appl Physiol, 2021. **121**(7): p. 1933–42.
60. Gutknecht, A.P., et al., *Maximizing anaerobic performance with repeated-sprint training in hypoxia: In search of an optimal altitude based on pulse oxygen saturation monitoring.* Front Physiol, 2022. **13**: p. 1010086.
61. Dennis, M.C., et al., *Repeated-sprint training in heat and hypoxia: Acute responses to manipulating exercise-to-rest ratio.* Eur J Sport Sci, 2023. **23**(7): p. 1175–85.
62. Raberin, A., et al., *The oxidative-glycolytic balance influenced by sprint duration is key during repeated sprint in hypoxia.* Med Sci Sports Exerc, 2023. **55**(2): p. 245–54.
63. Bouten, J., et al., *Effects of 2 different protocols of repeated-sprint training in hypoxia in elite female rugby sevens players during an altitude training camp.* Int J Sports Physiol Perform, 2023. **1**: p. 1–7.
64. Shi, Q., et al., *Repeated-sprint training in hypoxia boosts up team-sport-specific repeated-sprint ability: 2-week vs 5-week training regimen.* Eur J Appl Physiol, 2023. **123**(12): p. 2699–2710.
65. Brocherie, F., et al., *Effects of repeated-sprint training in hypoxia induced by voluntary hypoventilation on performance during ice hockey off-season.* Int J Sports Sci Coach, 2023. **18**(2): p. 446–52.

66. Fornasier-Santos, C., G.P. Millet, and X. Woorons, *Repeated-sprint training in hypoxia induced by voluntary hypoventilation improves running repeated-sprint ability in rugby players.* Eur J Sport Sci, 2018. **18**(4): p. 504–12.

67. Lapointe, J., et al., *Impact of hypoventilation training on muscle oxygenation, myoelectrical changes, systemic [k(+)], and repeated-sprint ability in basketball players.* Front Sports Act Living, 2020. **2**: p. 29.

68. Woorons, X., F. Billaut, and H. Vandewalle, *Transferable benefits of cycle hypoventilation training for run-based performance in team-sport athletes.* Int J Sports Physiol Perform, 2020. **15**(8): p. 1103–8.

69. McKee, J.R., et al., *Repeated-sprint training with blood-flow restriction improves repeated-sprint ability similarly to unrestricted training at reduced external loads.* Int J Sports Physiol Perform, 2023. **19**: p. 257–264.

70. Scott, B.R., et al., *Hypoxia and resistance exercise: A comparison of localized and systemic methods.* Sports Med, 2014. **44**(8): p. 1037–54.

71. Scott, B.R., et al., *Exercise with blood flow restriction: An updated evidence-based approach for enhanced muscular development.* Sports Med, 2015. **45**(3): p. 313–25.

72. Davids, C.J., et al., *Where does blood flow restriction fit in the toolbox of athletic development? A narrative review of the proposed mechanisms and potential applications.* Sports Med, 2023. **53**(11): p. 2077–2093.

73. Abe, T., et al., *Skeletal muscle size and circulating IGF-1 are increased after two weeks of twice daily KAATSU resistance training.* Int J Kaatsu Tran Res, 2005. **1**: p. 6–12.

74. Manimmanakorn, A., et al., *Effects of resistance training combined with vascular occlusion or hypoxia on neuromuscular function in athletes.* Eur J Appl Physiol, 2013. **113**(7): p. 1767–74.

75. Cook, C.J., L.P. Kilduff, and C.M. Beaven, *Improving strength and power in trained athletes with 3 weeks of occlusion training.* Int J Sports Physiol Perform, 2014. **9**(1): p. 166–72.

76. Barjaste, A., et al., *Concomitant aerobic- and hypertrophy-related skeletal muscle cell signaling following blood flow-restricted walking.* Science & Sports, 2021. **36**(2): p. e51–8.

77. Hosseini Kakhak, S.A., et al., *Performing soccer-specific training with blood flow restriction enhances physical capacities in youth soccer players.* J Strength Cond Res, 2022. **36**(7): p. 1972–77.

78. Friedmann, B., et al., *Effects of low-resistance/high-repetition strength training in hypoxia on muscle structure and gene expression.* Pflugers Arch, 2003. **446**(6): p. 742–51.

79. Scott, B.R., et al., *Acute physiological and perceptual responses to high-load resistance exercise in hypoxia.* Clin Physiol Funct Imaging, 2018. **38**(4): p. 595–602.

80. Benjanuvatra, N., et al., *How does multi-set high-load resistance exercise impact neuromuscular function in normoxia and hypoxia?* Eur J Sport Sci, 2023. **23**(7): p. 1223–32.

81. Mayo, B., et al., *The effect of resistance training in a hypoxic chamber on physical performance in elite rugby athletes.* High Alt Med Biol, 2018. **19**(1): p. 28–34.

82. Patterson, S.D., et al., *Blood flow restriction exercise: considerations of methodology, application, and safety.* Front Physiol, 2019. **10**: p. 533.

83. Brocherie, F., et al., *"Live high-train low and high" hypoxic training improves team-sport performance.* Med Sci Sports Exerc, 2015. **47**(10): p. 2140–9.

84. Wonnabussapawich, P., et al., *Living and training at 825 m for 8 weeks supplemented with intermittent hypoxic training at 3,000 m improves blood parameters and running performance.* J Strength Cond Res, 2017. **31**(12): p. 3287–94.

85. Zhang, Y., et al., *Effects of 'living high, training low' on the immune function of red blood cells and endurance performance in soccer players.* J Exerc Sci Fit., 2005. **3**(2): p. 81–6.

18

HYPOXIC TRAINING FOR STRENGTH ENHANCEMENT

Brendan R. Scott

18.1 Introduction

Physical activity guidelines recommend that adults incorporate resistance training on two days per week to improve or maintain muscle size and strength [1]. This is important across the lifespan and for different populations. Healthy young athletes are typically prescribed resistance training to improve muscular strength and power specific to their chosen sport. This practice not only increases exercise economy and sporting performance but also reduces the risk of injury [2]. Older adults should perform resistance training to attenuate age-related muscle mass loss, termed sarcopenia, and the reductions in functional abilities and independence that often accompany sarcopenia. Populations who experience chronic clinical conditions or are undertaking rehabilitation from an injury are also advised to undertake resistance training to help manage their diseases or accelerate recovery.

To enhance the adaptations to resistance training, researchers have investigated the application of a hypoxic stimulus during this exercise. This was initially examined using a localized hypoxic stimulus by wearing inflatable cuffs on the arms or legs to limit blood flow (and therefore oxygen delivery) to the limbs during exercise [3, 4]. Commonly referred to as blood flow restriction (BFR), this technique has been shown to substantially increase muscle size and strength when combined with low-load resistance training [5]. However, the BFR stimulus is limited to the muscles of the limbs, and so researchers have also implemented systemic hypoxia by having participants breathe hypoxic air during resistance training [6]. Resistance training in hypoxia (RTH) has demonstrated augmented muscular development in some studies [7, 8], though these adaptations are not as consistently observed as

DOI: 10.4324/9781003402879-27

for BFR training [9]. This chapter provides an overview of these different hypoxic methods to enhance responses to resistance training, explaining the typical adaptations, proposed mechanisms, and practical implications of these techniques.

18.2 Resistance training with localized hypoxia: Blood flow restriction

The use of BFR during resistance training was pioneered by Dr. Yoshiaki Sato during the 1960s in Japan [10]. This technique has been applied using specific methodologies in Japan, where it is referred to as Kaatsu training (translating to "additional pressure" in English). Since its inception, the methodologies for implementing BFR have evolved, with researchers now generally agreeing that cuffs should be inflated to a pressure which partially restricts, but does not occlude, blood flow [11]. Using BFR can cause substantial muscular adaptations when combined with low-load resistance training in the range of 20–40% of the one-repetition maximum (1RM). This is important for cohorts who cannot tolerate the mechanical demands associated with heavy resistance training (e.g., >70% 1RM), which has been traditionally prescribed to increase muscle size and strength [12].

18.2.1 Effects on muscular adaptations

The first English publication demonstrating that BFR training could augment muscle strength was from Shinohara et al. [3] in 1998. They reported that wearing inflatable cuffs (250 mmHg) during 4 weeks of low-load isometric knee extensor contractions (40% of maximal voluntary contraction torque, three times per week) resulted in larger improvements in strength than the same training without cuffs. Two years later, Takarada et al. [4] demonstrated the effect of BFR on muscle hypertrophy, showing larger increases in the cross-sectional area of the elbow flexor muscles following 16 weeks of low-load resistance training (ranging from 30% to 50% of 1RM) with BFR (pressure of ~110 mmHg), compared to equivalent exercise without BFR. These findings have been consistently replicated across different populations, including healthy older individuals [13], clinical populations [14], and athletes [15]. Even highly trained national-level powerlifters have successfully incorporated BFR during low-load front squat training sessions (30% 1RM, 120 mmHg) within a 6.5-week training program [16]. Significant increases in cross-sectional area of the *vastus lateralis* and *rectus femoris* muscles were observed, compared to no changes in a control group who continued normal high-load training (60–85% 1RM). Interestingly, these adaptations seemed to be driven by preferential hypertrophy in type I muscle fibers, with the BFR group experiencing ~12% increases in type I muscle fiber area, compared to ~0% change in the control group, while type II muscle fiber area was unchanged in both groups.

While low-load resistance training with BFR improves muscular strength, these improvements tend to be smaller than those observed following unrestricted high-load resistance training [17]. A possible explanation is the lack of current evidence for robust neural adaptations to low-load BFR resistance training. Heavy training is known to promote neural adaptations including increased agonist recruitment and reduced antagonist co-contraction [18]. However, these effects have not been comprehensively demonstrated for BFR exercise. While acute alterations in muscle activity [19] and corticomotor excitability [20] have been observed following low-load BFR resistance exercise, these findings should be expanded on. It is worth noting that some researchers have recently questioned the degree to which hypertrophy resulting from resistance training impacts strength improvements [21]. The larger increases in maximal strength following heavy compared to low-load BFR resistance training may be explained by a more specific "practice effect" from lifting heavy loads, making the training more aligned with the way maximal strength is tested [21]. Nevertheless, as there is currently limited evidence for neural adaptations to low-load BFR resistance training to improve muscle strength, it is likely that muscle growth contributes to some extent to improvements in strength.

18.2.2 Mechanisms for improved muscular development

Restricting blood flow to and from the exercising limbs during exercise creates a complex cascade of inter-related physiological responses which may increase muscle protein synthesis [6]. Throughout a BFR resistance training program, these acute responses are theoretically cumulative and result in muscle hypertrophy. Limiting blood delivery to working muscles during BFR creates a localized hypoxic environment, which is believed to increase the activation and proliferation of satellite cells [22]. These cells add myonuclei to muscle fibers, enhancing their potential for protein synthesis. The localized hypoxic environment also increases reliance on anaerobic metabolism, resulting in what researchers often term metabolic stress. This stress is often measured via increased concentrations of metabolites such as blood lactate or hydrogen ions, greater phosphocreatine depletion, and reductions in pH [23]. Increased intracellular metabolite concentration may draw fluid into muscle fibers to equilibrate the concentration gradient, which causes an acute muscle swelling proposed to trigger protein synthesis pathways [24]. This swelling is further augmented by altered hemodynamics during BFR exercise, as the technique imposes greater restrictions on venous outflow than arterial inflow [25]. Another consequence of heightened metabolic stress is a faster fatigue in recruited motor units, leading to the recruitment of additional higher-threshold motor units to maintain force production over multiple sets of resistance exercise. This increased muscle recruitment, observed via surface electromyography [19], indicates a larger portion of the muscle is stimulated to engage with exercise, likely contributing to adaptations when BFR is applied.

Perhaps the most important acute physiological response to BFR resistance exercise is intramuscular signaling for protein synthesis. Fujita et al. [26] reported increased phosphorylation ribosomal S6 kinase 1 (downstream regulator of the mechanistic target of rapamycin signaling pathway), following low-load resistance exercise with BFR. Significantly elevated muscle protein synthesis was also observed at 3 h following exercise, despite no changes in these physiological responses for the non-BFR control. These findings have been replicated by other researchers [27]. Reductions in the expression of myostatin, a negative regulator of muscle growth, have been reported following low-load BFR resistance exercise [28, 29]. Considering that these acute intramuscular signaling responses to low-load BFR exercise are conducive for muscle protein synthesis, it seems that the restriction of blood flow during low-load resistance training creates a cascade of biological events that can ultimately increase muscle growth, thereby improving strength [6].

18.3 Resistance training with systemic hypoxia

Classic research on the effects of prolonged exposure to altitude demonstrated muscle atrophy [30], possibly related to reductions in appetite and caloric intake. However, with more recent approaches to various live low–train high methodologies, innovative scientists have developed new hypoxic training techniques with the hope to confer even a small benefit to muscular adaptations. This has led to the application of a systemic hypoxic stimulus during resistance training [7, 8] as a novel application of live low–train high methods. As a BFR stimulus can only be applied to the limbs; the hip and trunk muscles cannot experience the same hypoxic conditions as the limb muscles. Resistance training in systemic hypoxia (RTH) could theoretically address this limitation while leveraging similar physiological benefits to BFR [6]. The research in this field is emerging, with some studies demonstrating larger improvements in muscle strength and hypertrophy [7, 8, 31–33] following a period of RTH compared to the equivalent training in normoxia. However, these benefits are not consistently reported by all studies [34, 35], and further research is needed to clarify the circumstances in which RTH may be advantageous for muscular development.

18.3.1 Effects on muscle hypertrophy and strength

One of the first studies to demonstrate benefits of RTH over normoxic training was from Nishimura et al. [7]. They reported significantly larger improvement in cross-sectional area and faster improvements in strength of the upper-arm muscles following 6 weeks of moderate-intensity resistance training (70% 1RM) in hypoxia (fraction of inspired oxygen [F_iO_2] = 0.16) compared to normoxia. Benefits of RTH for improving muscle hypertrophy or lean mass have since been reported by other researchers using various interventions such as moderate-load training (70% 1RM or 10RM) [32, 36], low-load training (20% 1RM) [8], and high-load circuit-style training (6RM) [37].

However, other studies have not reported the same promising effects. A 2018 meta-analysis, encompassing nine studies, concluded that RTH did not augment increases in muscle hypertrophy (measures of muscle cross-sectional area or lean mass) or 1RM strength [9]. This conclusion was supported by a more recent and extensive meta-analysis [38], which included 17 studies but still observed no greater benefit for RTH compared to normoxic resistance training for muscle hypertrophy or strength. It is important to acknowledge that the potential for hypoxia to enhance adaptations to an exercise stimulus may be highly individual, with some participants responding more strongly than others [39]. Additionally, no study has reported detrimental effects of RTH on muscle hypertrophy and strength adaptations. Ramos-Campo et al. [9] demonstrated improvements in muscle size and strength were observed from pre- to post-training in RTH research, indicating that hypoxia did not impair these adaptations compared to normoxic training [9]. The divergent findings in RTH literature are likely impacted by the differing methodologies across studies, including variations in exercise structure, severity of hypoxia used, and the training history of recruited participants [9] (see Section 18.3.5).

18.3.2 Effects on muscular power

An interesting consideration when designing hypoxic interventions is whether there is a difference between normobaric hypoxia (e.g., simulated altitude) and hypobaric hypoxia (e.g., terrestrial altitude). This becomes particularly pertinent to resistance training designed to improve muscular power, which typically involves lifting moderately heavy loads at high velocities. Feriche et al. [40] reported that bench press exercise performed in hypobaric hypoxia (2,320 m above sea level) resulted in faster lifting velocity and higher mean power compared to exercising in normoxia, especially for moderate and heavy loads (60–100% 1RM). Similar results were not observed for comparisons between normobaric hypoxia (F_iO_2 = 15.7%; corresponding to an altitude of ~2,300 m) and normoxia. This indicates that the effect is better explained by the reduced air density in hypobaric hypoxia rather than reduced oxygen availability having a physiological impact [40]. These acute responses have been expanded upon more recently [41], with greater improvements in jump height for combat athletes performing power-based training in hypobaric hypoxia (8.2%) compared with normoxic training (1.4%).

This may be attributed to the additive effects of several training sessions in hypobaric hypoxia with faster velocities compared to in normoxia.

18.3.3 Effects on muscular and cardiovascular endurance

Considering that hypoxia provides a physiological challenge for oxidative metabolism, some researchers have investigated whether this stimulus during resistance training could augment muscular endurance [8, 42]. Manimmana-korn et al. [8] trained netball athletes for five weeks using low loads (3 times per week, 3 sets of knee extension and flexion to failure at 20% 1RM, F_iO_2 adjusted to maintain arterial oxygen saturation at ~80%), and reported a larger increase in the number of repetitions that could be completed with 20% 1RM for a RTH group than for a normoxic training control [8]. Similar findings were reported by Kon et al. [42] for higher-load resistance training (3 times per week, 3×10 repetitions of bench press and leg press at 70% 1RM, F_iO_2 = 14.4%), where the RTH group outperformed a normoxic training group in an assessment of the maximal volume (repetitions × mass [kg]) possible with 70% 1RM after eight weeks of training.

Aside from muscular endurance, RTH may also benefit cardiorespiratory endurance. Eight weeks of high-load resistance circuit training (2 times per week, 6RM for several exercises) improved the fatigue index during a repeated-sprint ability test, along with running time to exhaustion and maximum oxygen uptake, when training was performed in hypoxia (F_iO_2 = 15.0%) but not in normoxia [43]. A small effect of high-load RTH ($d = 0.21$; F_iO_2 = 14.4%) compared to normoxic training for performance in the bronco 1,200 m shuttle run test has also been reported [44], though this small difference was not statistically significant. It should be noted that others have not reported RTH to benefit measures of cardiorespiratory endurance more than normoxic training [35]. Considering that the hypoxic stimulus challenges oxidative metabolism by limiting oxygen availability, it is likely that resistance training sessions designed to impose the greatest stress on aerobic metabolism may be most effective for eliciting changes in endurance. For example, the high-load circuit resistance training used in the research from Ramos-Campo et al. [43] may be a viable approach to targeting these adaptations.

18.3.4 Mechanisms for improved muscular development

Acute exposure to hypoxia during resistance exercise has been shown to up-regulate several physiological responses thought to be important for muscular adaptations [6]. Similarly to the mechanisms described for BFR exercise, performing resistance training in hypoxia augments metabolic stress [45], muscle activation [46], and responses related to satellite cells [47, 48].

However, the effects on mechanistic target of rapamycin signaling indicate hypoxia could in fact blunt the hypertrophic response [49]. It should be noted that there is substantially less research investigating the physiological responses of resistance training with systemic, compared to localized hypoxia. Considering that mixed evidence regarding the efficacy of RTH, it is likely that the physiological responses to systemic hypoxia are either slightly different or blunted compared to localized hypoxia.

18.3.5 Additional considerations

18.3.5.1 Training structure

Current RTH literature includes substantial heterogeneity in the exercise stimulus applied. Some studies have utilized heavy strength training sessions, typically targeting maximal strength (e.g., 2–4 sets of 3–6 repetitions with >75% 1RM and 180 s inter-set rest [31]), while others have included moderate-load hypertrophy-based training prescription (e.g., 4 sets of 10 repetitions with 70% 1RM and 60 s rest [7]), or even light-load exercise seemingly targeted at developing muscular endurance (e.g., 3 sets to failure with 20% 1RM and 30 s rest [8]). Given this diversity alone, the varied responses to RTH are not surprising. The most important factor to consider when designing the exercise program for RTH is likely the metabolic stress induced by the intervention [39]. The fundamental stimulus provided by hypoxia is a reduced oxygen availability, which acutely alters metabolic processes required for energy production. Therefore, exercise programs should be designed to capitalize on the metabolic challenge presented by hypoxia. Reducing the duration of rest periods between sets may be one simple way to achieve this [50], as it could take advantage of the altered time course of phosphocreatine resynthesis kinetics that accompany reduced systemic oxygen availability [51].

18.3.5.2 Hypoxic stimulus

Hypoxia can be considered an additional acute exercise variable that can be manipulated to target a desired physiological response or adaptation. However, there are no clear guidelines on the optimal range of hypoxia to promote beneficial responses to RTH. Endurance training literature indicates that an optimal hypoxic dose should be implemented for hypoxic interventions to enhance adaptations beyond those achieved with normoxic training [52]. However, the physiological effects of RTH are targeted at the muscle, rather than for improved oxygen-carrying capacity in endurance athletes. Even normoxic resistance exercise causes reductions in muscle oxygenation, and it may be difficult to further exaggerate the reduction in intramuscular oxygenation via a systemic hypoxic stimulus [39]. While Benavente et al. [38] reported no significant effects of moderate (F_iO_2 = 14.3–16.0%) versus severe (F_iO_2 = <14.2–11.0%) for the efficacy of RTH, practitioners should consider the severity of hypoxia in conjunction with the demands of the exercise stimulus in planning their RTH programs.

18.3.5.3 Status of participants

Considering the infrastructure required to undertake any hypoxic training intervention, the real-world application of RTH is likely to be focused on high-performance athletes who have access to hypoxic facilities. While some RTH research has recruited trained participants or athletes [8, 31, 44], most other evidence comes from untrained or recreationally active participants, and none have specifically compared the efficacy of RTH programs in well-trained versus untrained cohorts. It is not clear whether individuals who have already achieved substantial increases in muscle size and strength from resistance training could further potentiate these responses by including RTH into their program. Practitioners should also consider not only the substantial between-individual variation in the magnitude of adaptations to a resistance training program [53] but also the variability in responses to a given hypoxic stimulus [54]. Novel methods of controlling the hypoxic dose, such as adjusting the F_iO_2 to reach a consistent reduction in arterial oxygen saturation [8, 35], may help overcome this variability, though this is challenging to implement when training large groups together.

18.4 Practical implications

18.4.1 Prescribing resistance training with blood flow restriction (Figure 18.1)

Current guidelines for low-load BFR resistance training are to train 2–3 times per week for at least 3 weeks, using loads of 20–40% 1RM [11]. A common repetition scheme is performing 4 sets of 30-15-15-15 repetitions with 30–60 s rest, although variations to this (including sets to failure) can be used when appropriate [11]. The benefits of low-load BFR training are likely optimized if used as a supplementary stimulus in addition to normal high-load training for athletic populations. This has been demonstrated in well-trained American football athletes [55, 56] and power-lifters [16]. For populations who can tolerate traditional heavy strength training, additional improvements in muscle strength can be achieved by adding sets of low-load BFR resistance training as a supplementary stimulus toward the end of a training session. This is important, as low-load BFR resistance training alone is unlikely to facilitate neural adaptations to optimize maximal strength if used as the sole resistance

Injured tennis player

Athlete is recovering from anterior cruciate ligament reconstruction. Has commenced low-load rehabilitation exercises and sports doctor attempting to increase speed of recovery.

Hypoxic training strategy: BFR during rehabilitation.

Resistance training focus: Low-load resistance training to target muscles supporting the knee joint.

Training prescription:

- Cuff pressure: 60-80% AOP continuously across sets and rest periods. If poorly tolerated use intermittent pressure (deflate during rest).
- Volume: 2-4 sets of 10-30 repetitions (depending on exercise and stage of rehabilitation). 30-45 s rest between sets.
- Exercises: Dependant on stage of rehabilitation (e.g., isometric quadricep contractions, straight leg raises, unilateral leg press within pain-free range, wall sits, step-ups).
- Load: Can be difficult to prescribe based on 1RM in injured populations. Can prescribe based on effort (i.e., adjust load such that sets are difficult to complete, but failure is not reached).

Additional considerations: Passive BFR (i.e., cycles of inflation/deflation without exercise) can attenuate disuse atrophy in early stages of rehabilitation.

Bodybuilder

Training for upcoming competition, but believes more size is needed for biceps. Limited time to train each session and looking for approach to optimise effects of arm training.

Hypoxic training strategy: BFR as supplement.

Resistance training focus: Low-load resistance training as supplementary exercise following arm sessions.

Training prescription:

- Cuff pressure: 60% AOP continuously.
- Volume: 30/15/15/15 repetitions over 4 sets. Can perform final set to failure periodically. Rest only 30-45 s between sets (cuffs remain inflated).
- Exercises: With advanced training age, heavy resistance training (without BFR) is required. Include BFR during single-joint elbow flexion exercises, performed as last exercise/s of upper body sessions.
- Load: 20% 1RM (adjust load as necessary to enable close to the repetition scheme mentioned above).

Additional considerations: Higher cuff pressures (e.g., 80% AOP) can be more uncomfortable in arms compared to legs. Could progress exercise by increasing cuff pressure to 70% or 80% AOP over time, or instead by increasing load up to 40% 1RM.

FIGURE 18.1   Practical examples of implementing localized hypoxia during resistance training for athletes in different contexts.

BFR = blood flow restriction, AOP = arterial occlusion pressure, RM = repetition maximum.

training method [57]. Traditional heavy strength training should still be used to optimize these adaptations. Additionally, there is no strong evidence for applying BFR during heavier strength training to benefit muscular development [58, 59].

18.4.2 Prescribing resistance training with systemic hypoxia (Figure 18.2)

While results are not conclusive, there seem to be some circumstances where systemic hypoxia may augment adaptations to resistance training. Athletes aiming to use RTH to enhance muscular development should train 2–3 times per week for 5–8 weeks, at an F_iO_2 of 13–16%. Benefits have been observed using loads ranging from 20% to 90+% of individual 1RM, although the set and repetition structures should be targeted to the load lifted such that participants train with a high degree of effort (i.e., more repetitions per set for lighter loads and fewer required for heavier loads). Some sets to failure could be performed to ensure high effort but should be limited to the final set(s) of

Swimmer

Strength coach programming resistance training, but swimming coach instructs that it must be developed to elicit a large aerobic demand rather than just hypertrophy.

Hypoxic training strategy: RTH (normobaric hypoxia).

Resistance training focus: High-load circuit resistance training targeting whole-body exercises.

Training prescription:

- Hypoxia: F_iO_2 = 16-13% (reduce the F_iO_2 over sessions as athlete becomes accustomed to the hypoxic stimulus.
- Volume: 2-3 sets of 4-8 repetitions in circuit (3 exercises per circuit, 4-8 repetitions per exercise, 30 s rest between exercises, 2-3 minutes rest between sets of the circuit).
- Exercises: Large muscle mass (horizontal push and pull, squat and hip hinge patterns, trunk rotation).
- Load: targeted to elicit high degree of effort (e.g., 6-8RM loads for 4-6 repetitions; corresponding to 1-2 repetitions-in-reserve).

Additional considerations: Greater aerobic demands associated with circuit RTH may improve fatigue resistance and aerobic capacity, though the amount of load that can be lifted may be reduced in this format of training session.

Team sport athlete

Soccer team travelling to Sierra Nevada (Spain) for a 2-week altitude camp. Strength coaches are aiming to continue resistance training 2+ times per week during this training phase.

Hypoxic training strategy: RTH (hypobaric hypoxia).

Resistance training focus: High-velocity movements for power development.

Training prescription:

- Altitude: 2320 m above sea level (Sierra Nevada).
- Volume: 3-6 sets of 4-6 repetitions (2-3 minutes rest between sets).
- Exercises: dynamic exercises performed at high velocity (e.g., countermovement jump, broad jump, push jerk).
- Load: body weight or light to moderate loads that allow fast lifting velocity (30-50% 1RM).

Additional considerations: Rest periods may be slightly increased from normobaric RTH prescription, as the focus is high-velocity movements being augmented by low air resistance at altitude rather than eliciting a potent metabolic stimulus. Important to monitor athlete training responses (e.g., perceptual scales or lifting velocity) to ensure not too fatigued, especially with likely demands of other conditioning training undertaken during these camps.

FIGURE 18.2   Practical examples of implementing systemic hypoxia during resistance training for athletes in different contexts.

RTH = resistance training in hypoxia, F_iO_2 = fraction of inspired oxygen, RM = repetition maximum.

an exercise to avoid exaggerating recovery time following training. It seems that the exercise protocol should be designed with the aim to maximize the degree of metabolic stress achieved, meaning that rest periods between sets should be somewhat limited to ensure an incomplete recovery between sets; that is, 30–45 s for low-load training (20–40% 1RM), ~60 s for moderate-load training (60–70% 1RM), and ~120 s for high-load training (>80% 1RM) [39]. A novel RTH approach showing promising results is high-load circuit-style resistance training [37, 43, 45], which provides potent mechanical and neural stimuli while also exaggerating the metabolic demands of exercise in hypoxia.

Abbreviations

BFR   blood flow restriction
F_iO_2 fraction of inspired oxygen
RM   repetition maximum
RTH   resistance training in hypoxia.

References

1. Bull, F.C., et al., *World Health Organization 2020 guidelines on physical activity and sedentary behaviour.* British Journal of Sports Medicine, 2020. **54**(24): p. 1451–1462.
2. Suchomel, T.J., S. Nimphius, and M.H. Stone, *The importance of muscular strength in athletic performance.* Sports Medicine, 2016. **46**(10): p. 1419–1449.
3. Shinohara, M., et al., *Efficacy of tourniquet ischemia for strength training with low resistance.* European Journal of Applied Physiology and Occupational Physiology, 1998. **77**(1–2): p. 189–191.
4. Takarada, Y., et al., *Effects of resistance exercise combined with moderate vascular occlusion on muscular function in humans.* Journal of Applied Physiology, 2000. **88**(6): p. 2097–2106.
5. Perera, E., et al., *Effects of blood flow restriction therapy for muscular strength, hypertrophy, and endurance in healthy and special populations: a systematic review and meta-analysis* Clinical Journal of Sport Medicine, 2022. **32**(5): p. 531–545.
6. Scott, B.R., et al., *Hypoxia and resistance exercise: a comparison of localized and systemic methods.* Sports Medicine, 2014. **44**(8): p. 1037–1054.
7. Nishimura, A., et al., *Hypoxia increases muscle hypertrophy induced by resistance training.* International Journal of Sports Physiology and Performance, 2010. **5**(4): p. 497–508.
8. Manimmanakorn, A., et al., *Effects of low-load resistance training combined with blood flow restriction or hypoxia on muscle function and performance in netball athletes.* Journal of Science and Medicine in Sport, 2013. **16**(4): p. 337–342.
9. Ramos-Campo, D.J., et al., *The efficacy of resistance training in hypoxia to enhance strength and muscle growth: A systematic review and meta-analysis.* European Journal of Sport Science, 2018. **18**(1): p. 92–103.
10. Sato, Y., *The history and future of KAATSU training.* International Journal of KAATSU Training Research, 2005. **1**(1): p. 1–5.
11. Patterson, S.D., et al., *Blood flow restriction exercise: Considerations of methodology, application, and safety.* Frontiers in Physiology, 2019. **10**: p. 533.
12. Ratamess, N.A., et al., *American College of Sports Medicine position stand: Progression models in resistance training for healthy adults.* Medicine and Science in Sports and Exercise, 2009. **41**(3): p. 687–708.
13. Fabero-Garrido, R., et al., *Effects of low-load blood flow restriction resistance training on muscle strength and hypertrophy compared with traditional resistance training in healthy adults older than 60 years: Systematic review and meta-analysis.* Journal of Clinical Medicine, 2022. **11**(24).
14. Hughes, L., et al., *Blood flow restriction training in clinical musculoskeletal rehabilitation: A systematic review and meta-analysis.* British Journal of Sports Medicine, 2017. **51**(13): p. 1003–1011.
15. Davids, C.J., et al., *Where does blood flow restriction fit in the toolbox of athletic development? A narrative review of the proposed mechanisms and potential applications.* Sports Medicine, In Press.
16. Bjørnsen, T., et al., *Type 1 muscle fiber hypertrophy after blood flow-restricted training in powerlifters.* Medicine and Science in Sports and Exercise, 2019. **51**(2): p. 288–298.

17. Lixandrao, M.E., et al., *Magnitude of muscle strength and mass adaptations between high-load resistance training versus low-load resistance training associated with blood-flow restriction: A systematic review and meta-analysis.* Sports Medicine, 2018. **48**(2): p. 361–378.
18. Folland, J.P. and A.G. Williams, *The adaptations to strength training: Morphological and neurological contributions to increased strength.* Sports Medicine, 2007. **37**(2): p. 145–168.
19. Yasuda, T., et al., *Muscle activation during low-intensity muscle contractions with restricted blood flow.* Journal of Sports Sciences, 2009. **27**(5): p. 479–489.
20. Brandner, C.R., S.A. Warmington, and D.J. Kidgell, *Corticomotor excitability is increased following an acute bout of blood flow restriction resistance exercise.* Frontiers in Human Neuroscience, 2015. **9**: p. 652.
21. Loenneke, J.P., et al., *Exercise-induced changes in muscle size do not contribute to exercise-induced changes in muscle strength.* Sports Medicine, 2019. **49**(7): p. 987–991.
22. Nielsen, J.L., et al., *Proliferation of myogenic stem cells in human skeletal muscle in response to low-load resistance training with blood flow restriction.* The Journal of Physiology, 2012. **590**(Pt 17): p. 4351–4361.
23. Schoenfeld, B.J., *Potential mechanisms for a role of metabolic stress in hypertrophic adaptations to resistance training.* Sports Medicine, 2013. **43**(3): p. 179–194.
24. Loenneke, J.P., et al., *The anabolic benefits of venous blood flow restriction training may be induced by muscle cell swelling.* Medical Hypotheses, 2012. **78**(1): p. 151–154.
25. Scott, B.R., et al., *Exercise with blood flow restriction: An updated evidence-based approach for enhanced muscular development.* Sports Medicine, 2015. **45**(3): p. 313–325.
26. Fujita, S., et al., *Blood flow restriction during low-intensity resistance exercise increases S6K1 phosphorylation and muscle protein synthesis.* Journal of Applied Physiology, 2007. **103**(3): p. 903–910.
27. Fry, C.S., et al., *Blood flow restriction exercise stimulates mTORC1 signaling and muscle protein synthesis in older men.* Journal of Applied Physiology, 2010. **108**(5): p. 1199–1209.
28. Drummond, M.J., et al., *Human muscle gene expression following resistance exercise and blood flow restriction.* Medicine and Science in Sports and Exercise, 2008. **40**(4): p. 691–698.
29. Laurentino, G.C., et al., *Strength training with blood flow restriction diminishes myostatin gene expression.* Medicine and Science in Sports and Exercise, 2012. **44**(3): p. 406–412.
30. Hoppeler, H. and M. Vogt, *Muscle tissue adaptations to hypoxia.* The Journal of Experimental Biology, 2001. **204**(18): p. 3133–3139.
31. Inness, M.W., et al., *Heavy resistance training in hypoxia enhances 1RM squat performance.* Frontiers in Physiology, 2016. **7**: p. 502.
32. Yan, B., et al., *Effects of five-week resistance training in hypoxia on hormones and muscle strength.* Journal of Strength and Conditioning Research, 2016. **30**(1): p. 184–193.
33. Namboonlue, C., et al., *Optimal degree of hypoxia combined with low-load resistance training for muscle strength and thickness in athletes.* Journal of Physical Education and Sport, 2020. **20**(2): p. 828–838.

34. Ho, J.Y., et al., *Combining normobaric hypoxia with short-term resistance training has no additive beneficial effect on muscular performance and body composition.* Journal of Strength and Conditioning Research, 2014. 28(4): p. 935–941.

35. Törpel, A., B. Peter, and L. Schega, *Effect of resistance training under normobaric hypoxia on physical performance, hematological parameters, and body composition in young and older people.* Frontiers in Physiology, 2020. 11: p. 335.

36. Kurobe, K., et al., *Effects of resistance training under hypoxic conditions on muscle hypertrophy and strength.* Clinical Physiology and Functional Imaging, 2015. 35(3): p. 197–202.

37. Martinez-Guardado, I., et al., *Effects of high-intensity resistance circuit-based training in hypoxia on body composition and strength performance.* European Journal of Sport Science, 2019. 19(7): p. 941–951.

38. Benavente, C., et al., *Efficacy of resistance training in hypoxia on muscle hypertrophy and strength development: A systematic review with meta-analysis.* Scientific Reports, 2023. 13(1): p. 3676.

39. Deldicque, L., *Does normobaric hypoxic resistance training confer benefit over normoxic training in athletes? A narrative review.* Journal of Science in Sport and Exercise, 2022. 4: p. 306–314.

40. Feriche, B., et al., *Effect of acute exposure to moderate altitude on muscle power: hypobaric hypoxia vs. normobaric hypoxia.* PLoS One, 2014. 9(12): p. e114072.

41. Almeida, F., et al., *Effects of power-oriented resistance training during an altitude camp on strength and technical performance of elite judokas.* Frontiers in Physiology, 2021. 12: p. 606191.

42. Kon, M., et al., *Effects of systemic hypoxia on human muscular adaptations to resistance exercise training.* Physiological Reports, 2014. 2(6): p. e12033.

43. Ramos-Campo, D.J., et al., *Effect of high-intensity resistance circuit-based training in hypoxia on aerobic performance and repeat sprint ability.* Scandinavian Journal of Medicine and Science in Sports, 2018. 28(10): p. 2135–2143.

44. Mayo, B., et al., *The effect of resistance training in a hypoxic chamber on physical performance in elite rugby athletes.* High Altitude Medicine & Biology, 2018. 19(1): p. 28–34.

45. Ramos-Campo, D.J., et al., *Biochemical responses and physical performance during high-intensity resistance circuit training in hypoxia and normoxia.* European Journal of Applied Physiology, 2017. 117(4): p. 809–818.

46. Scott, B.R., et al., *Acute physiological responses to moderate-load resistance exercise in hypoxia.* Journal of Strength and Conditioning Research, 2017. 31(7): p. 1973–1981.

47. Britto, F.A., et al., *Acute environmental hypoxia potentiates satellite cell-dependent myogenesis in response to resistance exercise through the inflammation pathway in human.* FASEB J, 2020. 34(1): p. 1885–1900.

48. Gnimassou, O., et al., *Environmental hypoxia favors myoblast differentiation and fast phenotype but blunts activation of protein synthesis after resistance exercise in human skeletal muscle.* FASEB J, 2018. 32(10): p. 5272–5284.

49. Moberg, M., et al., *Acute normobaric hypoxia blunts contraction-mediated mTORC1- and JNK-signaling in human skeletal muscle.* Acta Physiologica (Oxford), 2022. 234(2): p. e13771.

50. Scott, B.R., K.M. Slattery, and B.J. Dascombe, *Intermittent hypoxic resistance training: is metabolic stress the key moderator?* Medical Hypotheses, 2015. 84(2): p. 145–149.

51. Haseler, L.J., M.C. Hogan, and R.S. Richardson, *Skeletal muscle phosphocreatine recovery in exercise-trained humans is dependent on* O_2 *availability.* Journal of Applied Physiology, 1999. **86**(6): p. 2013–2018.
52. Wilber, R.L., J. Stray-Gundersen, and B.D. Levine, *Effect of hypoxic "dose" on physiological responses and sea-level performance.* Medicine and Science in Sports and Exercise, 2007. **39**(9): p. 1590–1599.
53. Hubal, M.J., et al., *Variability in muscle size and strength gain after unilateral resistance training.* Medicine and Science in Sports and Exercise, 2005. **37**(6): p. 964–972.
54. Chapman, R.F., J. Stray-Gundersen, and B.D. Levine, *Individual variation in response to altitude training.* Journal of Applied Physiology, 1998. **85**(4): p. 1448–1456.
55. Yamanaka, T., R.S. Farley, and J.L. Caputo, *Occlusion training increases muscular strength in division IA football players.* Journal of Strength and Conditioning Research, 2012. **26**(9): p. 2523–2529.
56. Luebbers, P.E., et al., *The effects of a 7-week practical blood flow restriction program on well-trained collegiate athletes.* Journal of Strength and Conditioning Research, 2014. **28**(8): p. 2270–2280.
57. Centner, C. and B. Lauber, *A systematic review and meta-analysis on neural adaptations following blood flow restriction training: What we know and what we don't know.* Frontiers in Physiology, 2020. **11**: p. 887.
58. Laurentino, G., et al., *Effects of strength training and vascular occlusion.* International Journal of Sports Medicine, 2008. **29**(8): p. 664–667.
59. Teixeira, E.L., et al., *Blood flow restriction does not promote additional effects on muscle adaptations when combined with high-load resistance training regardless of blood flow restriction protocol.* Journal of Strength and Conditioning Research, 2021. **35**(5): p. 1194–1200.

SECTION 9

19

HEMATOLOGICAL AND DOPING ISSUES

*Antoine Raberin, Bastien Krumm and Raphael Faiss**

19.1 Hematological adaptations to acute exposures

Exposure to hypoxia induces hematological adaptations that depend on the hypoxic dose. Acutely, an increased hemoglobin concentration ([Hb]) occurs after brief hypoxic exposure, or even a short breath-hold period [1]. This initial increase in [Hb] results from two different mechanisms, spleen contraction and plasma volume (PV) shift.

The human spleen, among other functions, is a dynamic red blood cell reservoir that contains around 200 to 250 ml of blood, representing 10% of the human red cell volume. In other mammals like horse or seal, this storage capacity could reach 50% of the total red blood cell volume.

Spleen contraction, driven by sympathetic input and catecholamine release, is triggered by apnea, hypoxia, hypercapnia, and exercise. After maximal contraction, the red cell supply and volume of the spleen is restored in about 10 min.

Altitude exposure seems to impact spleen efficiency, with a greater spleen volume and contraction during exercise observed on return to low altitude after extreme altitude expeditions [2]. Consequently, top climbers have larger spleens and greater spleen contraction than recreational ones.

Due to the reduced spleen content in humans compared to other mammals, its physiological relevance during altitude exposure raises questions. Studies have demonstrated that an 18% reduction in spleen volume is accompanied by a 2.1% increase in both [Hb] and hematocrit (Hct) after breathing a gas

* A. Raberin and B. Krumm contributed equally to the work.

DOI: 10.4324/9781003402879-29

mixture with 12.8% of oxygen for 20 min [3]. While spleen volume is negatively correlated with [Hb] and Hct, spleen contraction was estimated to contribute to about 60% of the change in Hct during acute exposure to hypoxia. Therefore, PV contraction is responsible for the remaining Hct changes.

PV reduction increases with altitude duration, and a decrease over 10% can be observed within the first 24 h of exposure [4]. This initial steep decrease seems independent of altitude severity. PV contraction results from an imbalance between water loss and water intake and/or a fluid shift from the intravascular to extravascular compartment.

While a water loss was reported in altitude facilities where normal fluid and food intake are warranted [5] (usual confounding factor during trekking expeditions), the opposite was also shown [6]. However, in these latter cases, it is mostly associated to acute mountain sickness-related fluid retention. Water loss is attributed to a reduction in thirst sensation, increased diuresis, and higher respiratory fluid loss due to air conditioning. The magnitude of ventilatory adaptations is expected to impact respiratory fluid loss and diuresis through carbon dioxide elimination. Air temperature and humidity, generally decreased at altitude, may further impact this respiratory fluid loss.

Decreased renin angiotensin aldosterone axis activity, which promotes water reabsorption, and increase in atrial natriuretic peptide, a pro-natriuretic and diuretic hormone, during the first hours of exposure may contribute to greater diuresis. However, it is still unclear if hypoxia per se reduces thirst sensation and increases diuresis. Very recent studies controlling diet, water intake, physical activity, and temperature report a slight increase in diuresis during 4 days at 3,500 m only in women, not in men [7, 8]. These results suggest that acute PV reduction is driven by oncotic pressure and fluid redistribution to the extravascular medium. Indeed, a loss of plasma protein has been described in men and women during acute exposure to hypoxia. This could be explained by the hypoxia-related inflammatory response that increases vascular permeability, although this was not confirmed in a recent study [8]. On the other hand, a marked increase in diuresis after 6 h breathing 12% oxygen (O_2) (~4,300 m) was similarly reported in a well-controlled study [5]. This discrepancy has been proposed to be due to differences in hypoxic severity or to a normalization of diuresis upon longer periods.

Finally, an acute plasma contraction may ultimately lead to an initial decrease in blood volume that can be further balanced by long-term hematological adaptations, as summarized in Figure 19.1.

19.2 Hematological adaptations to prolonged exposures

The acute effects of hypoxic conditions on the human body at high altitudes have been described for over a century, primarily in mountain climbers and air force pilots exposed to high altitudes [9]. Altitude training strategies

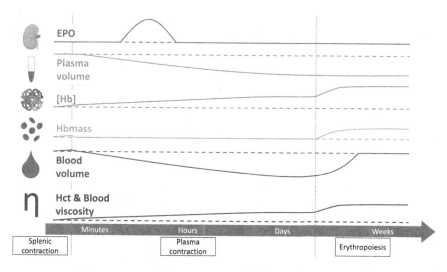

FIGURE 19.1 Time course of hematological and hemorheological changes during hypoxic exposure. Dashed lines represent baseline projection. Solid lines represent the changes over exposure. [Hb]: Hemoglobin concentration, Hbmass: Hemoglobin mass, Hct: Hematocrit.

The items in the figure from BioRender.com.

(i.e., prolonged hypoxic exposures) were then investigated in the last 50 years [10], following the 1968 Mexico Olympic Games at 2,300 m with hypoxia being an additional stimulus triggering robust physiological responses.

Undoubtably, hypoxic training or altitude exposure strategies have become popular ergogenic aids among competitive athletes, with a diverse array of possible combinations [11].

Despite substantial differences between the various forms of hypoxic training and/or exposure, their end goal remains to trigger physiological adaptations to improve exercise capacity.

While acute hypoxic exposure stabilizes hypoxia-inducible transcription factors (HIFs), playing a key role in the molecular cascade of angiogenic and metabolic adaptations, prolonged hypoxic exposure leads to a sustained stimulation of the sympathetic nervous system. This stimulation in turn increases resting metabolic rate and stimulates the bone marrow to rise the red blood cell production [12] through the release of erythropoietin (EPO), a glycoprotein hormone activating erythropoiesis. Hypoxia is the primary stimulus for serum EPO levels increasing up to several hundred-folds [13].

A subsequent increase in red blood cell mass may then improve O_2 carrying capacity to the working muscles if the hypoxic "dose" is sufficient.

However, EPO levels seem to decline gradually after an initial peak occurring during the first days [14]. The rate of decline may be affected by the hypoxic level, with evidence suggesting that EPO rises more significantly with a greater decline in partial pressure of oxygen in arterial blood [15]. To trigger hematological adaptions, an altitude level corresponding to 2,000–2,500 m for several weeks was hence recommended [16], at least in athletes.

The concept of hypoxic dose remains pivotal to support putative hematological adaptations through prolonged hypoxia. A meta-analysis suggests an approximate increase of 1% in total hemoglobin mass per 100 h of altitude exposure [17], and a simple metric combining time at altitude and actual altitude was proposed to estimate speculated gains [18]. However, the response to the hypoxic exposure is highly individual, and including O_2 saturation levels to evaluate hypoxic dose may provide a far better indication of ongoing responses to prolonged hypoxia [19]. Hence, hematological response may not be triggered if the altitude level is too low (i.e., if the individual response to the hypoxic stress is not strong enough) [14].

Nevertheless, HIFs may be considered as pivotal mediators of the adaptations to acute or prolonged hypoxia, independently of erythropoiesis as a beneficial consequence.

From a health perspective, HIFs were associated with the regulation of cellular responses to inflammation and hypoxia [20] and could be considered as central in the regulation of metabolism, acting as mediators of insulin resistance [21] and iron metabolism [22].

Voluntary exposure to hypoxia may trigger robust adaptive responses, improving HIFs signaling, with possible complications however in case of underlying metabolic diseases (e.g., diabetes) [23]. Moreover, HIFs function is inhibited by elevated fatty acid levels, while overweight status results in changes in fatty acid profiles [23]. In addition, cyclic hypoxia-reoxygenation has been shown to activate HIFs to preserve or enhance brain functions [24].

While the underlying mechanisms are still unresolved to date, this illustrates the potential of acute or prolonged hypoxic exposure alone or combined with exercise to trigger strong adaptive responses to improve health or exercise capacity.

19.3 Impact of hematological adaptations on O_2 transport and perfusion

Hemoconcentration starts rapidly after the initiation of hypoxic exposure, causing Hct and [Hb] to increase. The consequence is an increase in arterial O_2 carrying capacity to limit O_2 supply depletion. It also allows a decrease in cardiac output for a given O_2 supply, thereby limiting cardiovascular strain and increasing exercise tolerance [6].

Prolonged hematological adaptation with an increase in hemoglobin mass (Hbmass) further enhances arterial O_2 carrying capacity. This adaptation is particularly relevant for endurance performance upon return at sea level since a strong relationship between Hbmass and maximal O_2 uptake exists. An increase of 1 g in Hbmass is estimated to result in about 4 ml.min^{-1} enhancement of maximal O_2 uptake [25].

On the other hand, blood viscosity is highly dependent on Hct and is expected to increase with hypoxic exposure as soon as hemoconcentration is significant. According to the Poiseuille law, any increase in blood viscosity augments blood flow resistance and can impair perfusion. However, the expected rise in blood viscosity is not consistently observed due to the wide range of hypoxic stimuli across studies.

Hypoxia modifies other determinants of blood viscosity. A rise in fibrinogen concentration occurs during acute and chronic exposure, leading to a rise in plasma viscosity. Red blood cell (RBC) aggregation increases across various hypoxic conditions (acute to chronic exposure and moderate to severe hypoxia [26]), and the increased fibrinogen concentration is one of the causes. Changes in the deformability of RBC with hypoxia depend on the severity of the hypoxic stress. RBC are less deformable at moderate altitude, but their deformability increases with a severe hypoxic dose [27]. RBC deformability is partly mediated by nitric oxide produced by the RBC-nitric oxide synthase, and the blunt RBC-nitric oxide synthase activation under hypoxia could be compensated in severe hypoxia by the ability of deoxyhemoglobin to reduce nitrite to nitric oxide.

Considering that RBC deformability and aggregation alter capillaries perfusion, the balance between hematological and hemorheological adaptations to O_2 delivery must be considered (Figure 19.2). Excessive erythrocytosis reflects this delicate balance, as seen in chronic mountain sickness, which represents an extreme example that leads to cyanosis and impaired vascular function despite high [Hb] ([Hb] ≥ 21 g dl^{-1} and ≥ 19 g dl^{-1} for males and females, respectively).

However, nitric oxide synthase, which promotes vasodilation, is activated during hemoconcentration to balance shear rate increase. Hence, slight rise in blood viscosity stimulates nitric oxide synthase [28] and could be one mechanism for hypoxia compensatory vasodilation.

19.4 Doping issue: EPO use at altitude or in hypoxia as a confounding factor?

If the beneficial effects of hypoxia on hematological variables are not systematic and remain dependent on the individual responses to the hypoxic stimulus, blood doping is a shortcut that unfortunately offers similar and more assured benefits. With the primary aim of increasing blood volume and, therefore, convective oxygen transport to active muscles, blood transfusion is

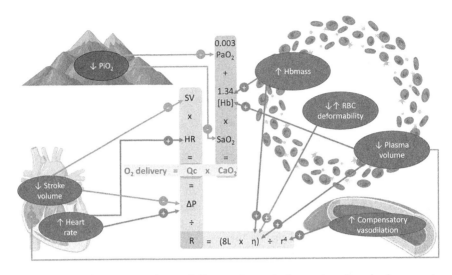

FIGURE 19.2 Alteration of O_2 delivery through hypoxia-related changes in hematological, hemorheological and cardiovascular parameters. Oxygen (O_2) delivery is defined by the product of cardiac output (Qc) and arterial oxygen content (CaO_2). Cardiac output can be defined by the product of stroke volume (SV) and heart rate (HR) or by the ratio between the delta blood pressure (ΔP) over vascular resistance (R). Poiseuille's law defined resistance as the product of 8 content length (L) and fluid viscosity (η) over the radius of the content exponent 4 (r^4). In this case, content and fluid refer to blood vessel and blood respectively. CaO_2 is defined by the sum of 0.003 arterial oxygen pressure (PaO_2) plus the product between 1.34 hemoglobin concentration ([Hb]) and arterial oxygen saturation (SaO_2).

Hbmass: Hemoglobin mass, PiO_2: nspired oxygen pressure, RBC: red blood cells.

The items in the figure from BioRender.com.

the first type of blood doping historically used by athletes to improve endurance performance [29].

First referred to as "blood boosting" [30], these blood manipulations for athletic purposes seem to have started in the late 60s. The 1968 Olympic Games in Mexico City, situated at 2,300 m, represented a major milestone in the liberation of this practice. The dominance of endurance races by athletes from high-altitude locations [31] emphasized the advantages of increased blood volume, particularly Hbmass, for endurance performance. While altitude training also had its early beginnings on this occasion [32], the use of blood transfusions, first in homologous form (exchange of blood between two individuals) and then autologous (reinfusion of blood from the same person), became particularly prevalent in endurance sports since the 1970s (e.g., cycling or cross-country skiing) [30]. A paradigm shift occurred following the development of recombinant EPO in the late 1980s. As the first hematopoietic growth factor synthesized and essentially administered for the treatment of renal insufficiency and subsequent anemia [33], recombinant EPO was commercialized in 1989 and quickly diverted from its original medical target for athletic use due to its key role in the erythropoiesis pathway [29]. Furthermore, the additive erythropoietic response obtained by combining hypoxic exposure and recombinant EPO injections [34] suggests that some athletes may have simultaneously used these two approaches to maximize their hematological adaptations and, consequently, their performance.

In the 2000s, the development of an electrophoretic method to discriminate recombinant EPO from endogenous hormones by Lasne and de Ceaurriz [35] represented a major turning point for antidoping efforts. This method, analyzing isoelectric patterns in urine samples, became a crucial tool in detecting recombinant EPO abuse and is still applied today. However, due to the relatively short half-life of recombinant EPO (~10 h by intravenous injection and twice this duration after subcutaneous injection) [33], direct detection methods have limitations. In this context, indirect detection has been investigated to support traditional detection methods. Rather than targeting the prohibited substance itself, this approach investigates the effects that the substance may have on specific biomarkers. First applied with population thresholds (e.g., "no-start" rule based on a cut-off level of hematocrit for cycling competitions) [29], this leads to the development of the Athlete Biological Passport (ABP) [36]. Based on a Bayesian approach, the ABP provides individual and longitudinal monitoring of blood markers sensible to altered erythropoiesis to identify nonphysiological patterns caused by prohibited substances (e.g., recombinant EPO) or methods (e.g., blood transfusion) (Figure 19.3). Since its first implementation in 2009, the ABP has repeatedly demonstrated its effectiveness [37], at least through its deterrent effect, illustrated by a significant reduction in the performance of several sports (e.g., running) [38].

However, due to its indirect approach, the ABP and its variables are susceptible to confounding factors [39], and altitude training is one of the most evident examples. Reported as a potential challenge since the introduction of the ABP, the confounding effect of altitude training on ABP variables has been repeatedly confirmed [40] (Figure 19.4). First, athletes often experience a rapid increase in [Hb] due to a plasma volume shift in the first days after arrival at

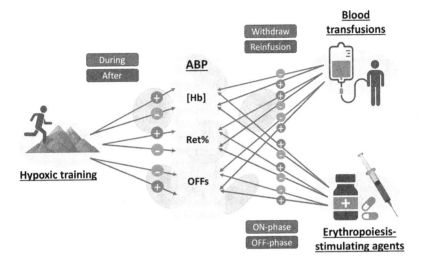

FIGURE 19.3 Athlete Biological Passport (ABP) of a male athlete tested on nine occasions for four biomarkers of blood doping: Hemoglobin concentration ([Hb]) and Off-score as primary biomarkers, Reticulocyte percentages (Ret%) and Abnormal Blood Profile Score as secondary biomarkers.

Blue lines represent actual test results for blood biomarkers. Red lines indicate two-tailed thresholds at which the test result is considered abnormal. Initial thresholds (e.g., 13.0–16.6 g·dL^{-1} for hemoglobin concentration) are based on population epidemiology and are adapted in the course of individual data acquisition by the Bayesian model to produce individual final thresholds. The Athlete Biological Passport aims to detect not only one single abnormal value but also a succession of abnormal values or abnormally high variance.

The items in the figure from BioRender.com.

altitude. Second, hypoxic exposure, by stabilizing HIFs and stimulating EPO, exerts a comparable influence to recombinant EPO on reticulocytes percentage (Ret%) and the related OFF-score (algorithm combining [Hb] and Ret%), a situation even more challenging with micro-dosing [41]. Finally, due to the reduction in endogenous EPO production when Hbmass levels exceed requirements at lower altitudes [42], a drop in Ret% comparable to the scenario after a blood transfusion is commonly observed upon return to sea level. Consequently, considering the occasionally similar trends observed in blood doping scenarios, these variations must be carefully considered by experts when evaluating longitudinal ABP profiles.

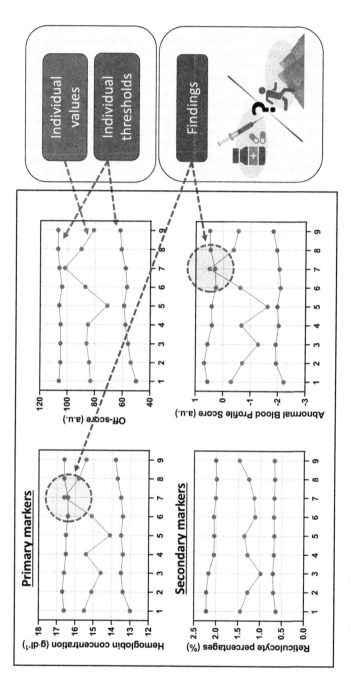

FIGURE 19.4 Impact of hypoxic training, erythropoiesis-stimulating agents abuse, or blood transfusion protocols on the main bio-markers of Athlete Biological Passport (ABP).

[Hb]: Hemoglobin concentration, Ret%: reticulocyte percentages, OFFs: OFF-score.

The items in the figure from BioRender.com.

Abbreviations

ABP   Athlete Biological Passport
EPO   erythropoietin;
[Hb]   hemoglobin concentration
Hbmass   hemoglobin mass
Hct   hematocrit
HIFs   hypoxia-inducible transcription factors
O_2 oxygen
PV   plasma volume
RBC   red blood cell
Ret%   reticulocytes percentage.

References

1. Lodin-Sundström, A. and E. Schagatay, *Spleen contraction during 20 min normobaric hypoxia and 2 min apnea in humans*. Aviat Space Environ Med, 2010. **81**(6): p. 545–9.
2. Engan, H.K., et al., *The effect of climbing Mount Everest on spleen contraction and increase in hemoglobin concentration during breath holding and exercise*. High Alt Med Biol, 2014. **15**(1): p. 52–7.
3. Richardson, M.X., et al., *Short-term effects of normobaric hypoxia on the human spleen*. Eur J Appl Physiol, 2008. **104**(2): p. 395–9.
4. Siebenmann, C., P. Robach, and C. Lundby, *Regulation of blood volume in lowlanders exposed to high altitude*. J Appl Physiol (1985), 2017. **123**(4): p. 957–66.
5. Swenson, E.R., et al., *Diuretic effect of acute hypoxia in humans: relationship to hypoxic ventilatory responsiveness and renal hormones*. J Appl Physiol (1985), 1995. **78**(2): p. 377–83.
6. Sawka, M.N., et al., *Blood volume: Importance and adaptations to exercise training, environmental stresses, and trauma/sickness*. Med Sci Sports Exerc, 2000. **32**(2): p. 332–48.
7. Schlittler, M., et al., *Regulation of plasma volume in male lowlanders during 4 days of exposure to hypobaric hypoxia equivalent to 3500 m altitude*. J Physiol, 2021. **599**(4): p. 1083–96.
8. Roche, J., et al., *Hypoxia briefly increases diuresis but reduces plasma volume by fluid redistribution in women*. Am J Physiol Heart Circ Physiol, 2022. **323**(6): p. H1068–79.
9. Barcroft, J., *The respiratory function of the blood*. 1914, Cambridge: University Press.
10. Millet, G.P., et al., *Combining hypoxic methods for peak performance*. Sports Med, 2010. **40**(1): p. 1–25.
11. Girard, O., F. Brocherie, and G.P. Millet, *Effects of altitude/hypoxia on single- and multiple-sprint performance: A comprehensive review*. Sports Med, 2017. **47**(10): p. 1931–49.
12. Grover, R.F., J.V. Weil, and J.T. Reeves, *Cardiovascular adaptation to exercise at high altitude*. Exerc Sport Sci Rev, 1986. **14**: p. 269–302.
13. Haase, V.H., *Hypoxic regulation of erythropoiesis and iron metabolism*. Am J Physiol Renal Physiol, 2010. **299**(1): p. F1–13.

14. Ploszczyca, K., J. Langfort, and M. Czuba, *The effects of altitude training on erythropoietic response and hematological variables in adult athletes: A narrative review.* Front Physiol, 2018. **9**: p. 375.

15. Eckardt, K.U., et al., *Rate of erythropoietin formation in humans in response to acute hypobaric hypoxia.* J Appl Physiol (1985), 1989. **66**(4): p. 1785–8.

16. Chapman, R.F., et al., *Defining the "dose" of altitude training: how high to live for optimal sea level performance enhancement.* J Appl Physiol (1985), 2014. **116**(6): p. 595–603.

17. Gore, C.J., et al., *Altitude training and haemoglobin mass from the optimised carbon monoxide rebreathing method determined by a meta-analysis.* Br J Sports Med, 2013. **47 Suppl 1**: p. i31–9.

18. Garvican-Lewis, L.A., K. Sharpe, and C.J. Gore, *Time for a new metric for hypoxic dose?* J Appl Physiol (1985), 2016. **121**(1): p. 352–5.

19. Millet, G.P., et al., *Commentaries on viewpoint: Time for a new metric for hypoxic dose?* J Appl Physiol (1985), 2016. **121**(1): p. 356–8.

20. Gaspar, J.M. and L.A. Velloso, *Hypoxia inducible factor as a central regulator of metabolism: Implications for the development of obesity.* Front Neurosci, 2018. **12**: p. 813.

21. Gabryelska, A., et al., *HIF-1α as a mediator of insulin resistance, T2DM, and its complications: Potential links with obstructive sleep apnea.* Front Physiol, 2020. **11**: p. 1035.

22. Peyssonnaux, C., V. Nizet, and R.S. Johnson, *Role of the hypoxia inducible factors HIF in iron metabolism.* Cell Cycle, 2008. **7**(1): p. 28–32.

23. Catrina, S.B. and X. Zheng, *Hypoxia and hypoxia-inducible factors in diabetes and its complications.* Diabetologia, 2021. **64**(4): p. 709–16.

24. Burtscher, J., et al., *Hypoxia and brain aging: Neurodegeneration or neuroprotection?* Ageing Res Rev, 2021. **68**: p. 101343.

25. Schmidt, W. and N. Prommer, *Impact of alterations in total hemoglobin mass on V̇O2max.* Exercise and Sport Sciences Reviews, 2010. **38**(2): p. 68–75.

26. Raberin, A., et al., *Hypoxia and hemorheological properties in older individuals.* Ageing Research Reviews, 2022. **79**: p. 101650.

27. Grau, M., et al., *Regulation of red blood cell deformability is independent of red blood cell-nitric oxide synthase under hypoxia.* Clinical Hemorheology and Microcirculation, 2016. **63**(3): p. 199–215.

28. Salazar Vázquez, B.Y., et al., *Cardiovascular benefits in moderate increases of blood and plasma viscosity surpass those associated with lowering viscosity: Experimental and clinical evidence.* Clinical Hemorheology and Microcirculation, 2010. **44**(2): p. 75–85.

29. Saugy, M. and N. Leuenberger, *Antidoping: From health tests to the athlete biological passport.* Drug Test Anal, 2020. **12**(5): p. 621–28.

30. Leigh-Smith, S., *Blood boosting.* Br J Sports Med, 2004. **38**(1): p. 99–101.

31. Atkinson, T.S. and M.J. Kahn, *Blood doping: Then and now. A narrative review of the history, science and efficacy of blood doping in elite sport.* Blood Rev, 2020. **39**: p. 100632.

32. Kasperowski, D., *Constructing altitude training standards for the 1968 Mexico Olympics: The impact of ideals of equality and uncertainty.* Int J History Sport, 2009. **26**(9): p. 1263–91.

33. Diamanti-Kandarakis, E., et al., *Erythropoietin abuse and erythropoietin gene doping: Detection strategies in the genomic era.* Sports Med, 2005. **35**(10): p. 831–40.

34. Bejder, J., et al., *Hematological adaptations and detection of recombinant human erythropoietin combined with chronic hypoxia.* Drug Test Anal, 2021. **13**(2): p. 360–68.

35. Lasne, F. and J. de Ceaurriz, *Recombinant erythropoietin in urine.* Nature, 2000. **405**(6787): p. 635.

36. Sottas, P.E., N. Robinson, and M. Saugy, *The athlete's biological passport and indirect markers of blood doping.* Handb Exp Pharmacol, 2010(195): p. 305–26.

37. Schumacher, Y.O., et al., *Detection of EPO doping and blood doping: The haematological module of the Athlete Biological Passport.* Drug Test Anal, 2012. **4**(11): p. 846–53.

38. Iljukov, S., et al., *Association between implementation of the athlete biological passport and female elite runners' performance.* Int J Sports Physiol Perform, 2020. **15**(9): p. 1231–1236.

39. Krumm, B. and R. Faiss, *Factors confounding the athlete biological passport: A systematic narrative review.* Sports Med Open, 2021. **7**(1): p. 65.

40. Lobigs, L.M., et al., *The athlete's hematological response to hypoxia: A meta-analysis on the influence of altitude exposure on key biomarkers of erythropoiesis.* Am J Hematol, 2018. **93**(1): p. 74–83.

41. Saugy, J.J., T. Schmoutz, and F. Botre, *Altitude and erythropoietin: Comparative evaluation of their impact on key parameters of the Athlete Biological Passport: A review.* Front Sports Act Living, 2022. **4**: p. 864532.

42. Bonne, T.C., et al., *Altitude training causes haematological fluctuations with relevance for the Athlete Biological Passport.* Drug Test Anal, 2015. **7**(8): p. 655–62.

20

POTENTIAL DOWNSIDES OF INTERMITTENT HYPOXIA

Immune function, inflammation, and oxidative stress

Marie Chambion-Diaz, Vincent Pialoux and Sébastien Baillieul

20.1 Introduction

Humans can experience systemic exposure to intermittent hypoxia (IH) in several conditions, such as environmental (e.g., altitude exposure) or pathological conditions (e.g., respiratory diseases, including sleep apnea). However, these conditions vary greatly in physiological terms [1]. The magnitude and qualitative effects of hypoxic exposure (either protective, beneficial, or pathologic) depend on individual susceptibility to hypoxia, which may vary throughout an individual's lifetime [2] and on the hypoxic dose [3–5]. The main determinants of the hypoxic dose are (1) the magnitude of hypoxia and the resulting hypoxemia, (2) the duration of exposure to hypoxia (acute versus chronic), (3) the pattern of hypoxic exposure (intermittent or sustained), and (4) in IH, the number of cycles/days [3]. Thus, high altitude residency [6], sustained severe hypoxia as experienced in respiratory insufficiency, or severe IH with high cycle frequency and/or severe hypoxic episodes as experienced in obstructive sleep apnea (OSA) are conditions where hypoxia is more likely to induce pathological effects [4]. Most of the organs can be damaged or their functions impaired in hypoxic conditions, through a cascade of detrimental mechanisms including, but not restricted to, inflammation, oxidative stress, and direct impact on immune function.

In animal models, chronic intermittent hypoxia (IH) causes different physiological dysfunctions depending on the hypoxic doses: cardiac hypertrophy, inflammation, fibrosis, and cardiac dysfunction as the first pathophysiological responses, and when the exposition is further expanded, cardiac apoptosis and oxidative stress appear [7, 8], although oxidative stress has been also shown to be responsible of these dysfunctions. In the majority of murine

DOI: 10.4324/9781003402879-30

models, chronic IH mimics the effects of OSA and can lead to liver fibrosis [9] and liver inflammation via oxidative stress [10], as well as melanoma lung metastasis [11], and also increases the risk of maternal and fetal complications [12].

20.2 Downsides of exposure to intermittent hypoxia: Evidence from studies in nonpathological populations

Worldwide, millions of healthy individuals travel to high altitudes for professional or recreational activities, exposing themselves to episodes of intermittent hypoxia. These activities include skydiving, extreme skiing, high-altitude trekking and mountaineering, traveling in commercial flights, or in more specific contexts such as for military or spatial flights [13].

Even if moderate intermittent hypoxic exposure is generally well tolerated by healthy individuals, it can sometimes trigger detrimental consequences, through a cascade of molecular mechanisms, with potential systemic consequences.

20.2.1 Oxidative stress

Oxygen sensing in cells is underpinned by many biochemical and molecular mechanisms, which can trigger adaptive or maladaptive transcriptional responses [14, 15]. Hypoxia-inducible factors 1 and 2 (HIF-1 and HIF-2, respectively) are key proteins for dioxygen sensing in most cells. Systemic oxygen sensing occurs primarily by peripheral chemosensors, especially those located in the carotid bodies, and depends on HIFs as well. The carotid bodies are chemoreceptors sensitive to oxygen variations in the arterial blood, adjusting ventilation on a cycle-to-cycle basis. In chronic hypoxia, their activation and coordinated regulation of downstream factors are critical for physiological adaptations. In chronic intermittent hypoxic conditions, an upregulation of HIF-1α and a downregulation of HIF-2α can be observed, causing an imbalance in the pro and antioxidant balance, thus leading to oxidative stress [16]. HIF-1 will activate genes encoding for the transcription of pro-oxidant enzymes, in particular NADPH oxidase 2, while HIF-2α downregulation will be associated with a decrease in gene transcription encoding antioxidant enzymes, as shown in several cell and animal models (for review, see [16]). By exposing 10 young healthy men to 4 days of intermittent hypoxia while awake (6 hours per day, cycling between 2 minutes at end-tidal $PO_2[P_{ET}O_2] = 45$ mmHg and 2 minutes at $P_{ET}O_2 = 88$ mmHg), Pialoux et al. [17] demonstrated that chronic intermittent hypoxia exposure in humans increased plasma oxidative stress through an increase in the production of reactive oxygen species (ROS) without a compensatory increase in antioxidant activity.

This was paralleled by significant increases in the acute hypoxic ventilatory response, with strong correlations between the changes in the acute hypoxic ventilatory response and DNA oxidation [17]. These results are in line with studies conducted in rats, indicating that oxidative stress through overproduction of superoxide from mitochondrial complex I is involved in the chemosensory response of the carotid bodies to hypoxia [18]. Additionally to the nitrosative and oxidative stress, the pro-inflammatory molecules may upregulate the hypoxic chemoreflex pathway. In this context, the cardiorespiratory alterations related to intermittent hypoxia may also depend on the glial-related neuroinflammation induced by the increased activation of the carotid bodies and the brainstem centers' chemosensory afferent input [19]. Interestingly, carotid bodies have also been shown to play a key role in the pathogenesis of hypertension associated with chronic intermittent hypoxic exposure [20], through the modulation of the activity of cardiorespiratory centers corresponding to a network of neurons located in the lower brainstem [21]. This has been demonstrated by Tamisier et al. [22], who showed in 12 healthy subjects a rise in arterial blood pressure (8 mmHg systolic and 5 mmHg diastolic) following 14 days of nocturnal intermittent hypoxic exposure (8 h of severe IH between 11:00 p.m. and 07:00 a.m., continuous fraction of inspired oxygen [FIO_2] of 0.13 in the tent, interspersed by 15-s bolus of oxygen every 120 s through a nasal cannula, i.e., 30 oxygen desaturation–resaturation sequences per hour). Interestingly, these changes in blood pressure were paralleled by an increase in muscle sympathetic nerve activity and a decline in baroreflex control of sympathetic outflow [22]. Thus, sympathetic nervous system activation and/or parasympathetic withdrawal [23, 24] may represent the mediating factors linking oxidative stress, carotid bodies activation, and cardiovascular consequences of intermittent hypoxic exposure. Veglio et al. [24] showed that moderate altitude increased heart rate and blood pressure without alteration of the cardiovascular response to the hypoxic test. The authors proposed that a sympathetic activation caused by hypoxia could lead to a concomitant blood pressure increase and a decrease in baroreceptor sensitivity [24].

Oxidative stress can also directly impair nitric oxide production, a mediator in the compensatory systemic vasodilation mediated by hypoxia [25]. In the study by Pialoux et al. [26], Losartan, an antihypertensive drug targeting type 1 angiotensin II receptor, prevented the increase in oxidative stress and peroxynitrite activity as well as the decrease in NO metabolism induced by intermittent hypoxic exposure (6 h of continuous cycles of 1 min of isocapnic hypoxia [$P_{ET}O_2$ nadir = 45.0 mmHg] and 1 min of normoxia [$P_{ET}O_2$ peak = 88.0 mmHg]). This result demonstrated the involvement of the renin–angiotensin system in the overproduction of ROS associated with intermittent hypoxia by upregulation of the actions of angiotensin II.

Concomitantly, Losartan prevented the BP increase induced by this specific IH exposure [27]. Taken together, these results suggest that the activation of the renin–angiotensin system may further contribute to hypertension induced by IH.

Moreover, several additional mechanisms have been proposed to explain the increase in ROS production during chronic intermittent hypoxia exposure, including electron leakage from complex I of the mitochondrial respiratory chain, activation of the xanthine oxidase pathway (similar to what can be observed during ischemia/reperfusion), and activation of the NADPH oxidase pathway [17].

20.2.2 Immune response and inflammation

Oxygen level variations may affect immune cells on a tissue-specific basis [28, 29]. It has been shown that physiological hypoxia exists in several primary and secondary lymphoid organs [28]. Hypoxia is an important regulator of the immune system and inflammation, with HIFs representing key mediators [30]. There is a link between the physiological hypoxia and the pathophysiological hypoxia and their effects on the immune system: All of the responses are mediated through the HIF pathway [30]. This activation of HIF in pathologies associated with hypoxia leads to an increase in epinephrine, cortisol, inflammatory cytokines, and immune checkpoints (PD-1, PD-L1, CTLA-4, Treg cells, and TGFβ) and results in immune suppression. In nonpathological populations, the most common situation in which IH occurs is during high intense intermittent physical exercise inducing repetitive bouts of hypoxia in muscular cells. Too high loads and/or too high intensities can be deleterious for performance, but especially for a person's health because it can lead to a decrease in immune function. The immune response is exercise-type dependent. Endurance exercise at moderate intensity likely improves immune defenses and decreases inflammation; on the contrary, exercise at high intensity or high volume decreases immune capacities but returns to baseline levels after a rest period of around 3 to 72 h. In this case, there is a production of ROS with an activation of the immune system. Resistance training can improve immune function if practiced at moderate intensity and in the long term.

Finally, it seems that exercise in hypoxia could be deleterious for the immune system. Their effects are dependent on the hypoxia severity, and the alpha and the beta-adrenergic systems seem to be the key factors with increasing inflammation and cytokines and through activation of immune cells. The acclimation phase is a necessity since the immune function is not affected when the exercise load is decreased under hypoxia, whereas the immune system is affected when the exercise load is maintained under hypoxia.

20.3 Downsides of exposure to intermittent hypoxia: Evidence from studies in pathological conditions

In some pathological conditions, intermittent hypoxia can be the overarching pathophysiological mechanism, triggering a cascade of molecular, cellular, and systemic consequences. If obstructive sleep apnea is the most frequent and the most studied pathological condition linked with intermittent hypoxia, cancer, and the tumoral environment, ischemia/reperfusion injury and heart disease are also characterized by episodes of intermittent or continuous hypoxia.

20.3.1 Obstructive sleep apnea

Obstructive sleep apnea (OSA) is part of sleep-disordered breathing as defined in the *International Classification of Sleep Disorders–Third version* [31, 32]. Sleep-disordered breathing encompasses a broad spectrum of sleep-related breathing disorders. Based on their underlying pathophysiological mechanisms, sleep-related breathing disorders are defined and categorized into four main groups: OSA, central sleep apnea [33], sleep-related hypoventilation disorder, and sleep-related hypoxemia disorder.

OSA is estimated to affect nearly one billion adults between the ages of 30 and 69 worldwide, making it the most common sleep-disordered breathing condition [34]. Its prevalence is probably underestimated due to the low specificity of symptoms (e.g., snoring, morning asthenia, daytime sleepiness, nocturia). OSA is currently considered a public health problem because of its major societal and economic consequences: excessive daytime sleepiness, road traffic accidents, cardiac and cerebrovascular morbidity and mortality, and cognitive repercussions with an impact on work performance and productivity [35, 36].

The pathophysiological mechanisms underlying cardiometabolic disease processes in OSA are complex and remain incompletely understood [37]. The cyclical, repeated episodes of apnea and hypopnea during sleep result in intermittent hypoxia, but also sleep fragmentation and fluctuations in intrathoracic pressure [35, 38, 39], which through intermediate cellular and molecular deleterious mechanisms such as oxidative stress and systemic inflammation as well as sympathetic nervous system activation, leads to metabolic and endothelial dysfunction, responsible for cardiometabolic comorbidities [35, 39–41]. Interestingly, in the joint analysis of four U.S. cohorts, higher C reactive protein was prospectively associated with increased OSA risk, particularly among younger individuals, underweight/normal-weight individuals, or premenopausal women, supporting the hypothesis of an inflammatory state associated with OSA [42].

Intermittent hypoxia seems to play a key role in this association as the recurrent nocturnal cycles of hypoxia/reoxygenation directly promote oxidative stress through an imbalance of the pro/antioxidant balance [43] and low-grade inflammation, which are the initiators of a pathophysiological cascade leading directly to sympathetic overactivity [35, 44–46]. Interestingly, it has been shown that oxidative stress levels were correlated with the severity of OSA7 and hypoxemia [47]. In addition, intermittent hypoxia also alters cerebrovascular regulation, which in addition to hypertension contributes to the pathogenesis of cerebrovascular diseases in patients with sleep apnea [47, 48] and may contribute to the pathogenesis of neurocognitive dysfunction related to OSA [46]. Part of these pathological responses are mediated by the IH-induced increased oxidative stress [17]. Thus, in patients with OSA, markers of oxidative stress are increased (including superoxide anion, NADPH oxidase, lipid peroxidation) and antioxidant defenses are reduced [43, 49].

Cardiovascular dysfunction can also be explained by lower circulating nitric oxide (NO) content, due to increased oxidative stress [45]. In addition, an NO synthase (which has vasoactive properties) uncoupling, that is, when electrons flowing from the reductase domain to the heme are diverted to molecular oxygen instead of to L-arginine results in the formation of superoxide and increased levels of oxidative stress. The beneficial properties on the cardiovascular system are then eliminated. The interactions between ROS, NO, and endothelial dysfunction in patients with sleep apnea remain complex, and not all mechanisms are yet known.

As OSA progresses, the sustained production of ROS, inflammation, and sympathetic overactivity may lead to early atherosclerosis (as reflected by an increase in carotid intima-media thickness and carotid plaques) [50] and elevated arterial stiffness [51]. Arterial stiffness is a strong predictor of late cardiovascular events and is associated with an increased risk of stroke. As OSA acts as a modulator of the occurrence, severity, and progression of chronic diseases/comorbidities, this result highlights the complex and often bidirectional relationship between OSA and its associated comorbidities, both potentially cause and consequence of each other. In line with this conclusion, a recent individual patient meta-analysis showed that the elevated arterial stiffness found in patients with OSA is driven by their comorbidities rather than by the hypoxic burden or OSA severity [52].

The impact of continuous positive airway pressure (CPAP), the first-line therapy of OSA, on metabolic or inflammatory markers is still debated [53]. In their systematic review and analysis of randomized studies comparing therapeutic versus sham CPAP intervention or CPAP withdrawal design, Jullian-Desayes et al. [53] concluded that well-designed studies failed to demonstrate any effect of CPAP on the alteration of metabolic or inflammatory markers in OSA, which contrasts with a positive and consistent impact of CPAP on sympathetic activity. The same was observed for mandibular advancement devices, with no impact on circulating biomarkers of inflammation

(C reactive protein, interleukin-6, tumor necrosis factor-α and its receptors, adiponectin, leptin, and P-selectin) in a randomized controlled trial conducted in 109 subjects free of cardiovascular comorbidity [54].

The detrimental consequences of intermittent hypoxia may also be mediated by microarousals that result in sleep fragmentation and are systematically associated with sympathetic surges, leading to elevated systolic blood pressure and a higher risk of hypertension [55]. Some other sleep-related factors potentially associated with the cardiometabolic repercussions of OSA are short sleep duration and circadian misalignment [37].

20.3.2 Cancer and other conditions

From a pathophysiological point of view, cancer is tightly linked to hypoxia, from increased cancer risk and tumor growth to metastasis. Thus, obstructive sleep apnea is an acknowledged risk factor for cancer [56, 57] and cancer mortality [58]. This association holds for several types of cancer, as highlighted in a recent meta-analysis by Wu and colleagues (Relative Risk [95% confidence interval], breast cancer = 1.32, [1.03–1.70]; central nervous system cancer = 1.71 [1.06–2.75]; kidney cancer = 1.81 [1.20–2.74]; liver cancer = 1.19, [1.10–1.29]; and pancreatic cancer = 1.23 [1.14–1.33]) [56]. In melanoma, efficient CPAP treatment for severe OSA was associated with improved melanoma outcomes when compared with untreated moderate to severe OSA [59].

The impact of chronic, sustained intermittent hypoxia has been confirmed in serval preclinical models of breast cancer [60] and melanoma [61, 62]. Thus, systemic intermittent hypoxia, through oxidative stress, impaired immune response and maintenance of a hypoxic tumor environment may promote cancer growth and malignancy [63]. Intermittent hypoxia is a key parameter of the solid tumor microenvironment [57, 64] being associated with increased angiogenesis and tumor necrosis, further promoting tumor growth and malignancy [63] as well as the metastatic potential of cancer cells [65].

Ischemia/reperfusion, or hypoxia/reoxygenation, is a phenomenon of intermittent hypoxia that occurs when a tissue deprived of blood supply (oxygen) regains its oxygen supply in a "brutal" way and causes reperfusion injuries, of which oxidative stress is one of the pathological mechanisms [66]. Ultimately, the period of ischemia/hypoxia leads to cell death caused by ROS via apoptosis, autophagy, inflammation, or cytotoxic effects. During reperfusion, a large number of free radicals are produced, which also leads to cell damage [46]. The main routes of ROS production on reperfusion are attributed to xanthine oxidase, mitochondria itself, endothelial NOS decoupling, and NADPH oxidase [17, 66]. Many studies now agree that reperfusion-related injuries are mostly due to ROS [7].

Finally, high-altitude diseases such as acute mountain sickness (AMS), high-altitude cerebral edema (HACE), and high-altitude pulmonary edema (HAPE) are linked to increases in proinflammatory cytokines and markers of oxidative stress and decreases in antioxidant markers [67]. Therefore, exposure to real altitude intermittently increases oxidative stress, and the onset of AMS appears to be correlated with this increase [67, 68]. Cytotoxic effects of ROS and inflammation are likely involved in the mechanisms that lead to AMS and HACE, whereas HAPE is caused by decreased bioavailability of NO and increased generation of ROS [69]. Some authors suggest that real altitude resulting from a reduction of the barometric pressure (hypobaric hypoxia) may induce more severe pathological responses (versus normobaric simulated normoxia) [70]. Environmental hypoxia results from a reduction of the barometric pressure (hypobaric hypoxia) or a reduction of the fraction of inspired oxygen (normobaric hypoxia). Indeed, it is known that OS is regulated differently in hypobaric and normobaric hypoxia, the former leading to lower levels of stimulation [71, 72].

20.4 Conclusion

Although IH can be used by athletes to improve performance, for cardiac preconditioning, or as therapy in obese people, it may also result in detrimental physiological responses leading to pathological conditions. This is particularly the case when the IH dose exceeds the adaptative characteristics of the

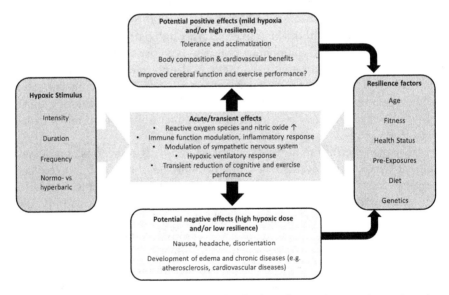

FIGURE 20.1 The hypoxic dose and individual resilience factors determine the outcomes of hypoxia exposures, including health risks.

subject/patient, especially in case of an impaired health status. In this context, oxidative stress and inflammation are likely the main mediators between the IH dose and the pathogenesis of these diseases. The U reverse nature of the oxidative stress and inflammation responses to a stimulus (here "intermittent hypoxia"), a phenomenon called hormesis, occurs at the cellular [73] or the body level [74]. This oxidative stress and inflammation hormesis fully corresponds to the wide spectrum of adaptive responses to IH, from bad to good adaptation, as a function of the dose of IH and the baseline health condition of the subjects, rendering them more or less susceptible to ROS and inflammatory mediators (Figure 20.1).

In conclusion, the follow-up of oxidative stress and inflammation status seems relevant to an early detection of maladaptation to IH, especially in people subjected directly or indirectly to this stimulus.

Abbreviations

AMS   acute mountain sickness
CPAP   continuous positive airway pressure
CTLA-4   cytotoxic T-lymphocyte associated protein 4
FIO_2 fraction of inspired oxygen
HACE   high-altitude cerebral edema
HAPE   high-altitude pulmonary edema
HIF   hypoxia-inducible factor
IH   intermittent hypoxia
mmHg   millimeter of mercury
NADPH   nicotinamide adenine dinucleotide phosphate
PD-1   programmed cell death protein 1
PD-L-1   programmed death-ligand 1
$P_{ET}O_2$ end-tidal PO_2
ROS   reactive oxygen species
TGFβ   transforming growth factor beta.

References

1. Viscor G, Ricart A, Pages T, et al. Intermittent hypoxia for obstructive sleep apnea? *High Alt Med Biol* 2014; 15: 520–521. DOI: 10.1089/ham.2014.1060
2. Richalet JP and Lhuissier FJ. Aging, tolerance to high altitude, and cardiorespiratory response to hypoxia. *High Alt Med Biol* 2015; 16: 117–124. DOI: 10.1089/ham.2015.0030
3. Navarrete-Opazo A and Mitchell GS. Therapeutic potential of intermittent hypoxia: A matter of dose. *Am J Physiol Regul Integr Comp Physiol* 2014; 307: R1181–1197. DOI: 10.1152/ajpregu.00208.2014
4. Verges S, Chacaroun S, Godin-Ribuot D and Baillieul S. hypoxic conditioning as a new therapeutic modality. *Front Pediatr* 2015; 3: 58. DOI: 10.3389/fped.2015.00058

5. Almendros I, Farre R, Planas AM, et al. Tissue oxygenation in brain, muscle, and fat in a rat model of sleep apnea: Differential effect of obstructive apneas and intermittent hypoxia. *Sleep* 2011; 34: 1127–1133. DOI: 10.5665/SLEEP.1176

6. West JB. Are permanent residents of high altitude fully adapted to their hypoxic environment? *High Alt Med Biol* 2017; 18: 135–139. DOI: 10.1089/ham.2016.0152

7. Yin X, Zheng Y, Liu Q, et al. Cardiac response to chronic intermittent hypoxia with a transition from adaptation to maladaptation: The role of hydrogen peroxide. *Oxid Med Cell Longev* 2012; 2012: 569520. DOI: 10.1155/2012/569520

8. Belaidi E, Khouri C, Harki O, et al. Cardiac consequences of intermittent hypoxia: A matter of dose? A systematic review and meta-analysis in rodents. *Eur Respir Rev* 2022. DOI: 10.1183/16000617.0269-2021

9. Mesarwi OA, Moya EA, Zhen X, et al. Hepatocyte HIF-1 and intermittent hypoxia independently impact liver fibrosis in murine nonalcoholic fatty liver disease. *Am J Respir Cell Mol Biol* 2021; 65: 390–402. DOI: 10.1165/rcmb.2020-0492OC

10. Li Y, Chen Y, Kuang J, et al. Intermittent hypoxia induces hepatic senescence through promoting oxidative stress in a mouse model. *Sleep Breath* 2023. DOI: 10.1007/s11325-023-02878-1

11. Li L, Ren F, Qi C, et al. Intermittent hypoxia promotes melanoma lung metastasis via oxidative stress and inflammation responses in a mouse model of obstructive sleep apnea. *Respir Res* 2018; 19: 28. DOI: 10.1186/s12931-018-0727-x

12. Badran M, Yassin BA, Lin DTS, et al. Gestational intermittent hypoxia induces endothelial dysfunction, reduces perivascular adiponectin and causes epigenetic changes in adult male offspring. *J Physiol* 2019; 597: 5349–5364. DOI: 10.1113/JP277936

13. Viscor G, Torrella JR, Corral L, et al. Physiological and biological responses to short-term intermittent hypobaric hypoxia exposure: From sports and mountain medicine to new biomedical applications. *Front Physiol* 2018; 9: 814. DOI: 10.3389/fphys.2018.00814

14. Lee P, Chandel NS and Simon MC. Cellular adaptation to hypoxia through hypoxia inducible factors and beyond. *Nat Rev Mol Cell Biol* 2020; 21: 268–283. DOI: 10.1038/s41580-020-0227-y

15. Baik AH and Jain IH. Turning the oxygen dial: Balancing the highs and lows. *Trends Cell Biol* 2020; 30: 516–536. DOI: 10.1016/j.tcb.2020.04.005

16. Prabhakar NR and Semenza GL. Adaptive and maladaptive cardiorespiratory responses to continuous and intermittent hypoxia mediated by hypoxia-inducible factors 1 and 2. *Physiol Rev* 2012; 92: 967–1003. DOI: 10.1152/physrev.00030.2011

17. Pialoux V, Hanly PJ, Foster GE, et al. Effects of exposure to intermittent hypoxia on oxidative stress and acute hypoxic ventilatory response in humans. *Am J Respir Crit Care Med* 2009; 180: 1002–1009. DOI: 10.1164/rccm.200905-0671OC

18. Peng YJ, Overholt JL, Kline D, et al. Induction of sensory long-term facilitation in the carotid body by intermittent hypoxia: Implications for recurrent apneas. *Proc Natl Acad Sci U S A* 2003; 100: 10073–10078. DOI: 10.1073/pnas.1734109100

19. Iturriaga R. Carotid body contribution to the physio-pathological consequences of intermittent hypoxia: Role of nitro-oxidative stress and inflammation. *J Physiol* 2023. DOI: 10.1113/JP284112

20. Iturriaga R, Oyarce MP and Dias ACR. Role of carotid body in intermittent hypoxia-related hypertension. *Curr Hypertens Rep* 2017; 19: 38. DOI: 10.1007/s11906-017-0735-0

21. Iturriaga R, Moya EA and Del Rio R. Inflammation and oxidative stress during intermittent hypoxia: The impact on chemoreception. *Exp Physiol* 2015; 100: 149–155. DOI: 10.1113/expphysiol.2014.079525

22. Tamisier R, Pepin JL, Remy J, et al. 14 nights of intermittent hypoxia elevate daytime blood pressure and sympathetic activity in healthy humans. *Eur Respir J* 2011; 37: 119–128. DOI: 10.1183/09031936.00204209

23. Meyer MJ, Mordukhovich I, Wellenius GA, et al. Changes in heart rate and rhythm during a crossover study of simulated commercial flight in older and vulnerable participants. *Frontiers in Physiology* 2019; 10: 1339. DOI: 10.3389/fphys.2019.01339

24. Veglio M, Maule S, Cametti G, et al. The effects of exposure to moderate altitude on cardiovascular autonomic function in normal subjects. *Clin Auton Res* 1999; 9: 123–127. DOI: 10.1007/BF02281624

25. Casey DP, Madery BD, Curry TB, et al. Nitric oxide contributes to the augmented vasodilatation during hypoxic exercise. *The Journal of Physiology* 2010; 588: 373–385. DOI: 10.1113/jphysiol.2009.180489

26. Pialoux V, Foster GE, Ahmed SB, et al. Losartan abolishes oxidative stress induced by intermittent hypoxia in humans. *J Physiol* 2011; 589: 5529–5537. DOI: 10.1113/jphysiol.2011.218156

27. Foster GE, Hanly PJ, Ahmed SB, et al. Intermittent hypoxia increases arterial blood pressure in humans through a renin-angiotensin system-dependent mechanism. *Hypertension* 2010; 56: 369–377. DOI: 10.1161/HYPERTENSIONAHA. 110.152108

28. Taylor CT and Scholz CC. The effect of HIF on metabolism and immunity. *Nat Rev Nephrol* 2022; 18: 573–587. DOI: 10.1038/s41581-022-00587-8

29. Zenewicz LA. Oxygen levels and immunological studies. *Front Immunol* 2017; 8: 324. DOI: 10.3389/fimmu.2017.00324

30. Burtscher J, Pasha Q, Chanana N, et al. Immune consequences of exercise in hypoxia: A narrative review. *J Sport Health Sci* 2023 DOI: 10.1016/j.jshs.2023. 09.007

31. Sateia MJ. International classification of sleep disorders–third edition: Highlights and modifications. *Chest* 2014; 146: 1387–1394. DOI: 10.1378/chest.14-0970

32. Medicine AAOS. International classification of sleep disorders, 3rd ed: *American Academy of Sleep Medicine*. Darien, IL 2014.

33. Baillieul S, Revol B, Jullian-Desayes I, et al. Diagnosis and management of central sleep apnea syndrome. *Expert Rev Respir Med* 2019; 13: 545–557. DOI: 10.1080/17476348.2019.1604226

34. Benjafield AV, Ayas NT, Eastwood PR, et al. Estimation of the global prevalence and burden of obstructive sleep apnoea: A literature-based analysis. *Lancet Respir Med* 2019; 7: 687–698. DOI: 10.1016/S2213-2600(19)30198-5

35. Levy P, Kohler M, McNicholas WT, et al. Obstructive sleep apnoea syndrome. *Nat Rev Dis Primers* 2015; 1: 15015. 20150625. DOI: 10.1038/nrdp.2015.15

36. Stepnowsky C, Sarmiento KF, Bujanover S, et al. Comorbidities, health-related quality of life, and work productivity among people with obstructive sleep apnea with excessive sleepiness: Findings from the 2016 US National Health and Wellness Survey. *J Clin Sleep Med* 2019; 15: 235–243. DOI: 10.5664/jcsm.7624

37. Ryan S, Cummins EP, Farre R, et al. Understanding the pathophysiological mechanisms of cardiometabolic complications in obstructive sleep apnoea: Towards personalised treatment approaches. *Eur Respir J* 2020 DOI: 10.1183/13993003.02295-2019

38. Javaheri S, Barbe F, Campos-Rodriguez F, et al. Sleep apnea: Types, mechanisms, and clinical cardiovascular consequences. *J Am Coll Cardiol* 2017; 69: 841–858. DOI: 10.1016/j.jacc.2016.11.069

39. Sanchez-de-la-Torre M, Campos-Rodriguez F and Barbe F. Obstructive sleep apnoea and cardiovascular disease. *Lancet Respir Med* 2013; 1: 61–72. DOI: 10.1016/S2213-2600(12)70051-6

40. Drager LF, McEvoy RD, Barbe F, et al. Sleep apnea and cardiovascular disease: Lessons from recent trials and need for team science. *Circulation* 2017; 136: 1840–1850. DOI: 10.1161/CIRCULATIONAHA.117.029400

41. McNicholas WT. Obstructive sleep apnoea and comorbidity - an overview of the association and impact of continuous positive airway pressure therapy. *Expert Rev Respir Med* 2019; 13: 251–261. DOI: 10.1080/17476348.2019.1575204

42. Huang T, Goodman M, Li X, et al. C-reactive protein and risk of OSA in four US cohorts. *Chest* 2021; 159: 2439–2448. DOI: 10.1016/j.chest.2021.01.060

43. Arnaud C, Bochaton T, Pepin JL and Belaidi E. Obstructive sleep apnoea and cardiovascular consequences: Pathophysiological mechanisms. *Arch Cardiovasc Dis* 2020. DOI: 10.1016/j.acvd.2020.01.003

44. Lavie L and Lavie P. Molecular mechanisms of cardiovascular disease in OSAHS: The oxidative stress link. *Eur Respir J* 2009; 33: 1467–1484. DOI: 10.1183/09031936.00086608

45. Lavie L. Oxidative stress in obstructive sleep apnea and intermittent hypoxia—revisited—the bad ugly and good: Implications to the heart and brain. *Sleep Med Rev* 2015; 20: 27–45. DOI: 10.1016/j.smrv.2014.07.003

46. Meliante PG, Zoccali F, Cascone F, et al. Molecular pathology, oxidative stress, and biomarkers in obstructive sleep apnea. *Int J Mol Sci* 2023; 24. DOI: 10.3390/ijms24065478

47. Foster GE, Brugniaux JV, Pialoux V, et al. Cardiovascular and cerebrovascular responses to acute hypoxia following exposure to intermittent hypoxia in healthy humans. *J Physiol* 2009; 587: 3287–3299. DOI: 10.1113/jphysiol.2009.171553

48. Beaudin AE, Hanly PJ, Raneri JK, et al. Impact of intermittent hypoxia on human vascular responses during sleep. *Exp Neurol* 2022; 347: 113897. DOI: 10.1016/j.expneurol.2021.113897

49. O'Halloran KD. Chronic intermittent hypoxia creates the perfect storm with calamitous consequences for respiratory control. *Respir Physiol Neurobiol* 2016; 226: 63–67. DOI: 10.1016/j.resp.2015.10.013

50. Baguet JP, Hammer L, Levy P, et al. The severity of oxygen desaturation is predictive of carotid wall thickening and plaque occurrence. *Chest* 2005; 128: 3407–3412. DOI: 10.1378/chest.128.5.3407

51. Pepin JL, Tamisier R, Baguet JP and Levy P. Arterial health is related to obstructive sleep apnea severity and improves with CPAP treatment. *Sleep Med Rev* 2013; 17: 3–5. DOI: 10.1016/j.smrv.2012.11.002

52. Joyeux-Faure M, Tamisier R, Borel JC, et al. Contribution of obstructive sleep apnoea to arterial stiffness: a meta-analysis using individual patient data. *Thorax* 2018; 73: 1146–1151. DOI: 10.1136/thoraxjnl-2018-211513

53. Jullian-Desayes I, Joyeux-Faure M, Tamisier R, et al. Impact of obstructive sleep apnea treatment by continuous positive airway pressure on cardiometabolic biomarkers: a systematic review from sham CPAP randomized controlled trials. *Sleep Med Rev* 2015; 21: 23–38. DOI: 10.1016/j.smrv.2014.07.004

54. Recoquillon S, Pepin JL, Vielle B, et al. Effect of mandibular advancement therapy on inflammatory and metabolic biomarkers in patients with severe obstructive sleep apnoea: a randomised controlled trial. *Thorax* 2019; 74: 496–499. DOI: 10.1136/thoraxjnl-2018-212609

55. Chouchou F, Pichot V, Pepin JL, et al. Sympathetic overactivity due to sleep fragmentation is associated with elevated diurnal systolic blood pressure in healthy elderly subjects: The PROOF-SYNAPSE study. *Eur Heart J* 2013; 34: 2122–2131. DOI: 10.1093/eurheartj/eht208

56. Wu D, Zhao Z, Chen C, et al. Impact of obstructive sleep apnea on cancer risk: A systematic review and meta-analysis. *Sleep Breath* 2023; 27: 843–852. DOI: 10.1007/s11325-022-02695-y

57. Almendros I and Gozal D. Intermittent hypoxia and cancer: Undesirable bed partners? *Respir Physiol Neurobiol* 2018; 256: 79–86. DOI: 10.1016/j.resp.2017.08.008

58. Nieto FJ, Peppard PE, Young T, et al. Sleep-disordered breathing and cancer mortality: Results from the Wisconsin Sleep Cohort Study. *Am J Respir Crit Care Med* 2012; 186: 190–194. DOI: 10.1164/rccm.201201-0130OC

59. Gomez-Olivas JD, Campos-Rodriguez F, Nagore E, et al. Role of sleep apnea and long-term CPAP treatment in the prognosis of patients with melanoma: A prospective multicenter study of 443 patients. *Chest* 2023. DOI: 10.1016/j.chest.2023.06.012

60. Minoves M, Kotzki S, Hazane-Puch F, et al. Chronic intermittent hypoxia, a hallmark of obstructive sleep apnea, promotes 4T1 breast cancer development through endothelin-1 receptors. *Sci Rep* 2022; 12: 12916. DOI: 10.1038/s41598-022-15541-8

61. Almendros I, Wang Y, Becker L, et al. Intermittent hypoxia-induced changes in tumor-associated macrophages and tumor malignancy in a mouse model of sleep apnea. *Am J Respir Crit Care Med* 2014; 189: 593–601. DOI: 10.1164/rccm.201310-1830OC

62. Almendros I, Montserrat JM, Torres M, et al. Intermittent hypoxia increases melanoma metastasis to the lung in a mouse model of sleep apnea. *Respir Physiol Neurobiol* 2013; 186: 303–307. DOI: 10.1016/j.resp.2013.03.001

63. Gozal D, Almendros I, Phipps AI, et al. Sleep apnoea adverse effects on cancer: True, false, or too many confounders? *Int J Mol Sci* 2020; DOI: 10.3390/ijms21228779

64. Matsumoto S, Yasui H, Mitchell JB and Krishna MC. Imaging cycling tumor hypoxia. *Cancer Res* 2010; 70: 10019–10023. DOI: 10.1158/0008-5472.CAN-10-2821

65. Rankin EB and Giaccia AJ. Hypoxic control of metastasis. *Science* 2016; 352: 175–180. DOI: 10.1126/science.aaf4405

66. Xiang M, Lu Y, Xin L, et al. Role of oxidative stress in reperfusion following myocardial ischemia and its treatments. *Oxid Med Cell Longev* 2021; 2021: 6614009. DOI: 10.1155/2021/6614009

67. Pena E, El Alam S, Siques P and Brito J. Oxidative stress and diseases associated with high-altitude exposure. *Antioxidants (Basel)* 2022; 11: 267. DOI: 10.3390/antiox11020267

68. Araneda OF, Garcia C, Lagos N, et al. Lung oxidative stress as related to exercise and altitude. Lipid peroxidation evidence in exhaled breath condensate: A possible predictor of acute mountain sickness. *Eur J Appl Physiol* 2005; 95: 383–390. DOI: 10.1007/s00421-005-0047-y

69. Berger MM, Macholz F, Mairbaurl H and Bartsch P. Remote ischemic preconditioning for prevention of high-altitude diseases: fact or fiction? *J Appl Physiol (1985)* 2015; 119: 1143–1151. DOI: 10.1152/japplphysiol.00156.2015

70. Millet GP, Faiss R and Pialoux V. Evidence for differences between hypobaric and normobaric hypoxia is conclusive. *Exerc Sport Sci Rev* 2013; 41: 133. DOI: 10.1097/JES.0b013e318271a5e1

71. Faiss R, Pialoux V, Sartori C, et al. Ventilation, oxidative stress, and nitric oxide in hypobaric versus normobaric hypoxia. *Med Sci Sports Exerc* 2013; 45: 253–260. DOI: 10.1249/MSS.0b013e31826d5aa2

72. Ribon A, Pialoux V, Saugy JJ, et al. Exposure to hypobaric hypoxia results in higher oxidative stress compared to normobaric hypoxia. *Respir Physiol Neurobiol* 2016; 223: 23–27. DOI: 10.1016/j.resp.2015.12.008

73. Ristow M and Schmeisser K. Mitohormesis: Promoting health and lifespan by increased levels of reactive oxygen species (ROS). *Dose Response* 2014; 12: 288–341. DOI: 10.2203/dose-response.13-035.Ristow

74. Goto S and Radak Z. Hormetic effects of reactive oxygen species by exercise: A view from animal studies for successful aging in human. *Dose Response* 2009; 8: 68–72. DOI: 10.2203/dose-response.09-044.Goto

SECTION 10

21

COMBINATION WITH TEMPERATURE CHANGES

Chris Esh, Sarah Carter, Bryna Chrismas and Lee Taylor

21.1 Introduction

Acute and chronic responses to hypoxic stimuli are well-defined in males, with applications in clinical [1] and athletic performance [2] settings across a range of exercise and health outcomes (as outlined within prior chapters). However, limited data exists for females and people with a disability/para-athlete populations [3, 4]. Understanding of combined hypoxic stimuli with other environmental extremes (e.g., heat [5, 6] and cold [7, 8]) is less well defined. Given the limited literature exploring the effects of hypoxia, heat, and cold on exercise or health is predominantly male-dominated, and extrapolating such data to female and/or people with a disability/para-athlete populations is challenging due to known physiological, psychological, and perceptual differences in these populations. Where available from the current literature, these differences are discussed within the chapter. However, further high-quality research is needed to determine female and people with a disability/para-athlete responses to hypoxia, heat, and cold. This research is essential to establish robust sex and disability-specific mechanisms and to create individualized best practice guidelines for health, safety, and performance within these populations [9].

Intriguing data demonstrates that acclimation or acclimatization to heat or cold can alter, often favorably, subsequent physiological and cellular responses to hypoxia and vice versa (reviewed here [9]; typically referred to as cross-tolerance). Limited data, particularly from a whole-body human perspective, exist on the specific combined effects of heat or cold stimuli with hypoxia [10, 11]. This is surprising given the variety of occupational (mine workers at ≥ 3,000 m [12]) and leisure (mountain climbing/ultramarathons [13]) pursuits

DOI: 10.4324/9781003402879-32

where individuals encounter a combination of stressors. Within such pursuits, individuals may experience myriad combinations of heat and cold exposure along with varying levels of hypoxia. From an extreme athletic perspective, during the Ultra Trail du Mont Blanc, competitors experience 10,000 m of total elevation gain (up to a peak altitude of ~2,500 m) in combination with temperatures ranging from below 0°C to 30°C [13, 14]. In the real world, it is rare that a stressor (i.e., heat, cold, hypoxia) is experienced in isolation [10, 11]. High altitude (i.e., hypoxic environment) mountain ranges are synonymous with cold temperatures while some mountainous regions in Southeast Asia experience a hot and humid climate [15]. Despite the intrigue surrounding cross-tolerance [9, 16, 17], the specific purpose of this chapter is to examine the combined effects of hypoxia and hot/cold stress on acclimation status or adaptations, exercise performance, and health.

The impact of hot/cold (e.g., air and water) alone on health, physiology, and exercise responses are well-characterized [10, 18–23]. The first section of this chapter will briefly describe these responses to temperature. However, the reader is directed to the following resources for in-depth descriptions, analysis, and review of the physiological and exercise responses to cold [10, 18–20] and heat [18, 21–23]. The subsequent focus will be on the combined effects of hypoxia and temperature. First, this includes a description on how to determine or quantify the effects of combined (hypoxia and temperature) versus individual (hypoxia/temperature alone) stressors on exercise and health. Second, the current knowledge surrounding the combined impact of hypoxia-and-cold and hypoxia-and-heat on exercise and health will be reviewed. Finally, a discussion of the future research required in this space will be provided.

21.2 Passive exposure to individual stressors

For hypoxia specific implications on physiology, health, and performance, the reader is referred to previous chapters where these have been extensively outlined. Thus, this section will focus solely on exposure to hot and cold stressors (see Figure 21.1 for an overview).

21.2.1 Temperature

Both increases or decreases in body temperature (discrete and/or repeated) can have either beneficial [24–27] or detrimental [27, 28] impacts on health. The impacts can be transient, enduring, and inconsistent within and between individuals, depending on the degree of stimulus, application, and morphology [29, 30]. Human core temperature (Tc) homeostasis is maintained at ~37°C [31], with a typical oscillation of ~1°C across 24 h [31]. Maintaining homeostasis between heat gain/loss (i.e., thermal balance) is imperative for

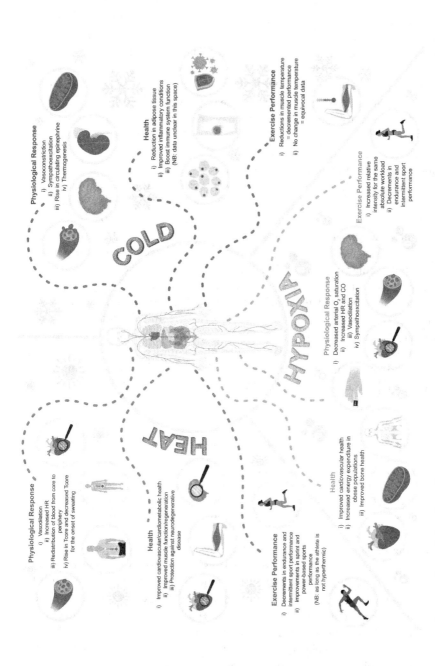

FIGURE 21.1   An overview of the physiological responses to environmental stress and the impact on health and exercise performance.

optimal health, performance (bodily functions and exercise), and survival [32]. Exposure to cold or hot temperatures challenges Tc homeostasis, with human Tc survival limits said to be between 27°C and 42°C [27, 33, 34]. However, even a relatively small change in Tc (~±2.5°C) can, in certain circumstances, have severe detrimental effects (i.e., sustained hypo- and hyperthermia can lead to death) [27, 28].

In contrast, acute, well-controlled (i.e., defined temperature and duration of exposure) and intentional (i.e., research and/or health-based interventions) exposure to cold and hot can have positive health impacts [27, 35]. For example, repeated cold water immersion [(CWI) from ice water as low as −2°C to cold water up to 20°C] has demonstrated benefits in reducing and/or transforming adipose tissue and thus, may be protective against various global health concerns associated with excess body fat and obesity (e.g., diabetes and cardiovascular disease) [26]. While there is a hypothesis that CWI may positively impact inflammatory conditions and boost immune system function, the data are equivocal in this space [27]. In terms of heat, sauna bathing [24] or passive heat therapy [35] have shown improvements in cardiovascular/cardiometabolic health [24, 25], muscle function, regeneration from injury, and/or age-related detriments [36, 37] and may protect against certain neurodegenerative diseases [38]. Essentially, well-controlled exposure to cold/hot, when informed by evidence and aligned with a specific rationale, can be safe and beneficial to health. However, when sustained exposure to cold/hot temperatures are unintentional or unavoidable (e.g., prolonged cold/hot weather) population-specific detrimental impacts on health can occur, often with notable variation within and between participants.

21.3 Exercise responses to individual stressors

21.3.1 Cold

Acute cold exposure induces various physiological responses depending on the severity of the exposure. These include cutaneous vasoconstriction, sympathoexcitation (i.e., activation of the sympathetic nervous system), and a rise in circulating epinephrine [39, 40]. The physiological response to cold is influenced by individual characteristics (e.g., sex, age, body composition) [39]. Exposure to extreme cold such as CWI can induce "cold shock," which is associated with gasping and hyperventilation [41]. Sustained exposure to cold initiates thermogenesis (e.g., increases metabolic processes and shivering) to increase heat production and prevent/reduce decreases in Tc [39]. Repeated exposure to cold elicits cold acclimation adaptations (~6 exposures are required to observe acclimation adaptations [39, 42, 43]) that invoke three distinct physiological adjustments: habitual, metabolic, and insulative (for a full review, see [39]).

Exercise capacity in the cold requires further investigation, and it is currently debated whether cold decreases exercise capacity [20]. Where cold produces decreases in muscle temperature, there are decrements in maximal oxygen uptake ($\dot{V}O_2$max), exercise duration and power, and/or sprint capabilities [10], with a 4% to 6% decrease in these performance parameters per 1°C decrease in muscle temperature [44–46]. In cold temperatures that do not influence muscle temperature, there is no consensus on the impact it may have on aerobic performance, primarily due to a lack of a standardized approach (i.e., temperature, test used to assess performance, etc.) for assessing exercise performance in the cold [20]. Studies have observed decreases [47–50], improvements [51, 52], and no change [53, 54] in aerobic exercise performance.

21.3.2 Heat

Unlike cold, exercise in the heat has been extensively studied in males (with females being underrepresented in exercise thermoregulation research [55]). Exercise in the heat exacerbates physiological and perceptual strain [56–58], which can have detrimental impacts on physical endurance-type performance [56, 59, 60]. Conversely, sprint and power-based physical performance can be improved in the heat if the athlete is not hyperthermic [61]. In response to heat stress at rest, increased heart rate drives elevated cardiac output, as stroke volume does not change significantly in response to acute heat stress [35, 62]. The body attempts to dissipate heat from the core to the periphery (i.e., core to skin and subsequently the environment) and results in a significant increase in skin blood flow [29, 63]. Sustained exposure to heat will inevitably lead to a rise in Tc that is generally synonymous with the onset of sweating [63]. Similar to repeated cold exposure, repeated exposure to heat induces physiological acclimation adaptations, including but not limited to a decrease in resting and exercising heart rate and Tc (for a given task), an increase in plasma volume, and enhanced sweat rates [64, 65]. Adaptations to heat tend to occur more rapidly in males; however, no sex differences are seen at ~10 days of heat exposure [66].

21.4 Determining the magnitude of effect: Combined versus individual stressors

When investigating the effect of an individual stressor compared to a control condition, it is relatively simple to determine what effect the experimentally

TABLE 21.1 The definition of terms that describe and the calculation of the magnitude of the effect when comparing combined stressors to individual stressors

Term	Definition	Calculation
Additive	The effect of the combined stressor is equal to the sum of the effect of the individual stressors.	Hypoxia & heat/cold combined = hypoxia + heat/cold individually
Synergistic	The effect of the combined stressor is greater than the sum of the effect of the individual stressors.	Hypoxia & heat/cold combined > hypoxia + heat/cold individually
Antagonistic	The effect of the combined stressor is less than the sum of the effect of the individual stressors.	Hypoxia & heat/cold combined < hypoxia + heat/cold individually
Nullifying	The effect of the combined stressor is equal to the effect of one individual stressor.	Hypoxia & heat/cold combined = hypoxia or heat/cold individually
Multiplicative	The effect of the combined stressor is equal to the multiplication of the effect of the individual stressors.	Hypoxia & heat/cold combined = hypoxia × heat/cold individually

manipulated interventional stressor has had, enabling identification and quantification of the responsible biological processes. For example, in response to hypoxia/heat/cold, exercise performance may be positively (i.e., improved), negatively (i.e., decremented), or not impacted at all. Investigators then determine if a change in performance is statistically significant, whether the magnitude of change has meaningful real-world applications and consider the integrated biological processes responsible.

Investigating combined stressors is evidently more complex. Such interactions are placed into five categories: (1) additive; (2) synergistic; (3) antagonistic; (4) nullifying; and (5) multiplicative (see Table 21.1 for an overview of these terms [67]). These definitions will be used throughout the remainder of the chapter to classify the effects of combined hypoxia and temperature stress on exercise responses.

21.5 Combined hypoxia and temperature: passive responses

21.5.1 Cold

Limited data exist on the combined effects of hypoxia and cold (Figure 21.2 provides an overview of this data), mainly focused on cutaneous blood flow and thermoregulatory responses [15]. Exposure to hypoxia and cold in isolation induce sympathoexcitation, but conflicting cardiovascular responses

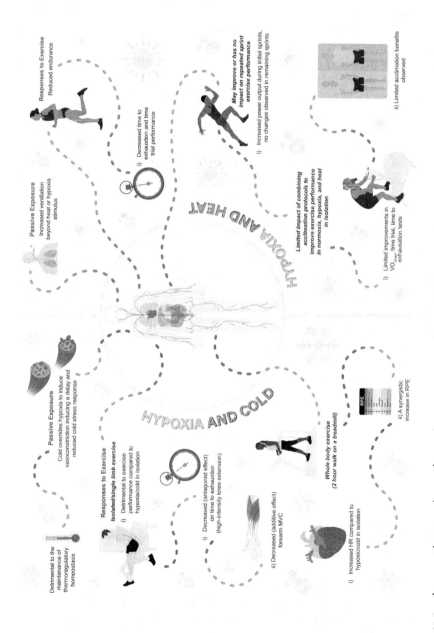

FIGURE 21.2 An overview passive and exercise responses to the combination of hypoxia and temperature stress.

(e.g., hypoxia = vasodilation, cold = vasoconstriction in most vascular beds) are observed [15]. An early study investigating the acute impact of hypoxia/cold on thermoregulatory responses observed a quicker decline and plateauing of Tc during a 2-hour exposure at 15.5°C at 5,000 m compared to 2,500 m and sea level, with end Tc similar between the two hypoxic conditions [68]. The authors suggested that this was due to an increase in distribution of blood from the core to the periphery [68]. In support, hypoxic cutaneous vasodilation was maintained during acute cooling (using a whole-body water-perfused suit cooled from 34°C to 14°C across 10 min) at simulated altitude (F_iO_2: 0.11, ~4,900 m) [69]. Contrastingly, during a longer duration and more severe cold stress (cooling from 36°C to 23°C over 30 min, followed by 45 min cold exposure at 10°C) in the presence of hypoxia (F_iO_2 was manipulated to induce a reduction in arterial oxygen saturation to 80%), cutaneous vasoconstriction was augmented compared to cold alone [70]. Eucapnic hypoxia (12% O_2 in N_2) has been observed to delay the onset of vasoconstriction during mild cold stress (passive cooling after 25 min cycling at 50% maximum workload in 28°C water until Tc dropped below 35.5°C or vigorous shivering), likely because hypoxia lowers the Tc threshold for vasoconstriction by ~0.14°C [71]. Due to varying study methodologies, determining the combined magnitude of effects of hypoxia/cold on these physiological/thermoregulatory responses is challenging. While human responses to hypoxic/cold are variable, current evidence suggests that during prolonged exposure, the cold stress response tends to override the hypoxic stress response [68, 70, 71]. However, due to conflicting cardiovascular responses, the timeline of the cold response is delayed and its magnitude is reduced, which results in a greater disruption to homeostasis [15].

21.5.2 Hot

Research on physiological responses to combined hypoxia and heat are also sparse [15] (Figure 21.2 provides an overview of this data). In combined hypoxia/hot, ventilatory responses were increased compared to normothermic hypoxia [72, 73]. Specifically, there was an increase in ventilation of 7.2 L·min^{-1} (Tc: ~38.2°C, 12% O_2 in N_2) compared to 4.1 L·min^{-1} in normothermic hypoxia (Tc: ~36.7°C, 12% O_2 in N_2) [72]. This aligns with previous data showing an increase in ventilation and mean inspiratory flow (specific data not provided) following a Tc increase of ~1.4°C (hypoxic exposure variable from moderate to severe), though there was considerable individual variability in respiratory sensitivity to hypoxia [73]. Without investigating heat, hypoxia, and thermoneutral-normoxia, the magnitude of the effect of the combined stressors cannot be determined [72, 73]. However, increases in ventilation suggest that a combination of stressors likely induces greater physiological stress than one stressor alone [15].

21.6 Combined hypoxia and temperature: Exercise responses

21.6.1 Cold

Combined hypoxia/cold has the propensity to compromise exercise capacity by reducing muscle blood flow (i.e., oxygen transport) and arterial oxygen content (or hypoxemia) [74–76] (Figure 21.2 provides an overview of this data). However, studies investigating the impact of combined hypoxia and cold stress on exercise responses are limited [8, 77, 78]. A recent American College of Sports Medicine (ACSM) consensus statement [10] and other commentaries [7, 11, 17] highlight the paucity of knowledge in this space. The majority of literature has focused on the crosstalk [79] and cross-adaptation [9, 80] between hypoxia and cold (and vice versa) at rest despite the frequency with which these stressors are experienced simultaneously in real-world athletic and occupational pursuits [7, 11, 17].

21.6.1.1 Isolated/single limb exercise responses

Current research on combined hypoxia and cold stress has demonstrated an undesirable impact on exercise capacity and performance, specifically observed in male participants [8, 77] (see Table 21.2). A reduction in high-intensity dynamic knee extension time to exhaustion is observed when cold and hypoxic stress are combined compared to each stressor in isolation [77]. After 40 min of rest in the respective conditions [thermoneutral normoxic (25°C), thermoneutral hypoxia (F_iO_2 0.125, equivalent to ~4100 m), cold (5°C) and hypoxic-cold], time to exhaustion, assessed via dynamic knee extension (~50 W at 60 extensions per min) until exhaustion, was reduced by 505 s in hypoxia and 190 s in cold compared to thermoneutral normoxia [77]. However, when hypoxia and cold were combined, time to exhaustion was further reduced by 589 s [77], demonstrating a clear antagonistic effect (~106 s). Similarly, forearm muscle maximal isometric voluntary contraction (MVC) force is reduced when hypoxia and cold are combined compared to each stressor individually [8]. Following 70 min of rest in the respective conditions [normoxic-thermoneutral (23°C), hypoxic-thermoneutral (F_iO_2 = 0.13, ~4,000 m), normoxic-cold (5°C), and hypoxic-cold], participants completed 8 × 5 min exercise bouts (dynamic grip clenches every 2 s at 15% MVC) with 110 s rest between bouts. MVC force, assessed at the end of every second 5 min bout, decreased in hypoxic-thermoneutral (–8.1%) and normoxic-cold (–13.9%) alone and had a small additive effect (~0.6%; although likely ~synergistic when considering measurement error) in hypoxic-cold (–21.4%) compared to thermoneutral normoxia [8].

TABLE 21.2 Effects of combined hypoxia and temperature vs hypoxia and temperature alone

Study	Exercise protocol (number of participants)	Impact of stressor on exercise performance parameters compared to thermoneutral-normoxic conditions					Magnitude of combined effect
		H	T	Sum of H + T	H & T combined	Difference (H + T) – H & T combined	
Hypoxia & Cold							
Lloyd et al. (2015) [8]	Intermittent dynamic forearm exercise at 15% MVC (n = 8)	–8.1%	–13.9%	–22%	–21.4%	–0.6%	Additive/ synergistic
Lloyd et al. (2016) [7]	High intensity dynamic knee extension TTE (n = 9)	–505 s	–190 s	–695 s	–589 s	–106 s	Antagonistic
Robinson and Haymes (1990) [78]	RPE during 30 min cycling at 50% HR reserve (n = 7)	+3	–1	+2	+3	+1	Synergistic
Hypoxia & Heat							
Girard and Racinais (2014) [5]	TTE: cycling at 66% PO at V̇O₂max (n = 11)	–36%	–35%	–71%	–51%	–20%	Antagonistic
Lee et al. (2014) [87]	90 min cycling at 50% normoxic V̇O₂max–TTE (n = 12)	–8 min	–11 min	–19 min	–16 min	–3 min	Antagonistic

Study	Protocol						Outcome
Bradbury et al. (2019) [86]	TT (work done kJ) (n = 12, 10 male, 2 female)	-24.1 kJ	-15.4 kJ	-39.5 kJ	-33.1 kJ	-6.4	Antagonistic
Levine and Buono (2019) [88]	2 hr treadmill walking (n = 10, 5 male, 5 female)	HR: +3 RPE: 0	HR: +25 RPE: +1.9	HR: +28 RPE: +1.9	HR: +32 RPE: +3.3	HR: +4 RPE: +1.4	Synergistic Synergistic
Yamaguchi et al. (2020) [6]	Cycling: 3 sets 3 × 10 s max sprints, 40 s rest (n = 10)	aPPO: 0	aPPO: +3%	aPPO: +3%	aPPO: +2.3%	aPPO:-0.7%	Antagonistic
Yamaguchi et al. (2021) [89]	Cycling: 3 sets 5 × 6 s max sprints, 30 s rest (n = 11)	PO: 0	PO: 0	PO: 0	PO: 0	PO: 0	Nullifying

[a] differences only observed during the first two sprints, all other sprints saw no differences. **NB:** all participants are male unless stated otherwise. Abbreviations: H (hypoxia), T (temperature), MVC (maximal voluntary contraction), TTE (time to exhaustion), RPE (rate of perceived exertion), HR (heart rate), PO (power output), TT (time trial), PPO (peak power output).

21.6.2 Whole body exercise response

Limited evidence, primarily from male participants [78], is available regarding the whole-body exercise response to combined hypoxia and cold compared to either condition alone. Compared to thermoneutral-normoxia, normoxia-cold, and thermoneutral-hypoxia heart rate (specific data unavailable to determine magnitude of this effect) and perceived exertion (a synergistic effect, see Table 21.2) were increased [78] during a 30 min cycle ergometer protocol at 50% heart rate reserve (8°C and breathing 12% O_2 in N_2, ~4,000–4,500 m) [78].

When hypoxia and cold are combined, exercise capacity/performance appears to be impaired (see Table 21.2), although evidence is limited [8, 77, 78]. The effects range from approximately additive (e.g., –21.4% reduction in MVC in hypoxic/cold versus the sum of hypoxia and cold alone = –22% [8]) to modestly synergistic [e.g., +3 units rate of perceived exertion (RPE) in hypoxic/cold versus the sum of hypoxia and cold alone = +2 [78]]. Considerably more research is required to fully elucidate the combined effects of these stressors, with a particular focus on differences between the sexes, both acutely and chronically, and considering within and between participant variation. Attention to measurement error is crucial, especially when nuanced biological interactions are being considered, across a variety of sport/exercise/health domains.

21.6.3 Possible causes of impaired exercise performance in combined hypoxia and cold

Comparing the physiological responses to exercise (e.g., treadmill walking and isolated/single limb) in hypoxia [81] and cold [20, 44, 82] separately to the combined hypoxia/cold studies [8, 77, 78] may provide insights into why exercise performance/capacity is further impaired in hypoxic/cold compared to either hypoxia or cold alone. In cold alone, Tc reductions from 0.5°C to 2°C lead to a decrease in maximal heart (–10 to –30 b·min^{-1}), conspiring to reduce $\dot{V}O_2$max [82]. Submaximal exercise heart rate is lower at any given power output or %$\dot{V}O_2$max, declining linearly with decreases in Tc [20, 44]. Cardiac output between cold and temperate environments during exercise tends to remain unchanged due to increases in stroke volume in the cold [20, 82]. Conversely, during submaximal exercise in hypoxia, cardiac output is higher than in normoxic exercise, achieved through an increased heart rate, resulting in a similar $\dot{V}O_2$ at the same intensity as in normoxia [81]. In summary, exercise in the cold can reduce $\dot{V}O_2$max [82], while hypoxia results in an increased heart rate to achieve the same $\dot{V}O_2$ relative to normoxia [81]. However, the responses are dependent on specific design or environmental factors (e.g., muscle temperature maintenance/decrease and hypoxic dose).

During forearm MVC, heart rate was significantly lower in cold (by up to 15 beats per min ($b \cdot min^{-1}$)) compared to all other conditions (see Table 21.1 in [8]), as expected based on current literature [10, 20]. Interestingly, heart rate was lower throughout the MVC protocol in hypoxic/cold (mean: 80.3 $b \cdot min^{-1}$) compared to hypoxia alone (mean: 86.9 $b \cdot min^{-1}$), with significance ($p < 0.05$) observed at only one time point (MVC 3, hypoxic/cold: 81.3 $b \cdot min^{-1}$; hypoxia alone: 90.4 $b \cdot min^{-1}$) [8]. Similarly, during the high-intensity dynamic knee extension protocol [dynamic knee extension (~50 W at 60 extensions per min) until exhaustion], heart rate at exhaustion was significantly lower ($p < 0.05$) during hypoxic/cold (116.4 $b \cdot min^{-1}$, 326 s) compared to cold alone (124.2 $b \cdot min^{-1}$, 725 s), hypoxic neutral (141 $b \cdot min^{-1}$, 410 s), and neutral (132.6 $b \cdot min^{-1}$, 915 s) [77]. This suggests that the stress of cold may override or nullify the stress of hypoxia when the two stressors are combined, and that humans respond to multiple simultaneous stressors on a "worst-strain-take-precedence" model based on current evidence [77].

Finally, the hypoxic conditions used in the described studies [8, 77] could be described as extreme (F_iO_2 of 0.125–0.13, ~4,000 m). It is unlikely that common sporting competitions will take place at such altitudes (e.g., the highest altitude for the winter Olympics has been ~2,800 m for the men's downhill at Salt Lake City in 2002 [83]). Without evidence in athletes who compete in combined hypoxic/cold conditions, it is difficult to ascertain the generalizability of the findings from the current studies. However, the data does present opportunities for hypotheses and debate surrounding how exercise in combined hypoxia/cold could enhance and/or detriment exercise capacity and be of benefit and/or detriment to health, some of which will be discussed later in this chapter.

21.6.4 Chronic exposure to combined hypoxia and cold

Despite the prevalence of hypoxic-cold environments in the natural world, there is limited evidence on chronic exposure to these conditions, the potential adaptations, and their impact on exercise capacity/performance [10, 20]. Existing studies are predominantly conducted on male samples, even within the cross-adaptation/tolerance space where data are also limited [9]. Studies have investigated the impact of hypoxia and cold on basal metabolism [84] and oral temperature [85]. Native highlanders' basal metabolism was higher than that of native lowlanders across a 5-week exposure to a mix of hypoxia/cold (~3,300 m, 6°C to 11°C) or hypoxia/thermoneutral (~3,300 m, 25°C to 28°C, $n = 10$ lowlanders, 3 weeks hypoxia/cold then 2 weeks hypoxia/thermoneutral, $n = 10$ lowlanders vice versa) [84]. In a similar study design, oral temperature fell continuously in native lowlanders (and native highlanders) across a 6-week exposure to cold/hypoxia (~36.8°C to ~36.4°C) [85]. Without other physiological/hematological data, it is difficult to determine whether exposure to chronic combined hypoxia and cold is detrimental to achieve full acclimation to one or both stressors, or whether adaptation/acclimation to both hypoxia and cold can be achieved simultaneously. Such data would be important to athletes who are frequently exposed to hypoxic/cold environments (e.g., cross country skiers). Understanding whether "live-high train-high" or "live-high train-low" (LHTL) interventions are optimal, or perhaps confounded by conflict between hypoxia/cold adaptations, for inducing desired adaptations and subsequent improvements in exercise performance as well as any sex differences would be interesting.

21.6.5 Heat

The literature in this space covers two distinct research questions (Figure 21.2 provides an overview of this data):

1. How the combination of hypoxia/heat impacts exercise performance/capacity
2. Whether training in the combination of heat/hypoxia (i.e., an acclimation intervention) can induce greater adaptations than either hypoxia or heat alone and improve subsequent exercise performance/capacity in normoxia, hypoxia, and/or heat.

21.6.6 Endurance exercise responses

Endurance-type exercise is negatively impacted by combined hypoxia/heat at moderate to high intensity [5, 86] (see Table 21.2). Cycling at 66% power output at $\dot{V}O_2$max, time to exhaustion was reduced by 36% (hypoxia, F_iO_2 = 0.15, ~2,500 m), 35% (heat, 35°C), and 51% (hypoxia/heat) compared to temperate normoxia (22°C), inducing an antagonistic effect (~20%) [5]. In a 90-min cycling session at 50% normoxic $\dot{V}O_2$max, only two participants completed the whole exercise in temperate normoxia (18°C), hypoxia (F_iO_2 = 0.14, ~3,000 m), heat (40°C), and hypoxia/heat [87], with time to exhaustion of 89 min (temperate normoxia), 81 min (hypoxia), 78 min (heat), and 73 min (hypoxia/heat), also showing an antagonistic effect (~3 min) [87]. Time trial performance (total work done, kJ) was decreased compared to temperate-normoxia (20°C) by 15.4 kJ (heat, 35°C), 24.1 kJ (hypoxia, F_iO_2 = 0.14, ~3,000 m), and 33.1 kJ (hypoxia/heat), demonstrating another antagonistic effect (~6.4 kJ) [86]. During low intensity exercise (2 hr walking on a treadmill) heart rate increased by 32 b·min⁻¹ (synergistic effect, 4 b·min⁻¹) in hypoxia/heat compared to temperate normoxia (23°C), with increases of 25 b·min⁻¹ (heat, 38°C) and 3 b·min⁻¹ (hypoxia, F_iO_2 = 0.15, ~2,500 m) [88]. Rate of perceived exertion (RPE) was increased synergistically (~1.4 units) in hypoxic/heat by 3.3 units compared to 1.9 (heat) and no change in hypoxia [88].

The concomitant increases in physiological (heart rate), perceptual (RPE, thermal sensation) and thermal (Tc) stress impair oxygen delivery to the working muscles and exacerbate cardiovascular strain are cited as the inter-related mechanisms of impaired (antagonistic and synergistic effects seen) exercise performance in combined hypoxia/heat [5, 86–88]. Whether these multiple stressors combine equally to impair exercise performance, or if one element has significantly greater implications in hypoxia/heat, is unclear.

21.6.7 Repeated sprint exercise responses

Combined hypoxia/heat does not appear to impair repeated sprint exercise [6, 89] (see Table 21.2). Indeed, a positive antagonistic (0.7%) impact on repeated sprint exercise across 3 sets of 3×10 s max sprints with 40 s recovery compared to temperate-normoxia has been observed [6]. Average peak power output was improved by 2.3% across the first two sprints in hypoxia/heat compared to temperate normoxia (20°C) [6]. In heat alone (35°C), the improvement was 3%, and there were no differences in hypoxia (F_iO_2 = 0.14, ~3,000 m); no differences existed after the second sprint [6]. In another study by the same group, involving 5×6 s maximal sprints with 30 s recovery, there were no changes in peak or mean power output compared to normoxia (23°C) in hypoxia (23°C; F_iO_2 = 0.14, ~3,000 m) and heat/hypoxia (35°C; F_iO_2 = 0.14, ~3,000 m) [89].

Hypoxia alone is known to negatively impact repeated sprint performance [90], whereas heat has been shown to improve [91] and impair [92] repeated sprint performance, potentially depending on the severity of heat stress (and Tc, skin temperature, and muscle temperature observed) and modality of exercise (i.e., treadmill running versus cycle ergometer) [59]. Similar to endurance exercise, repeated sprint performance in hypoxia is impaired via decreased muscle oxygen delivery and increases in heart rate (alongside other potential mechanisms reviewed here [90]). In the heat, increases in muscle temperature may improve muscle fiber contraction velocity and anaerobic ATP turnover in fast-twitch fibers [59]. This may explain improved performance in the initial sprints during repeated sprint exercise in the heat and hypoxia/heat (positive antagonistic effect). Nevertheless, this potential benefit is abolished if the individual becomes hyperthermic (reviewed in-depth here [59]). Thus, speculatively, during hypoxia/heat, the benefits of heat on repeated sprint performance may override the negative impact of hypoxia (at least in early sprints of a set). When hypoxia and heat are combined, exercise capacity/performance can be improved (antagonistic effect in repeated sprint exercise) or decreased (antagonistic effect during endurance exercise) dependent on exercise modality, intensity, and the environmental conditions. Endurance exercise at moderate intensity also appears to be impaired, and the effect is antagonistic in nature [5, 86, 87]. Contrastingly, repeated sprint exercise performance may improve or is not negatively impacted by combined hypoxia/heat [6, 89]. Again, it should be noted that such conclusions are drawn from a limited evidence base.

21.6.8 Exercise responses to chronic hypoxic/heat exposure

As described in previous chapters, repeated/chronic exposure to and exercise in hypoxic environments (i.e., acclimation) are employed to induce beneficial physiological adaptations to exercise [2]. It is reported that acclimation to heat can improve exercise performance/responses in hypoxia, and vice versa (i.e., cross-adaptation/cross-tolerance) [9, 17]. Therefore, it is a plausible hypothesis that combining hypoxia and heat across an acclimation protocol could elicit a greater magnitude of physiological adaptation and subsequently benefit exercise performance. To date, there have been mixed results, albeit from a variety of different hypoxic/heat protocols [duration (days) of heat/hypoxic exposure, type of heat/hypoxic exposure (see Table 21.3 for an overview of methodologies used)] and assessments of success (exercise performance in normothermic/heat/hypoxia) [93–97].

21.6.9 Performance outcomes

Hypoxia/heat acclimation did not increase $\dot{V}O_2$max in thermoneutral normoxia (23°C, 47% RH), hypoxia or hot, although peak power output improved in thermoneutral normoxia [93]. Time to exhaustion (constant load at 80% of peak Watts at $\dot{V}O_2$max) was improved in hot (12.9% increase in time to exhaustion), but no changes were observed in normoxia or hypoxia (Study 1, Table 21.3) [93]. Heat acclimation only (Study 2, Table 21.3), compared to heat acclimation and overnight hypoxia and a control condition (no heat, no hypoxia), improved 3 km running time trial performance (3.3%) in temperate normoxia (two different outdoor locations: 13.5°C, 55.2% RH and 19.5°C, 53.3% RH) [96]. Cycling time trial performance (15 min total distance covered) improved by ~5.5% following LHTL, LHTL/heat acclimation, and heat acclimation alone compared to a control with no differences between environmental interventions (Study 4, Table 21.3) [97].

Study designs required participants to perform a high number of maximal (i.e., $\dot{V}O_2$max) and performance (i.e., time trial, time to exhaustion) tests either side of an intense training intervention. Often, post-intervention performance tests were performed within days of completing the training intervention, alongside the physiological stress of being exposed to two environmental stressors [93, 95–97]. Plausibly, the burden placed on participants, even those well-trained [95, 96], was too high and may have masked any potential performance effects of the training intervention. Intense post-intervention testing in similar studies has been suggested to impact an athlete's performance [96, 98].

TABLE 21.3 Overview of chronic hypoxia/heat study methodologies

Study	Duration	Hypoxia	Heat	Training stimulus
(1) Sotiridis et al. (2019) [93]	10 days (n = 8)	$F_iO_2 = 0.14$, ~3,000 m (22 hours per day)	37°C 39% RH	LHTL: 90 min daily at 50% normoxic W_{peak}
(2) Mccleave et al. (2017) [96]	21 days (n = 26, 17 M, 9 F)	$F_iO_2 = 0.14$, ~3,000 m (13 hours per day)	32.5°C 59% RH	LHTL: 9 × 90 min treadmill 6 × interval, 6 × moderate continuous run session
(3) Mccleave et al. (2019) [95]	21 days (n = 25, 16 M, 9 F)	$F_iO_2 = 0.14$, ~3,000 m (14 hours per day)	32.7°C 59% RH	LHTL: 9 × 90 min treadmill 6 × interval, 6 × moderate continuous run session
(4) Hanson et al. (2022) [97]	12 days (n = 21, 17 M, 4 F)	$F_iO_2 = 0.16$, ~2,500 m (12 hours per day)	30°C, 80% RH	LHTL: 60 min ~58% of normoxic $\dot{V}O_2$max PPO

NB: all training occurred during heat exposure and participants are male unless stated otherwise. Abbreviation: M (male), F (female), F_iO_2 (fraction of inspired oxygen), RH (relative humidity), LHTL (live-high train-low), W_{peak} (Watts at peak oxygen consumption), $\dot{V}O_2$max (maximal oxygen uptake), PPO (peak power output).

Additionally, studies tended to investigate performance in the heat alone and not across hypoxia, thermoneutral-normoxia, or combined hypoxia/heat. Thus, the results cannot be interpreted as additive, antagonistic, and so forth as previously done in this chapter.

21.6.10 Acclimation adaptations

Varied acclimation adaptations have been observed between studies and the different methodologies implemented. Study (1) from Table 21.3 saw the combined hypoxia/heat intervention induce significant increases in hemoglobin concentration at day 10 (162 g dL^{-1}) compared to baseline (149 g dL^{-1}), plasma volume (PV) significantly decreased (−15.1%), and resting Tc and heart rate remained unchanged [93]. In Study (2) from Table 21.3, PV increased by 3.8% during heat acclimation alone with no change in the hypoxic/heat intervention or control group [96]. Hemoglobin mass was increased by 3.8% during the hypoxic/heat exposure but not in heat acclimation alone or the control group [96]. During Study (3) from Table 21.3 there were no clear differences in physiological adaptions (Tc, HR, sweat rate) but PV which increased (~4%) in hot alone [95]. In Study (4), heat acclimation alone decreased hemoglobin concentration by 2.9% and increased PV by 3.8%, while there was a 4.1% decrease and 2% increase in hemoglobin concentration and PV respectively during the hypoxic/heat exposure [97]. The physiological/hematological adaptations to hypoxia and/or heat training observed (e.g., changes in PV, aemoglobin mass and concentration) are evidenced to be beneficial for exercise performance in the respective conditions (i.e., hypoxia or heat), although limited benefits during exercise performance are observed [93, 96, 97]. As seen with combined hypoxia/cold [8, 77], a "worst-strain-takes-precedence" principle appears to apply to combined chronic hypoxia/heat exposure. Accordingly, hypoxia driven acclimation adaptations were seen compared to heat acclimation when participants were exposed to hypoxia and heat in combination (e.g., decreased PV, increased hemoglobin concentration with limited reduction in Tc, heart rate, sweat rate) [93, 96, 97].

To summarize, the adaptations invoked by protocols outlined in Table 21.3 have not been observed to be ergogenic to exercise performance in hypoxia, heat, and thermoneutral normoxia alone. The current evidence suggests that there is little benefit in increasing the physiological burden on athletes by exposing them to combined hypoxia and heat to improve exercise performance within conditions where only one environmental stress is experienced. Albeit this evidence is limited to a small number of studies with low sample sizes and study designs that lack ecological validity (e.g., high density of training intervention and temporality of performance tests). Furthermore, it remains unexplored whether chronic exposure to hypoxia/heat improves exercise performance in hypoxic/hot conditions, and there is insufficient data to inform female specific responses to hypoxia/heat.

Abbreviations

CWI	cold water immersion
F_iO_2	fraction of inspired oxygen
HR	heart rate
LHTL	live-high train-low
MVC	maximal voluntary contraction
PV	plasma volume
RH	relative humidity
RPE	rate of perceived exertion
Tc	core temperature
$\dot{V}O_2max$	maximal oxygen uptake.

References

1. Pouyssegur, J. and J. López-Barneo, *Hypoxia in health and disease.* Molecular Aspects of Medicine, 2016. **47–48**: p. 1–2.
2. Girard, O., et al., *"Living high-training low" for Olympic medal performance: What have we learned 25 years after implementation?* The International Journal of Sports Physiology and Performance, 2023. **18**(6): p. 563–572.
3. West, J.B., *Physiological effects of chronic hypoxia.* New England Journal of Medicine, 2017. **376**(20): p. 1965–1971.
4. Michiels, C., *Physiological and pathological responses to hypoxia.* The American Journal of Pathology, 2004. **164**(6): p. 1875–1882.
5. Girard, O. and S. Racinais, *Combining heat stress and moderate hypoxia reduces cycling time to exhaustion without modifying neuromuscular fatigue characteristics.* European Journal of Applied Physiology, 2014. **114**: p. 1521–1532.
6. Yamaguchi, K., et al., *Acute performance and physiological responses to repeated-sprint exercise in a combined hot and hypoxic environment.* Physiological Reports, 2020. **8**(12): p. e14466.
7. Lloyd, A. and G. Havenith, *Interactions in human performance: An individual and combined stressors approach.* Temperature, 2016. **3**(4): p. 514–517.
8. Lloyd, A., S. Hodder, and G. Havenith, *The interactive effect of cooling and hypoxia on forearm fatigue development.* European Journal of Applied Physiology, 2015. **115**: p. 2007–2018.
9. Gibson, O.R., et al., *Cross-adaptation: Heat and cold adaptation to improve physiological and cellular responses to hypoxia.* Sports Medicine, 2017. **47**(9): p. 1751–1768.
10. Castellani, J.W., et al., *ACSM expert consensus statement: Injury prevention and exercise performance during cold-weather exercise.* Current Sports Medicine Reports, 2021. **20**(11): p. 594–607.
11. Tipton, M., *A case for combined environmental stressor studies.* Extreme Physiology & Medicine, 2012. **1**(1): p. 1–2.
12. Vinnikov, D. and V. Krasotski, *Healthy worker survival effect at a high-altitude mine: Prospective cohort observation.* Scientific Reports, 2022. **12**(1): p. 13903.
13. Hurdiel, R., et al., *Combined effects of sleep deprivation and strenuous exercise on cognitive performances during The North Face® Ultra Trail du Mont Blanc® (UTMB®).* Journal of Sports Sciences, 2015. **33**(7): p. 670–674.
14. Suter, D., et al., *Even pacing is associated with faster finishing times in ultramarathon distance trail running—the "ultra-trail du Mont Blanc" 2008–2019.* International Journal of Environmental Research and Public Health, 2020. **17**(19): p. 7074.
15. Wait, S.O., et al., *Combining hypoxia with thermal stimuli in humans: Physiological responses and potential sex differences.* American Journal of Physiology-Regulatory, Integrative and Comparative Physiology, 2023. **324**(6): p. R677–R690.
16. Ely, B.R., et al., *Heat acclimation and cross tolerance to hypoxia: Bridging the gap between cellular and systemic responses.* Temperature, 2014. **1**(2): p. 107–114.
17. Lee, B.J., et al., *Cross adaptation and cross tolerance in human health and disease.* Frontiers in Physiology, 2019. **9**: p. 1827.
18. Cheung, S., *Advanced environmental exercise physiology.* 2010: Human Kinetics.

19. Nakamura, K. and S.F. Morrison, *Central efferent pathways for cold-defensive and febrile shivering.* The Journal of Physiology, 2011. **589**(Pt 14): p. 3641–3658.

20. Castellani, J.W. and M.J. Tipton, *Cold stress effects on exposure tolerance and exercise performance.* Comprehensive Physiology, 2015. **6**(1): p. 443–469.

21. Wendt, D., L.J. van Loon, and W.D. Lichtenbelt, *Thermoregulation during exercise in the heat: Strategies for maintaining health and performance.* Sports Medicine, 2007. **37**(8): p. 669–682.

22. Périard, J. and S. Racinais, *Heat stress in sport and exercise.* Cham, Switzerland: Springer, 2019.

23. Travers, G., et al., *Physiological function during exercise and environmental stress in humans—An integrative view of body systems and homeostasis.* Cells, 2022. **11**(3): p. 383.

24. Heinonen, I. and J.A. Laukkanen, *Effects of heat and cold on health, with special reference to Finnish sauna bathing.* American Journal of Physiology-Regulatory, Integrative and Comparative Physiology, 2018. **314**: pp. R629–8.

25. Price, B.S., et al., *Does heat thermotherapy improve cardiovascular and cardio-metabolic health? A systematic review and narrative synthesis of the literature.* medRxiv, 2020: p. 2020.05. 19.20106666.

26. Espeland, D., L. de Weerd, and J.B. Mercer, *Health effects of voluntary exposure to cold water: A continuing subject of debate.* International Journal of Circumpolar Health, 2022. **81**(1): p. 2111789.

27. Tipton, M.J., et al., *Cold water immersion: Kill or cure?* Experimental Physiology, 2017. **102**(11): p. 1335–1355.

28. Leon, L.R. and A. Bouchama, *Heat stroke.* Comprehensive Physiology, 2015. **5**(2): p. 611–647.

29. Cramer, M.N. and O. Jay, *Biophysical aspects of human thermoregulation during heat stress.* Autonomic Neuroscience, 2016. **196**: p. 3–13.

30. Kakitsuba, N., I.B. Mekjavic, and T. Katsuura, *Individual variability in the peripheral and core interthreshold zones.* Journal of Physiological Anthropology, 2007. **26**(3): p. 403–408.

31. Refinetti, R., *The circadian rhythm of body temperature.* Frontiers in Bioscience (Landmark Ed), 2010. **15**: p. 564–594.

32. Morrison, S.F. and K. Nakamura, *Central mechanisms for thermoregulation.* Annual Review of Physiology, 2019. **81**: p. 285–308.

33. Bierens, J.J., et al., *Physiology of drowning: A review.* Physiology (Bethesda), 2016. **31**(2): p. 147–1366.

34. Gagge, A.P. and L.P. Herrington, *Physiological effects of heat and cold.* Annual Review of Physiology, 1947. **9**(1): p. 409–428.

35. Brunt, V.E. and C.T. Minson, *Heat therapy: Mechanistic underpinnings and applications to cardiovascular health.* Journal of Applied Physiology, 2021. **130**(6): p. 1684–1704.

36. Kim, K., et al., *Skeletal muscle adaptations to heat therapy.* Journal of Applied Physiology, 2020. **128**(6): p. 1635–1642.

37. Rodrigues, P., et al., *Effects of passive heating intervention on muscle hypertrophy and neuromuscular function: A preliminary systematic review with meta-analysis.* Journal of Thermal Biology, 2020. **93**: p. 102684.

38. Hunt, A.P., et al., *Could heat therapy be an effective treatment for Alzheimer's and Parkinson's diseases? A narrative review.* Frontiers in Physiology, 2020. **10**: p. 1556.

39. Castellani, J.W. and A.J. Young, *Human physiological responses to cold exposure: Acute responses and acclimatization to prolonged exposure*. Auton Neurosci, 2016. **196**: p. 63–74.
40. Stocks, J.M., et al., *Human physiological responses to cold exposure*. Aviat Space Environ Med, 2004. **75**(5): p. 444–457.
41. Tipton, M.J., *The initial responses to cold-water immersion in man*. Clinical Science, 1989. **77**(6): p. 581–588.
42. Blondin, D.P., et al., *Increased brown adipose tissue oxidative capacity in cold-acclimated humans*. J Clin Endocrinol Metab, 2014. **99**(3): p. E438–E446.
43. Brazaitis, M., et al., *Time course of physiological and psychological responses in humans during a 20-day severe-cold–acclimation programme*. PLoS One, 2014. **9**(4): p. e94698.
44. Bergh, U. and B. Ekblom, *Physical performance and peak aerobic power at different body temperatures*. Journal of Applied Physiology, 1979. **46**(5): p. 885–889.
45. Bergh, U., *Human power at subnormal body temperatures*. Acta Physiologica Scandinavica. Supplementum, 1980. **478**: p. 1–39.
46. Bergh, U. and B. Ekblom, *Influence of muscle temperature on maximal muscle strength and power output in human skeletal muscles*. Acta Physiologica Scandinavica, 1979. **107**(1): p. 33–37.
47. Galloway, S.D. and R.J. Maughan, *Effects of ambient temperature on the capacity to perform prolonged cycle exercise in man*. Medicine & Science in Sports & Exercise, 1997. **29**(9): p. 1240–1249.
48. Patton, J.F. and J.A. Vogel, *Effects of acute cold exposure on submaximal endurance performance*. Medicine and Science in Sports and Exercise, 1984. **16**(5): p. 494–497.
49. Sandsund, M., et al., *Effect of cold exposure (–15° C) and Salbutamol treatment on physical performance in elite nonasthmatic cross-country skiers*. European Journal of Applied Physiology and Occupational Physiology, 1998. **77**: p. 297–304.
50. Savourey, G. and J. Bittel, *Cold thermoregulatory changes induced by sleep deprivation in men*. European Journal of Applied Physiology and Occupational Physiology, 1994. **69**(3): p. 216–220.
51. Carling, C., G. Dupont, and F. Le Gall, *The effect of a cold environment on physical activity profiles in elite soccer match-play*. International Journal of Sports Medicine, 2011. **32**: p. 542–545.
52. Parkin, J., et al., *Effect of ambient temperature on human skeletal muscle metabolism during fatiguing submaximal exercise*. Journal of Applied Physiology, 1999. **86**(3): p. 902–908.
53. Cheuvront, S.N., et al., *Hypohydration impairs endurance exercise performance in temperate but not cold air*. Journal of Applied Physiology, 2005. **99**(5): p. 1972–1976.
54. Renberg, J., et al., *Effect of ambient temperature on female endurance performance*. Journal of Thermal Biology, 2014. **45**: p. 9–14.
55. Hutchins, K.P., et al., *Female (under) representation in exercise thermoregulation research*. Sports Med Open, 2021. **7**(1): p. 43.
56. Nybo, L., P. Rasmussen, and M.N. Sawka, *Performance in the heat-physiological factors of importance for hyperthermia-induced fatigue*. Comprehensive Physiology, 2014. **4**(2): p. 657–689.

57. Tyler, C.J., et al., *The effects of heat adaptation on physiology, perception and exercise performance in the heat: A meta-analysis.* Sports Medicine, 2016. **46**(11): p. 1699–1724.

58. Périard, J.D., T.M.H. Eijsvogels, and H.A.M. Daanen, *Exercise under heat stress: thermoregulation, hydration, performance implications, and mitigation strategies.* Physiological Reviews, 2021. **101**(4): p. 1873–1979.

59. Girard, O., F. Brocherie, and D.J. Bishop, *Sprint performance under heat stress: A review.* The Scandinavian Journal of Medicine & Science, 2015. **25**(S1): p. 79–89.

60. Racinais, S., et al., *Consensus recommendations on training and competing in the heat.* British Journal of Sports Medicine, 2015. **49**(18): p. 1164–1173.

61. Racinais, S. and J. Oksa, *Temperature and neuromuscular function.* Scandinavian Journal of Medicine & Science in Sports, 2010. **20**: p. 1–18.

62. Crandall, C.G. and T.E. Wilson, *Human cardiovascular responses to passive heat stress.* Comprehensive Physiology, 2015. **5**(1): p. 17–43.

63. Schlader, Z.J., et al., *Orderly recruitment of thermoeffectors in resting humans.* The American Journal of Physiology—Regulatory, Integrative and Comparative Physiology, 2018. **314**(2): p. R171–R180.

64. Taylor, N.A., *Human heat adaptation.* Comprehensive Physiology, 2011. **4**(1): p. 325–365.

65. Taylor, N.A.S., S.R. Notley, and M.I. Lindinger, *Heat adaptation in humans: The significance of controlled and regulated variables for experimental design and interpretation.* European Journal of Applied Physiology, 2020. **120**: p. 2583–2595.

66. Kelly, M.K., et al., *Heat adaptation for females: A systematic review and meta-analysis of physiological adaptations and exercise performance in the heat.* Sportsmed Mumbai, 2023. **53**(7): p. 1395–1421.

67. Folt, C., et al., *Synergism and antagonism among multiple stressors.* Limnology and Oceanography, 1999. **44**(3part2): p. 864–877.

68. Cipriano, L.F. and R.F. Goldman, *Thermal responses of unclothed men exposed to both cold temperatures and high altitudes.* Journal of Applied Physiology, 1975. **39**(5): p. 796–800.

69. Simmons, G.H., et al., *Hypoxic cutaneous vasodilation is sustained during brief cold stress and is not affected by changes in CO2.* Journal of Applied Physiology, 2010. **108**(4): p. 788–792.

70. Simmons, G.H., et al., *Cutaneous vascular and core temperature responses to sustained cold exposure in hypoxia.* Experimental Physiology, 2011. **96**(10): p. 1062–1071.

71. Johnston, C.E., et al., *Eucapnic hypoxia lowers human cold thermoregulatory response thresholds and accelerates core cooling.* Journal of Applied Physiology, 1996. **80**(2): p. 422–429.

72. Curtis, A.N., M.L. Walsh, and M.D. White, *Influence of passive hyperthermia on human ventilation during rest and isocapnic hypoxia.* Applied Physiology, Nutrition, and Metabolism, 2007. **32**(4): p. 721–732.

73. Petersen, E.S. and H. Vejby-Christensen, *Effects of body temperature on ventilatory response to hypoxia and breathing pattern in man.* Journal of Applied Physiology: Respiratory, Environmental and Exercise Physiology, 1977. **42**(4): p. 492–500.

74. Amann, M. and J.A. Calbet, *Convective oxygen transport and fatigue.* Journal of Applied Physiology, 2008. **104**(3): p. 861–870.
75. Gregson, W., et al., *Influence of cold water immersion on limb and cutaneous blood flow at rest.* The American Journal of Sports Medicine, 2011. **39**(6): p. 1316–1323.
76. Yanagisawa, O., et al., *Magnetic resonance imaging evaluation of cooling on blood flow and oedema in skeletal muscles after exercise.* European Journal of Applied Physiology, 2004. **91**: p. 737–740.
77. Lloyd, A., et al., *Interaction between environmental temperature and hypoxia on central and peripheral fatigue during high-intensity dynamic knee extension.* Journal of Applied Physiology, 2016. **120**(6): p. 567–579.
78. Robinson, K.A. and E.M. Haymes, *Metabolic effects of exposure to hypoxia plus cold at rest and during exercise in humans.* Journal of Applied Physiology, 1990. **68**(2): p. 720–725.
79. Mugele, H., et al., *Integrative crosstalk between hypoxia and the cold: Old data and new opportunities.* Experimental Physiology, 2021. **106**(1): p. 350–358.
80. Lunt, H.C., et al., *"Cross-adaptation": Habituation to short repeated cold-water immersions affects the response to acute hypoxia in humans.* The Journal of Physiology, 2010. **588**(18): p. 3605–3613.
81. Mazzeo, R.S., *Physiological responses to exercise at altitude.* Sports Medicine, 2008. **38**(1): p. 1–8.
82. Pendergast, D.R., *The effect of body cooling on oxygen transport during exercise.* Medicine and Science in Sports and Exercise, 1988. **20**(5 Suppl): p. S171–6.
83. Chapman, R.F., J.L. Stickford, and B.D. Levine, *Altitude training considerations for the winter sport athlete.* Experimental Physiology, 2010. **95**(3): p. 411–421.
84. Nair, C., M. Malhotra, and P. Gopinath, *Effect of altitude and cold acclimatisation on the basal metabolism in man.* Aerospace Medicine, 1971. **42**(10): p. 1056–1059.
85. Nair, C. and S. George, *The effect of altitude and cold on body temperature during acclimatization of man at 3,300 m.* International Journal of Biometeorology, 1972. **16**: p. 79–84.
86. Bradbury, K.E., et al., *Separate and combined influences of heat and hypobaric hypoxia on self-paced aerobic exercise performance.* Journal of Applied Physiology, 2019. **127**(2): p. 513–519.
87. Lee, B.J., et al., *The impact of submaximal exercise during heat and/or hypoxia on the cardiovascular and monocyte HSP72 responses to subsequent (post 24 h) exercise in hypoxia.* Extreme Physiology & Medicine, 2014. **3**(1): p. 15.
88. Levine, A. and M.J. Buono, *Rating of perceived exertion increases synergistically during prolonged exercise in a combined heat and hypoxic environment.* Journal of Thermal Biology, 2019. **84**: p. 99–102.
89. Yamaguchi, K., et al., *Effects of combined hot and hypoxic conditions on muscle blood flow and muscle oxygenation during repeated cycling sprints.* European Journal of Applied Physiology, 2021. **121**(10): p. 2869–2878.
90. Girard, O., F. Brocherie, and G.P. Millet, *Effects of altitude/hypoxia on single- and multiple-sprint performance: A comprehensive review.* Sports Medicine, 2017. **47**(10): p. 1931–1949.

91. Girard, O., D. Bishop, and S. Racinais, *Hot conditions improve power output during repeated cycling sprints without modifying neuromuscular fatigue characteristics.* European Journal of Applied Physiology, 2013. **113**: p. 359–369.

92. Girard, O., et al., *Running mechanical alterations during repeated treadmill sprints in hot versus hypoxic environments. A pilot study.* Journal of Sports Sciences, 2016. **34**(12): p. 1190–1198.

93. Sotiridis, A., et al., *No ergogenic effects of a 10-day combined heat and hypoxic acclimation on aerobic performance in normoxic thermoneutral or hot conditions.* European Journal of Applied Physiology, 2019. **119**(11–12): p. 2513–2527.

94. Buchheit, M., et al., *Adding heat to the live-high train-low altitude model: A practical insight from professional football.* British Journal of Sports Medicine, 2013. **47**(Suppl 1): p. i59–i69.

95. McCleave, E.L., et al., *Impaired heat adaptation from combined heat training and "live high, train low" hypoxia.* International Journal of Sports Physiology and Performance, 2019. **14**(5): p. 635–643.

96. McCleave, E.L., et al., *Temperate performance benefits after heat, but not combined heat and hypoxic training.* Medicine and Science in Sports and Exercise, 2017. **49**(3): p. 509–517.

97. Hanson, E.D., et al., *Heat acclimation with or without normobaric hypoxia exposure leads to similar improvements in endurance performance in the heat.* Sports, 2022. **10**(5): p. 69.

98. Karlsen, A., et al., *Heat acclimatization does not improve VO2max or cycling performance in a cool climate in trained cyclists.* Scandinavian Journal of Medicine & Science in Sports, 2015. **25**: p. 269–276.

22

INTERMITTENT HYPOXIA–HYPEROXIA

Mechanisms and clinical application

*Oleg S. Glazachev, Martin Burtscher, Lutz Schega,
Tom Behrendt and Robert T. Mallet*

22.1 Introduction

The effectiveness of hypoxia conditioning (HC) for augmenting physical performance in athletes and the clinical dynamics of HC-enhanced exercise tolerance in patients with different pathologies depends on several aspects of
the HC protocols: the durations of the hypoxia exposures and, in the case of
intermittent HC (IHC), the interspersed reoxygenation periods, the intensity
(i.e., reduction in atmospheric partial pressure of oxygen, PO_2) of each
hypoxia exposure, the number of hypoxia–reoxygenation cycles per session,
the number of sessions per week and the duration of the HC program.
Among the myriad HC protocols that have undergone preclinical and clinical testing, short-term hypoxia exposures with normoxic intervals of about
5–8 min for 4–7 cycles per session (Figure 22.1) were first implemented in
the former Soviet Union for high-altitude acclimatization of Soviet pilots,
and subsequently employed by clinicians for treatment of respiratory and
neurological disorders, hypertension, diabetes mellitus, radiation toxicity,
and other conditions [1].

Passive, short-term IHC programs (also termed interval hypoxic exposures, IHE) have proven beneficial and well tolerated by both healthy elderly
people and patients with various diseases. To improve the efficacy of IHC
regimens and to facilitate patients' tolerance to hypoxic stimuli, a modification of the IH protocol in which the normoxic intervals between hypoxic
stimuli are replaced by moderately hyperoxic ones (intermittent hypoxia–
hyperoxia conditioning, IHHC, also termed interval hypoxic–hyperoxic
exposures, IHHE), has been empirically proposed [2].

DOI: 10.4324/9781003402879-33

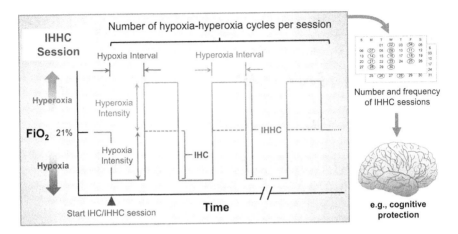

FIGURE 22.1 Key features of clinically efficacious intermittent hypoxia-hyperoxia programs. The factors determining the capacity of IHHC programs to protect cognitive function include intensities and durations of hypoxic and hyperoxic exposures, number of hypoxia–hyperoxia cycles per IHHC session, number of sessions per week, and duration of IHHC regimen.

FiO_2: inspired O_2 fraction; IHC: intermittent hypoxia–normoxia exposures; IHHC: intermittent hypoxia–hyperoxia exposures.

22.2 Rationale for combining hypoxia with hyperoxia

The potential benefits of both IHC and IHHC protocols are effected by molecular mechanisms mobilized by the multiple, abrupt transitions from hypoxia to normoxia or hyperoxia, that is, reoxygenation, and the associated production of reactive oxygen species (ROS). Although excessive ROS formation, for instance, that engendered by abrupt reperfusion of ischemic tissue, is destructive to cells and organelles, more moderate ROS concentrations are known to trigger adaptive redox signaling cascades, imparting resistance to damage at the cellular, organ, and organismal levels [3, 4]. Redox signaling activates transcription factors, most notably NF-κB, Nrf2, activator protein 1 (AP-1), and HIF-1α, which induce expression of myriad protective molecules, such as antioxidant, anti-inflammatory, glycolytic and repair enzymes, vascular endothelial growth factor, erythropoietin, heat shock proteins, and iron-regulating proteins [2, 5]. Thus, in IHC and to an even greater extent IHHC regimes, mitochondrial ROS production during the hypoxic phase is supplemented by additional moderate ROS generation upon reoxygenation [6]. When hypoxia is followed by hyperoxia instead of normoxia, ROS-induced signaling may be reinforced without having to impose more severe hypoxia [7]. Additional benefits of IHHC may result from increased O_2-independent ATP production during hypoxia by augmented glycolytic enzymes, followed by rapid reactivation of the highly efficient oxidative phosphorylation machinery by hyperoxia, which quickly restores ATP resources and promotes clearance of blood lactate and other metabolites during hyperoxic recovery [5].

22.3 Studies of hypoxia–normoxia and hypoxia–hyperoxia in rodents

Preclinical testing of IHHC protocols began with the studies of Arkhipenko et al. [2], who demonstrated improved exercise tolerance, increased rates of ROS detoxification, and augmented antioxidant enzyme activities in the heart, liver, and brain of rats completing 15 consecutive daily 60 min sessions alternating 5 min hypoxia (10% FiO_2) and 3 min hyperoxia (30% FiO_2). This approach was more effective than a traditional IHC protocol, alternating 10% and 21% FiO_2. Rats completing eight swimming sessions combined with eight sessions of IHHC showed attenuated brain and myocardial lipid peroxidation during acute stress imposed by swimming to exhaustion, versus rats completing swim training alone or combined with IHC [7]. Training and IHHC also attenuated, more effectively than training alone or combined with IHC, over-activation of heat shock proteins and the antioxidant enzymes superoxide dismutase (SOD) and catalase during acute stress. The authors concluded that IHHC, more efficiently than IHC, augmented training-induced adaptations limiting oxidative damage to heart and brain.

In rats, a two-week program of daily, moderate IHHC (5 cycles alternating 5 min 10% FiO_2 and 5 min 30% FiO_2) produced greater upregulation of adaptive ROS signaling than an IHC protocol alternating 10% and 21% FiO_2 [8]. The IHHC regimen was associated with decreased basal and Fe^{2+}/ascorbate-induced lipid peroxidation and formation of protein carbonyls and H_2O_2 in liver mitochondria during subsequent severe hypoxia (7% FiO_2 for 60 min). IHHC also induced a more robust induction of the antioxidant enzymes Mn-SOD and glutathione peroxidase which likely contributed to the IHHC-enhanced antioxidant protection.

Bigdeli et al. [9] demonstrated in rats that a 6-day program of 4 h/d severe hyperoxia (95% FiO_2) increased cerebral resistance to 60 min middle cerebral artery occlusion, indicated by decreased neurologic deficit and infarct volume, as effectively as a 10-min preconditioning occlusion. Both hyperoxic conditioning and ischemic preconditioning increased cerebral contents of excitatory amino acid transporters and tumor necrosis factor-α converting enzyme, suggesting enhanced capacity to remove excitotoxic glutamate and inflammatory cytokines from the extracellular milieu. Although Bigdeli et al. [9] employed 4 h uninterrupted, severe hyperoxia, their findings suggest possible mechanisms of brain benefits afforded by the more moderate (30–33% FiO_2), intermittent hyperoxia used clinically [10].

Studies in mice identified important limitations of continuous hyperoxia and hypoxia. Benderro et al. [11] demonstrated a progressive decline in capillary density in the parietal cortex over 21 days of continuous exposure to 50% FiO_2. The hyperoxic mice failed to gain body weight, and hematocrit fell from ~46% to ~35% over the 3 weeks of chronic hyperoxia. Also in mice, Terraneo et al. [12] reported that 28 days of uninterrupted hypoxia (FiO_2 10%) or hyperoxia (FiO_2 30%) increased cerebral lipid peroxidation and neuronal apoptosis; thus, both hyperoxia and hypoxia imposed cerebral oxidative stress. Hypoxia but not hyperoxia increased the cerebral content of subunit 4 of NAD(P)H oxidase, a major ROS generator in the brain, and only hypoxia elicited cerebral angiogenesis. Both sustained hypoxia and hyperoxia-inflicted cerebral injury likely ascribable, at least in part, to an imbalance between ROS formation and antioxidant defenses. Ortet et al. [13] studied the impact of prolonged hyperoxia (3 weeks of continuous exposure to 50% O_2) on cognitive function (Y-maze test) and motor function (grip strength and rotarod tests) in mice. Hyperoxia lowered hematocrit from 50 ± 5 to $38 \pm 1\%$ and impaired cognitive but not motor function. Thus, moderately severe hyperoxia uninterrupted by normoxia or hypoxia impaired cognitive function in mice. Collectively, these reports strongly suggest that the benefits of IHHC result from adaptations triggered by periodic transitions between hypoxia and hyperoxia, while severe, continuous changes of O_2 availability in both directions (hypoxia and hyperoxia) can be detrimental.

22.4 Studies using hypoxia and/or hyperoxia in humans

Table 22.1 summarizes clinical studies of IHHC intervention for cognitive impairment, cardiometabolic disorders, and physical rehabilitation. Those studies demonstrated improved exercise capacity/tolerance and beneficial effects on cardiometabolic parameters after IHHC intervention in elderly patients, especially in those suffering from cardiometabolic diseases [14–20]. IHHC was also shown to improve cognition by itself or in combination with other interventions in patients (with cognitive impairment) undergoing multimodal training interventions [14, 18, 21].

The first clinical pilot study of IHHC was performed on track and field athletes with overtraining syndrome [23]. A 4-week program of repeated hypoxic–hyperoxic exposures (6–8 cycles alternating 4–6 min 10% FiO_2 and 1–3 min 35% FiO_2) combined with low-intensity sport-specific exercise improved physical working capacity, autonomic balance, and hypoxia tolerance without hematological changes in athletes with overtraining syndrome [7, 23].

Bayer et al. [14] demonstrated the cognitive benefits of IHHC when combined with physiotherapy training. Elderly adults (ages 64–92) underwent 15–20 days of multimodal training physiotherapy either alone or combined

TABLE 22.1 Studies evaluating intermittent hypoxia-hyperoxia conditioning in adult patients

Reference	Study population	Intervention	Main outcomes
Bayer et al. [14]	34 geriatric (64–92 years) patients: 8 MTI + IHHC, 16 MTI + sham IHHC	5–7 weeks MTI + IHHC vs. MTI + sham IHHC	Additional IHHC contributed significantly to improved cognitive function and functional exercise capacity following MTI.
Behrendt et al. [22]	30 geriatric (72–94 years) patients: 16 cycling training + IHHC, 14 cycling training + sham IHHC	6 weeks cycling training + IHHC vs. training + sham IHHC	Additional IHHC lowered systolic blood pressure and showed some influence on the acute exercise-related increases in LDL-C concentration.
Behrendt et al. [18]	25 geriatric (77–94 years) patients: 14 aerobic training + IHHC, 11 aerobic training + sham IHHC	6 weeks aerobic training + IHHC vs. training + sham IHHC	Additional IHHC improved global cognitive functions and physical performance, which may help to preserve functional mobility in geriatric patients.
Bestavashvili et al. [19]	65 patients with metabolic syndrome: 32 IHHC, 33 sham IHHC	3 weeks IHHC vs. sham IHHC	IHHC improved components of metabolic syndrome, which improved the arterial stiffness lipid profile and liver functional state.
Dudnik et al. [15]	29 cardiac patients with comorbidities: 15 IHHC, 14 sham IHHC	5 weeks IHHC vs. sham IHHC	IHHC significantly improved cardiorespiratory fitness
Glazachev et al. [16]	46 CAD patients: 27 IHHC, 19 sham IHHC	3 weeks IHHC vs. sham IHHC	IHHC improved exercise tolerance, cardiometabolic risks factors profile, and quality of life.
Glazachev et al. [17]	36 cardiac patients: 17 IHHC, 19 sham IHHC	3 weeks IHHC vs. sham IHHC	IHHC improved exercise tolerance, cardiometabolic risk factor profile, perception of the quality of life and psycho-emotional status.

(Continued)

TABLE 22.1 (Continued)

Reference	Study population	Intervention	Main outcomes
Serebrovska et al. [21]	21 patients (51–74 years) with mild cognitive impairment: 8 IHHC, 6 sham IHHC, 7 controls	3 weeks IHHC in MCI, vs. sham IHHC in MCI	IHHC improved cognitive function; decreased Aβ serum concentration and NETs formation.
Serebrovska et al. [20]	55 pre-diabetic patients: 17 IHHC, 16 IHT, 22 controls	3 weeks IHHC vs. IHC and vs. sham IHHC	IHHC and IHC improved glucose and lipid metabolism; IHHC was suggested to require shorter sessions vs IHC.
Susta et al. [23]	34 field and track athletes (with and without over-training syndrome): 15 IHHC, 19 controls	4 weeks IHHC + light exercise vs. healthy controls	Adding IHHC to low-intensity exercise, facilitated functional recovery in athletes with overtraining syndrome.

Aβ, amyloid beta (Aβ); CAD, coronary artery disease; IHC, intermittent hypoxia conditioning; IHHC, intermittent hypoxia-hyperoxia conditioning; LDL-C, low-density lipoprotein cholesterol; MCI, mild cognitive impairment; MTI, multimodal training intervention; NETs, neutrophil extracellular traps.

with 12–15 sessions of 30–40 min IHHC (10–14% FIO_2 for 4–7 min + 30-40% FIO_2 for 2–4 min). Multimodal training with IHHC, but not training alone, increased cognitive performance evaluated by dementia detection and clock-drawing tests, and IHHC + multimodal training effected a greater increase in functional exercise capacity assessed by 6-minute walking distance than did multimodal training alone. Thus, IHHC, which was well tolerated by the elderly adults, improved cognitive performance and functional exercise capacity.

Serebrovska et al. [21] studied IHHC treatment (4 cycles/session of 5 min 12% FiO_2 + 3 min 33% FiO_2, 5 sessions/week for 3 weeks) in older adults (51–74 years) with mild cognitive impairment (MCI). IHHC but not sham training improved cognitive function and lowered circulating amyloid-β concentrations, platelet aggregation, and neutrophil extracellular traps (NETS) produced by adhesion molecules released by aggregated platelets. Suppression of amyloid-β production and NETs formation persisted at least for one month post-IHHC. More recently, a cross-over study evaluating the safety of IHC/IHHC versus risk of excessive oxidative stress induction assessed oxidative stress and antioxidant capacity in healthy adults after acute exposure to IHC or IHHC [24]. Neither IHC nor IHHC increased oxidative stress measures or lowered antioxidant capacity versus the respective baselines. The results suggest that single IHC or IHHC sessions do not elicit excessive ROS production or deplete antioxidant defenses in healthy individuals.

Serebrovska et al. [25] evaluated the impact of IHHC (4 cycles/session of 5 min 12% FiO_2 and 3 min 33% FiO_2, 5 sessions/week for 3 weeks) on pro-inflammatory factors in 29 healthy older adults and 16 MCI patients. IHHC but not sham training improved cognitive function (Montréal Cognitive Assessment score), shortened latency of cognitive evoked potentials, and lowered circulating NETS and amyloid-β in the MCI patients. The authors proposed that IHHC-induced elevation of circulating inflammatory markers may trigger cellular adaptations culminating in cognitive improvement and decreased neuropathology in cognitively impaired elderly adults.

Behrendt et al. [22] evaluated the effects of IHHC (4–8 cycles of 10–14% FIO_2 for 1–5 min + 30-40% FiO_2 for 1–3 min, 3 sessions/week for 6 weeks) before 30 min aerobic cycling on cognitive and physical performance in geriatric patients. IHHC and cycling produced greater increases in cognitive function and physical performance than cycling alone and better preserved functional mobility.

Behrendt et al. [26] analyzed clinical evidence that IHHC may be an effective, noninvasive strategy to increase peak O_2 uptake (VO_{2peak}), exercise tolerance, and cognitive function while lowering serum glucose. Eight studies were examined: one in geriatric patients, three in older adults with cardiovascular disease, two with metabolic disease, one with cognitive impairment, and one in young athletes with overtraining syndrome. These trials applied 4–8 IHHC cycles/session of 10–12% O_2 for 2–7 min and 30–40% O_2 for 1–6 min, 2–5 sessions/week for 3–6 weeks. IHHC increased exercise tolerance, VO_{2peak} and cognitive performance, and lowered serum glucose concentrations. IHHC also proved beneficial in patients with mild cognitive impairment.

Tessema et al. [27] reviewed 38 clinical studies of IHC, IHHC and obstructive sleep apnea. Most studies showed IHC and IHHC produced similar benefits (e.g., improved cognitive function, decreased systolic blood pressure, serum glucose, and cholesterol), while the intermittent hypoxia associated with obstructive sleep apnea was detrimental. IHC and IHHC improved quality of life, cognitive function, and physical performance; lowered serum glucose, cholesterol, and LDL concentrations, systolic arterial pressure, and inflammation; and increased red cell mass and resistance to apoptotic stimuli while delaying aging-associated increases in senescence markers and β-galactosidase. In contrast, obstructive sleep apnea-associated intermittent hypoxia was associated with hypertension, metabolic syndrome, vascular dysfunction, decreased quality of life and cognitive function, accelerated brain aging, increased insulin resistance, and elevated serum IL-6, C-reactive protein, and H_2O_2.

22.5 Is IHHC superior to IHC?

Although studies in rodents support the hypothesis that IHHC could induce more beneficial adaptations than IHC, this superiority of IHHC in humans needs still to be established convincingly. At this time, there is only one study (utilizing one protocol) directly comparing the effects of IHC and IHHC in humans [20]. These authors found a similar positive impact of both interventions on selected metabolic parameters in prediabetic patients but referred to some reduction in the duration of the sessions due to shortening reoxygenation periods, which could represent an advantage of IHHC application [20]. Well-designed studies comparing the physiological effects and clinical outcomes of different protocols are needed to decipher potential differences between adaptations initiated by IHHC compared to IHC programs.

Abbreviations

AP-1	activator protein-1
$A\beta$	amyloid-β
CAD	coronary artery disease
FiO_2	O_2 fraction of inspired air
HC	hypoxia conditioning
HIF	hypoxia inducible factor
IHC	intermittent hypoxia conditioning
IHE	interval hypoxic exposure
IHHC	intermittent hypoxia–hyperoxia conditioning
IHHE	interval hypoxic–hyperoxic exposure
IL-6	interleukin-6
LDL-C	low density lipoprotein (LDL) cholesterol
MCI	mild cognitive impairment
MTI	multimodal training intervention
NETS	neutrophil extracellular traps
NF-κB	nuclear factor-κB
Nrf2	nuclear factor erythroid 2-related factor 2
ROS	reactive oxygen species
SOD	superoxide dismutase
VO_{2peak}	peak O_2 uptake.

References

1. Serebrovskaya, T.V., *Intermittent hypoxia research in the former Soviet Union and the Commonwealth of Independent States: History and review of the concept and selected applications.* High Alt Med Biol, 2002. **3**(2): p. 205–221.
2. Arkhipenko, Y.V., T.G. Sazontova, and A.G. Zhukova, *Adaptation to periodic hypoxia and hyperoxia improves resistance of membrane structures in heart, liver, and brain.* Bull Exp Biol Med, 2005. **140**(3): p. 278–281.

3. Sazontova, T.G. and I.V. Arkhipenko, *[The role of free radical processes and redox-signalization in adaptation of the organism to changes in oxygen level].* Ross Fiziol Zh Im I M Sechenova, 2005. **91**(6): p. 636–655.

4. Roy, J., et al., *Physiological role of reactive oxygen species as promoters of natural defenses.* FASEB J, 2017. **31**(9): p. 3729–3745.

5. Burtscher, J., et al., *Adaptive responses to hypoxia and/or hyperoxia in humans.* Antioxid Redox Signal, 2022. **37**(13–15), p. 887–912.

6. Sazontova, T.G., et al., *Adaptation to hypoxia and hyperoxia improves physical endurance: the role of reactive oxygen species and redox-signaling.* Rossiiskii fiziologicheskii zhurnal imeni I.M. Sechenova, 2012. **98**(6): p. 793–807.

7. Sazontova, T., et al., Adaptation to intermittent hypoxia/hyperoxia enhances efficiency of exercise training, in *Intermittent hypoxia and human diseases*, L. Xi and T. Serebrovskaya, Editors. 2012, Springer: Heidelberg New York London, p. 191–205.

8. Gonchar, O. and I. Mankovska, *Moderate hypoxia/hyperoxia attenuates acute hypoxia-induced oxidative damage and improves antioxidant defense in lung mitochondria.* Acta Physiol Hung, 2012. **99**(4): p. 436–446.

9. Bigdeli, M.R., *Preconditioning with prolonged normobaric hyperoxia induces ischemic tolerance partly by upregulation of antioxidant enzymes in rat brain tissue.* Brain Res, 2009. **1260**: p. 47–54.

10. Bigdeli, M.R., M. Asheghabadi, and A. Khalili, *Time course of neuroprotection induced by normobaric hyperoxia in focal cerebral ischemia.* Neurol Res, 2012. **34**(5): p. 439–446.

11. Benderro, G.F., et al., *Decreased VEGF expression and microvascular density, but increased HIF-1 and 2α accumulation and EPO expression in chronic moderate hyperoxia in the mouse brain.* Brain Res, 2012. **1471**: p. 46–55.

12. Terraneo, L., et al., *Brain adaptation to hypoxia and hyperoxia in mice.* Redox Biol, 2017. **11**: p. 12–20.

13. Ortet, G., et al., *Impaired cognitive performance in mice exposed to prolonged hyperoxia.* Adv Exp Med Biol, 2022. **1395**: p. 69–73.

14. Bayer, U., et al., *Intermittent hypoxic–hyperoxic training on cognitive performance in geriatric patients.* Alzheim DementTranslat Res Clin Intervent, 2017. **3**(1): p. 114–122.

15. Dudnik, E., et al., *Intermittent hypoxia-hyperoxia conditioning improves cardiorespiratory fitness in older comorbid cardiac outpatients without hematological changes: A randomized controlled trial.* High Alt Med Biol, 2018. **19**(4): p. 339–343.

16. Glazachev, O., et al., *Adaptations following an intermittent hypoxia-hyperoxia training in coronary artery disease patients: A controlled study.* Clin Cardiol, 2017. **40**(6): p. 370–376.

17. Glazachev, O.S., et al., *[Adaptation to dosed hypoxia-hyperoxia as a factor in improving the quality of life of elderly patients with cardiac pathology.]* Adv Gerontol, 2019. **32**(1-2): p. 145–151.

18. Behrendt, T., et al., *Effects of intermittent hypoxia-hyperoxia exposure prior to aerobic cycling exercise on physical and cognitive performance in geriatric patients: A randomized controlled trial.* Front Physiol, 2022. **13**: p. 899096.

19. Bestavashvili, A., et al., *Intermittent hypoxic–hyperoxic exposures effects in patients with metabolic syndrome: Correction of cardiovascular and metabolic profile.* Biomedicines, 2022. **10**(3): p. 566.

20. Serebrovska, T.V., et al., *Intermittent hypoxia/hyperoxia versus intermittent hypoxia/normoxia: Comparative study in prediabetes.* High Alt Med Biol, 2019. **20**(4): p. 383–391.

21. Serebrovska, Z.O., et al., *Intermittent hypoxia-hyperoxia training improves cognitive function and decreases circulating biomarkers of Alzheimer's disease in*

patients with mild cognitive impairment: A pilot study. Int J Mol Sci, 2019. 20(21): p. 5405.

22. Behrendt, T., et al., *Influence of acute and chronic intermittent hypoxic-hyperoxic exposure prior to aerobic exercise on cardiovascular risk factors in geriatric patients: A randomized controlled trial.* Front Physiol, 2022. **13**: p. 1043536.

23. Susta, D., E. Dudnik, and O.S. Glazachev, *A programme based on repeated hypoxia–hyperoxia exposure and light exercise enhances performance in athletes with overtraining syndrome: A pilot study.* Clin Physiol Funct Imaging, 2017. **37**(3): p. 276–281.

24. Susta, D., et al., *Redox homeostasis in humans exposed to intermittent hypoxia-normoxia and to intermittent hypoxia-hyperoxia.* High Alt Med Biol, 2020. **21**(1): p. 45–51.

25. Serebrovska, Z.O., et al., *Response of circulating inflammatory markers to intermittent hypoxia-hyperoxia training in healthy elderly people and patients with mild cognitive impairment.* Life (Basel), 2022. **12**(3): 432.

26. Behrendt, T., et al., *Effects of intermittent hypoxia-hyperoxia on performance- and health-related outcomes in humans: A systematic review,* in *Sports Med Open.* 2022,p. 70.

27. Tessema, B., et al., *Effects of intermittent hypoxia in training regimes and in obstructive sleep apnea on aging biomarkers and age-related diseases: A systematic review.* Front Aging Neurosci, 2022. **14**: p. 878278.

INDEX

Pages in *italics* refer to figures and pages in **bold** refer to tables.

Printed in the United States
by Baker & Taylor Publisher Services